Escherichia coli O157 in Farm Animals

Escherichia coli O157 in Farm Animals

Edited by

C.S. Stewart

and

H.J. Flint
Rowett Research Institute
Aberdeen, UK

CABI *Publishing*

CABI *Publishing* is a division of CAB *International*

CABI Publishing
CAB International
Wallingford
Oxon OX10 8DE
UK

Tel: +44 (0)1491 832111
Fax: +44 (0)1491 833508
Email: cabi@cabi.org

CABI Publishing
10 E. 40th Street
Suite 3203
New York, NY 10016
USA

Tel: +1 212 481 7018
Fax: +1 212 686 7993
Email: cabi-nao@cabi.org

A catalogue record for this book is available from the British Library, London, UK.

Library of Congress Cataloging-in-Publication Data
Escherichia coli O157 in farm animals / edited by C.S. Stewart and H.J. Flint.
p. cm.
Includes bibliographical references and index.
ISBN 0-85199-332-X (alk. paper)
1. Escherichia coli O157:H7. 2. Escherichia coli infections. 3. Escherichia coli infections in animals. I. Stewart, C. S. (Colin S.) II. Flint, H. J.
QR201.E82E834 1999
579.3′42--dc21 99-20673
CIP

ISBN 0 85199 332 X

Typeset in 10/12pt Garamond by Columns Design Ltd, Reading
Printed and bound in the UK by the University Press, Cambridge

Contents

Contributors

L. Beutin, Robert Koch Institute, Division of Emerging Bacterial Pathogens, Nordufer 20, D-13353 Berlin, Germany

I.R. Booth, Department of Molecular and Cell Biology, Institute of Medical Sciences, University of Aberdeen, Foresterhill, Aberdeen AB25 2ZD, UK

B.T. Bosworth, Enteric Diseases and Food Safety Research Unit, National Animal Disease Center, ARS–USDA, Ames, IA 50010, USA

C.A. Brown, Centre for Food Safety and Quality Enhancement, College of Agricultural and Environmental Sciences, Griffin, GA 30223–1797, USA

P. Carter, Department of Medical Microbiology, Institute of Medical Sciences, University of Aberdeen, Foresterhill, Aberdeen AB25 2ZD, UK

T.A. Casey, National Animal Disease Center, ARS–USDA, Ames, IA 50010, USA

P.A. Chapman, Public Health Laboratory, Herries Road, Sheffield, South Yorkshire S5 7BQ, UK

W.C. Cray, Jr, National Animal Disease Center, ARS–USDA, Ames, IA 50010, USA

E.A. Dean-Nystrom, Enteric Diseases and Food Safety Research Unit, National Animal Disease Center, ARS–USDA, Ames, IA 50010, USA

M.P. Doyle, Centre for Food Safety and Quality Enhancement, College of Agricultural and Environmental Sciences, Griffin, GA 30223–1797, USA

S.H. Duncan, Rowett Research Institute, Greenburn Road, Bucksburn, Aberdeen AB21 9SB, UK

H.J. Flint, Rowett Research Institute, Greenburn Road, Bucksburn, Aberdeen AB21 9SB, UK

V.P.J. Gannon, Food Directorate, Health Canada, c/o Animal Disease Research Institute, Lethbridge, Alberta, Canada T1J 3Z4

J. Glover, Department of Molecular and Cell Biology, Institute of Medical Sciences, University of Aberdeen, Foresterhill, Aberdeen AB25 2ZD, UK

C.L. Gyles, Department of Pathobiology, University of Guelph, Guelph, Ontario, N1G 2W1, Canada

B.G. Harmon, Department of Veterinary Pathology, College of Veterinary Medicine, The University of Georgia, Athens, GA 30602–7388, USA

C.A. Hart, Department of Medical Microbiology, University of Liverpool, Liverpool, Merseyside L69 3BX, UK

K. Jacobsen, Department of Veterinary Pathology, College of Veterinary Medicine, The University of Georgia, Athens, GA 30602–7388, USA

R.P. Johnson, Health Canada, Guelph Laboratory, 110 Stone Road West, Guelph, Ontario, N1G 3W4, Canada

S. Jordan, Department of Microbiology, Institute of Food Research, Whiteknights Road, Reading RG6 6BZ, UK

A.J. McCarthy, School of Biological Sciences, University of Liverpool, Liverpool, Merseyside L69 3BX, UK

L. Malcolm, Department of Molecular and Cell Biology, Institute of Medical Sciences, University of Aberdeen, Foresterhill, Aberdeen AB25 2ZD, UK

T.S. Marks, Centre for Applied Microbiology Research, Porton Down, Salisbury, Wiltshire SP4 0JG, UK

P. Michel, Health Canada, Guelph Laboratory, 110 Stone Road West, Guelph, Ontario, N1G 3W4, Canada

K.J. Mobbs, School of Biological Sciences and Department of Medical Microbiology, University of Liverpool, Liverpool, Merseyside L69 3BX, UK

H.W. Moon, Veterinary Medical Research Institute, College of Veterinary Medicine, Iowa State University, Ames, IA 50011, USA

E. Mueller, Department of Veterinary Pathology, College of Veterinary Medicine, The University of Georgia, Athens, GA 30602–7388, USA

A.D. O'Brien, Department of Microbiology and Immunology, F. Edward Hebert School of Medicine, Uniformed Services University of the Health Sciences, Bethesda, MD 20814, USA

S. Park, Department of Microbiology, Institute of Food Research, Whiteknights Road, Reading RG6 6BZ, UK

A.H. Parks, Department of Large Animal Medicine, College of Veterinary Medicine, The University of Georgia, Athens, GA 30602–7388, USA

T.H. Pennington, Department of Medical Microbiology, University of Aberdeen, Foresterhill, Aberdeen AB25 2ZD, UK

K. Rahn, Health Canada, Guelph Laboratory, 110 Stone Road West, Guelph, Ontario, N1G 3W4, Canada

M.A. Rasmussen, National Animal Disease Center, ARS–USDA, Ames, IA 50010, USA

S.A. Renwick, Science Division, Canadian Food Inspection Agency, 3851 Fallowfield Road, Nepean, Ontario, K2H 8P9, Canada

J.R. Saunders, School of Biological Sciences, University of Liverpool, Liverpool, Merseyside L69 3BX, UK

K.P. Scott, Rowett Research Institute, Greenburn Road, Bucksburn, Aberdeen AB21 9SB, UK

M.J. Sergeant, School of Biological Sciences, University of Liverpool, Liverpool, Merseyside L69 3BX, UK

R.J. Sharp, Centre for Applied Microbiology Research, Porton Down, Salisbury, Wiltshire SP4 0JG, UK

J.S. Spika, Bureau of Infectious Diseases, Health Canada, Laboratory Centre for Disease Control, Tunney's Pasture, Ottawa, Ontario, K1A 0L2, Canada

C.S. Stewart, Rowett Research Institute, Greenburn Road, Bucksburn, Aberdeen AB21 9SB, UK

B.A. Synge, SAC, Veterinary Science Division, Drummond Hill, Stratherrick Road, Inverness IV2 4JZ, UK

F. Thomson-Carter, Scottish Reference Laboratory for *E. coli* O157 and *Campylobacter*, Department of Medical Microbiology, University of Aberdeen, Foresterhill, Aberdeen AB25 2ZD, UK

S. Tkalcic, Department of Veterinary Pathology, College of Veterinary Medicine, The University of Georgia, Athens, GA 30602–7388, USA

J.S. Wallace, Department of Life Sciences, University of East London, Romford Road, London E15 4LZ, UK

T.L. Wickman, National Animal Disease Center, ARS–USDA, Ames, IA 50010, USA

J.B. Wilson, Bureau of Infectious Diseases, Health Canada, Laboratory Centre for Disease Control, Department of Population Medicine, University of Guelph, Guelph, Ontario, N1G 2W1, Canada

T. Zhao, Centre for Food Safety and Quality Enhancement, College of Agricultural and Environmental Sciences, Griffin, GA 30223–1797, USA

Preface

In April 1998, a workshop was held at the Rowett Research Institute, Bucksburn, Aberdeen, to discuss the occurrence of *Escherichia coli* O157 in farm animals and the factors affecting the spread of this bacterium in the environment and to humans. Scotland has suffered the worst single outbreak of disease caused by this bacterium to date and it seemed particularly appropriate that some of the scientific problems and challenges raised should be discussed here, by an international group. This volume contains the papers on which the contributions were based, together with two extra reviews, which Victor Gannon and Roger Johnson and his colleagues kindly agreed to provide. The editors are very grateful to the contributors for their forbearance in responding to numerous questions; any mistakes that remain may be ascribed to our editorial shortcomings, for which of course we apologize in advance.

For their help with organizing and operating the workshop, we thank Dr. Andrew Chesson, Sylvia Duncan, Vera Smith, Margaret Davidson, Kate Mason, Hilary Robertson, Tony Richardson and Kenneth Young. We are also grateful for additional financial assistance provided by Marks and Spencer plc and Tesco Stores Ltd. We thank Professor W.P.T. James, Director of the Rowett Research Institute, for his creative input and support. The Rowett Research Institute is funded by the Scottish Office Agriculture, Environment and Fisheries Department.

Colin Stewart and Harry Flint
Aberdeen, December 1998

1

Genetics and Molecular Ecology of *Escherichia coli* O157

J.R. Saunders,[1] M.J. Sergeant,[1] A.J. McCarthy,[1] K.J. Mobbs,[1, 2] C.A. Hart,[2] T.S. Marks[3] and R.J. Sharp[3]

[1]*School of Biological Sciences and* [2]*Department of Medical Microbiology, University of Liverpool, Liverpool, UK;* [3]*Centre for Applied Microbiology Research, Porton Down, Salisbury, UK*

INTRODUCTION

Escherichia coli O157 is the most notorious serogroup of verotoxigenic *E. coli* (VTEC) and belongs to a subgroup of VTEC that is associated with human disease and referred to as enterohaemorrhagic *E. coli* (EHEC). Relatively recent acquisition of verotoxin (VT)-converting phages is believed to be largely responsible for the recent emergence of *E. coli* O157:H7 as a new pathogen created from more mildly pathogenic O55:H7 and O127:H6 progenitors (Whittam, 1995). Many virulence determinants, including toxin production, attachment to the intestinal surface and enterocyte damage, are shared and widely distributed genetic characters among *E. coli* isolates of varying disease-producing phenotypes isolated from both humans and animals. The pathogenesis of *E. coli* O157, other EHEC and VTEC is complex and encoded by a variety of plasmid, bacteriophage and chromosomal genes. Like enteropathogenic *E. coli* (EPEC), EHEC contain virulence plasmids that promote non-intimate attachment, and a pathogenicity island encoding both intimate attachment and the signalling apparatus to induce attaching effacement of the mammalian enterocyte (Table 1.1). This chapter will review the molecular genetics of pathogenicity and ecology in *E. coli* O157 and, in particular, the role of toxin-converting bacteriophages in the biology of VTEC.

Table 1.1. Principal virulence determinants in *E. coli* O157 and VTEC.

O antigen – LPS
Virulence plasmid (~60 MDa/90 kbp)
Bundle-forming (type IV) pili (Bfp)
Ehx haemolysin
KatP catalase
Regulators of virulence genes (Per)
Chromosomal pathogenicity island
Enterocyte effacement locus (LEE) (35 kbp)
Signal transduction (EspA, EspB, EspD)
Intimin (EaeA – 94 kDa) (colonic specificity?)
Translocated intimin receptor (Tir – 78 kDa → Hp90)
Type III secretion system (Sep, Cfm)
Toxin-converting phages
Enterohaemolysin (Ehly1, 2)
VT1/VT2 (SLT)

PATHOLOGY CAUSED BY VTEC

EHEC can produce asymptomatic infections, cause non-bloody diarrhoea, bloody diarrhoea or haemorrhagic colitis (HC), haemolytic uraemic syndrome (HUS) and thrombocytic thrombocytopenic purpura (TTP) (Griffin, 1995) (Fig. 1.1). Haemorrhagic colitis caused by EHEC is characterized by severe abdominal cramps, bloody stools, little or no fever and evidence of colonic mucosal oedema (Griffin and Tauxe, 1991). Approximately 2–7% of patients affected by VTEC develop systemic complications, most commonly HUS, which is characterized by microangiopathic haemolytic anaemia, thrombocytopenia, renal failure and central nervous system symptoms. TTP is considered to be a manifestation of HUS where renal failure is normally mild but neurological involvement is greater (Griffin, 1995).

The majority of the untoward consequences of VTEC infection stem from production of one or both types of verotoxin, VT1 and VT2; verotoxins are also known as shiga-like toxins (SLT). Throughout this chapter, the terms VT and VTEC are therefore used interchangeably for SLT and SLTEC, respectively. There is little evidence for the presence of circulating VT in the blood of patients with systemic VTEC infections. Direct detection of the toxin is difficult, as only minute amounts are needed to cause disease. Also, the globo-series globotriaosylceramide (G3b) receptor targeted by VT is part of blood-group antigens Pk and P1, which bind VT2 readily, lowering the amount available for detection. Binding of VT to P antigen may also explain why patients who express low levels of this antigen are more likely to progress to HUS or TTP when infected with EHEC (Taylor *et al.*, 1990).

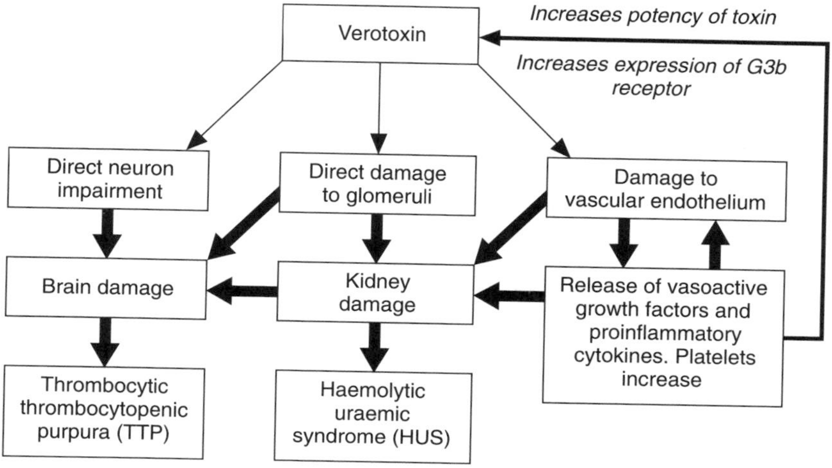

Fig. 1.1. Role of verotoxin in disease caused by *E. coli* O157.

Patients with HUS may have circulating antibodies to VT (Karmali *et al.*, 1983). VT2 is also considered a poor immunogen *per se*: for example, an antibody response to VT2 could not be detected in cows experimentally infected with O157:H7 strains expressing both VT1 and VT2 (Johnson *et al.*, 1996). The B-lymphocyte marker CD77 can function as a receptor for VT (Maloney and Lingwood, 1994) and is involved in signal transduction and regulation in B-cell proliferation and differentiation. By targeting lymphocytes expressing CD77, verotoxins could suppress the humoral arm of the immune response. This would inhibit the antibody response to VT1 and VT2 and enable evasion of host antibody response (Maloney and Lingwood, 1994). Indeed, gnotobiotic pigs persistently infected with *E. coli* O111-expressing VT1 have been shown to become immunocompromised, with lower peripheral lymphocyte counts and lower proliferative responses to mitogens (Christopher-Hennings *et al.*, 1993). It is clear that malnourishment in both humans and animals may also play a role in rendering hosts susceptible to VT (Kurioka *et al.*, 1998).

Biologically active VT1 is able to move across intact polarized intestinal epithelial cells without apparent cellular disruption (Acheson *et al.*, 1996). The presence of VT receptors on the apical surface of intestinal epithelial cells might offer some protection against absorption of luminal VT1, explaining greater virulence associated with VT2-expressing strains. Since VT2 binds to its receptor much less readily than VT1, it can be absorbed from the lumen more easily. Once in the bloodstream, VT2 can again escape inactivation by binding less efficiently to P blood-group antigens. However, upon reaching the cortex of the kidney, where G3b is abundant, VT2 can bind more readily and exert its damaging effects, even in minute quantities.

The VT gene has been found in over 100 serotypes of *E. coli* (Rietra *et al.*, 1989; Mobbs, 1997), in *Citrobacter freundii* (Schmidt *et al.*, 1993), *Enterobacter cloacae* (Paton and Paton, 1996) and *Aeromonas* spp. (Haque *et al.*, 1997). O157:H7 is by far the most commonly isolated serotype from symptomatic patients and O157 strains are frequently encountered in farm environments (Porter *et al.*, 1997). Of the non-O157 serogroups, O26:H11, O103:H2, O111:NM and O113:H21 are most frequently isolated (Griffin and Tauxe, 1991). Non-O157 VTEC cause less severe symptoms, but illness is often more protracted, and many non-O157 VTEC strains are not human pathogens (Ramotar *et al.*, 1995). The proportion of healthy persons whose stools harbour non-O157 VTEC is similar to that reported for those with diarrhoea (Gunzer *et al.*, 1992). Non-O157 VTEC are isolated from food samples and cattle faeces far more frequently than O157 (Griffin, 1995). Non-O157 VTEC isolated from humans with HC or HUS are much more likely to contain key virulence determinants encoded by the 60 MDa (90 kbp) EHEC plasmid and *eae*A gene (see below) than those from animals. This suggests that many non-O157 VTEC isolated from animals are not human pathogens (Beutin *et al.*, 1995) and that only a subset of VTEC strains is pathogenic for humans (Paton *et al.*, 1996, 1997). It is clear also, from gene probing (Table 1.2), that populations of *E. coli* can carry various combinations of genes associated with EHEC pathogenesis (Mobbs, 1997). Only when strains carry a full, or at least nearly complete, complement of the appropriate genes may severe disease become apparent. Also, the entire *E. coli* population in humans and animals may be regarded as an extended gene pool that acts as a reservoir for the creation of new combinations of virulence determinants and new epidemic clones of importance in human and animal medicine. Indeed, *Shigella* spp., the apparent source of verotoxins, are considered to be part of that gene pool.

DETERMINANTS OF EHEC PATHOGENICITY

EHEC tend to produce attaching–effacing (att/eff) lesions in the colon that are very similar to those produced in the proximal small intestine by EPEC, and which provide the model for producing this type of pathology. In EPEC, the bacteria become intimately attached to the enterocyte membrane, which becomes cupped around the bacterium and is frequently raised beneath adherent bacteria to form characteristic pedestal structures. The microvilli become effaced and the brush border disintegrates into vesicles containing enterocyte enzymes. Polymerized actin from cytoskeletal microfilaments becomes concentrated in the apical cytoplasm beneath adherent bacteria to produce att/eff. The loss of microvilli and rearrangement of the cytoskeleton, together with loss of brush-border enzyme activity, reduces the absorptive surface and in itself leads to an osmotic diarrhoea (Hart *et al.*, 1993). Coupled to this, *E. coli* O157 and other EHEC produce a variety of

Table 1.2. Distribution of virulence-determining gene sequences in selected VTEC isolates.

Isolate	Serogroup	EHEC	VT1	VT2	*eae*A
C409	O4	−	+	−	−
C415	O26	+	+	−	+
D172	O26	+	+	−	+
D175	O111	+	+	+	−
C412	O111	+	+	−	+
D167	O113	+	−	+	−
D176	O113	−	−	+	+
D166	O121	+	−	−	+
D165	O126	−	−	+	−
D177	O145	+	+	−	+
C877	O157	+	+	+	+
D420	O157	+	−	+	+
C410	O160	−	+	−	−
D178	ROUGH	+	−	+	+
D149	ND	+	+	+	+
D152	ND	+	+	−	+
D156	ND	−	−	+	+
D157	ND	+	−	+	+
D160	ND	−	+	−	+
D161	ND	+	−	−	+

+, Hybridization (Mobbs, 1997) with labelled gene probes specific for the genes concerned; −, no hybridization; ND, not determined. Probes: VT1, verotoxin 1 (Willshaw *et al.*, 1985); VT2, verotoxin 2 (Willshaw *et al.*, 1987); *eae*A (Jerse *et al.*, 1990); EHEC (Levine *et al.*, 1985).

toxins, which damage gut tissue and, on gaining access to the bloodstream, may cause lesions of varying severity. The attributes that lead to the pathogenesis of *E. coli* O157 (Table 1.1) are numerous and their interplay is complex.

Adherence factors

A 60-MDa non-self-transmissible plasmid designated EAF (EPEC adherence factor), present in many EPEC strains and analogous plasmids in EHEC (Hales *et al.*, 1992), encodes type IV bundle-forming pili (Bfp) (Donnenberg *et al.*, 1992). Aggregation of Bfp from different individual bacteria leads to a unique attachment pattern, called localized adherence (LA), where bacterial cells adhere to tissue-culture cells in distinct microcolonies (Nataro *et al.*, 1985). Many EPEC strains are also able to adhere to HEp-2 cells, a property rare in enterotoxigenic *E. coli* (ETEC) or enteroinvasive *E. coli* (EIEC) strains.

Loss of the EAF plasmid eliminates both the LA phenotype and adherence to HEp-2 cells. However, the EAF plasmid alone is not sufficient to produce fully functional Bfp, and chromosomal loci are also involved (Donnenberg and Kaper, 1992). EPEC lacking EAF plasmids are less pathogenic when fed to volunteers, but are still capable of causing att/eff lesions *in vitro* (Levine *et al.*, 1985). The EAF plasmid encodes a gene designated *per*, which enhances expression of the chromosomal *eae*A gene (see below) and is related in sequence to *env*Y, a gene involved in the thermoregulation of protein expression (Jerse and Kaper, 1991). The *sep*B (secretion of EPEC proteins) gene is involved in the export of at least five proteins involved in att/eff lesion formation (McDaniel *et al.*, 1995).

The 60 MDa plasmid present in most strains of EHEC encodes a haemolysin, fimbrial colonization antigens and other virulence determinants (Table 1.1). The plasmid may have a role in initial attachment to mucosal surfaces (Karch *et al.*, 1987), since O157:H7 strains cured of such plasmids failed to express fimbriae and lost the ability to adhere to intestinal cells. Conversely, *E. coli* K-12 strains transformed with the 60-MDa plasmid produced fimbriae and were able to adhere to intestinal cells. In contrast, Junkins and Doyle (1989) showed that adherence of a plasmidless derivative O157:H7 to Henle 407 cells was threefold greater than the parental strain. Also, only one in five O157:H7 strains possessing the 60-MDa plasmid were piliated and yet all adhered to Henle 407 and HEp-2 cells (Sherman *et al.*, 1987). Surprisingly, O157:H7 strains are unable to adhere to Caco-2 cells, derived from human colon carcinoma (Knutton *et al.*, 1989), and yet the colon is believed to be the main site of infection by EHEC in humans and animals. A 60-MDa plasmid transferred to K-12 strains conferred weak adherence, but also induced formation of a pedestal-like structure and actin polymerization in the cells adjacent to the point of adhesion (Toth *et al.*, 1990). When the wild-type EHEC strain 933 and its plasmid-cured derivative, 933-cu, were fed to streptomycin-treated mice, the plasmid-containing wild-type strain always outcompeted the plasmid-cured derivative (Waldolkowski *et al.*, 1990a, b), although the cured strain was still capable of colonizing the mouse gut.

EHEC strains have been shown to adhere to human ileocaecal epithelial cells (HCT8) in a pattern designated as log-jam (McKee and O'Brien, 1995). This pattern was not observed on HEp-2 cells, was independent of the EHEC *eae*A gene (see below) and was shared with non-pathogenic strains, but not *E. coli* K-12. The log-jam phenotype may represent an additional means by which EHEC strains initially interact with enterocytes. EPEC strains cured of their EAF plasmids may be less pathogenic because of their reduced ability to infect the proximal small intestine (Tzipori *et al.*, 1989, 1995). Conversely, experiments by Waldolkowski *et al.* (1990b) showed a cured EHEC strain (933-cu-rev) that, unlike other EHEC, was able to colonize the distal small intestine and was lethal to mice.

Genetics of att/eff formation

All the genes necessary for att/eff formation are encoded on a large chromosomal locus (pathogenicity island) called LEE (locus of enterocyte effacement), which is conserved in other intestinal pathogens causing att/eff lesions, including EPEC, EHEC, *Hafnia alvei* and *Citrobacter freundii* (McDaniel *et al.*, 1995). The *eae*A (enterocyte attaching and effacing) gene in the LEE encodes a 94-kDa outer membrane protein (intimin), which shows homology to the invasins of *Yersinia* spp. (Jerse *et al.*, 1990). The gene is present in all EPEC isolates, and homologues exist in most EHEC strains (McDaniel *et al.*, 1995). The EHEC *eae*A gene, which seems to confer attachment specificity for the colonic epithelium, as opposed to the specificity for the proximal small intestine exhibited by EPEC intimin (Griffin, 1995), differs somewhat in sequence from that found in classical (O111) EPEC, particularly at the 3′ end (Yu and Kaper, 1992). Att/eff in EHEC is not always associated with intimin: an O113:H21 EHEC strain produces clinical features comparable to those associated with infection by strains inducing att/eff lesions, and yet it is negative for *eae*A (Dytoc *et al.*, 1994). However, F-actin adhesion pedestals on the host plasma membrane and recruitment of other cytoskeletal elements below foci of bacterial adhesion are absent. Figure 1.2 shows the 'classical' three-stage model for att/eff formation, proposed originally by Donnenberg and Kaper (1992). This model involves initial interaction between Bfp and receptors on the enterocyte, followed by more intimate attachment mediated by intimin (EaeA) and other LEE-encoded genes specifying signal transduction to cause actin accumulation and cytoskeletal rearrangement. The signal-transduction pathway that leads to att/eff lesion formation in EPEC involves the phosphorylation of a 90-kDa protein (Hp90) by host-cell tyrosine kinase (Rosenshine *et al.*, 1992). Although originally believed to be a host protein, it is now clear that this protein, the translocated intimin receptor (Tir) is specified by the attaching–effacing bacteria as a gene product of the LEE (Wolff *et al.*, 1998). This extraordinary behaviour thus involves the bacterial pathogen producing and transporting its own receptor into the mammalian host enterocyte as a prelude to formation of the characteristic att/eff lesion (Wolff *et al.*, 1998).

The signal-transduction apparatus for att/eff is complex and involves a contact-dependent type III secretion apparatus and the involvement of secreted proteins EspA, EspB and EspD. EspA forms filamentous structures, similar morphologically to the invasomes of *Salmonella*, which may act as primary adhesins and, more importantly, form the delivery apparatus for the type III secretion system (Knutton *et al.*, 1998). By means of EspA filaments, EspB, EspD and other components, such as the Tir protein (alias Hp90), may be delivered from the bacterium to the enterocyte (Wolff *et al.*, 1998). It is now clear that the classical model (Fig. 1.2) may not account for all of the adhesive properties of EPEC and EHEC. Thus, a modified four-stage model

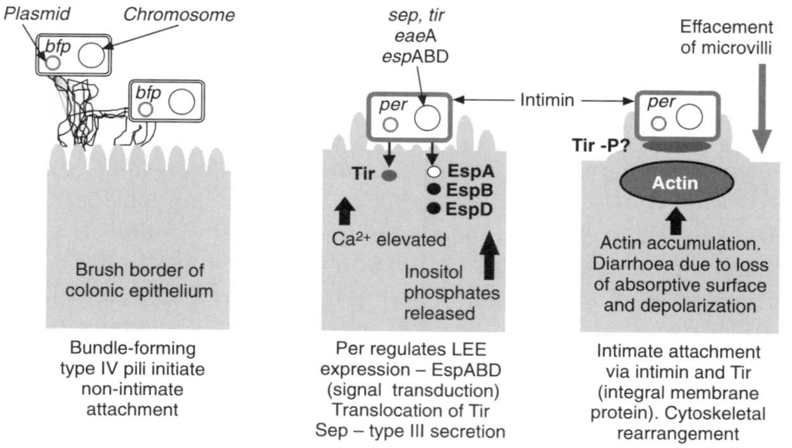

Fig. 1.2. Classical three-stage model for attaching and effacement in *E. coli* O157.

for EPEC pathogenesis has been proposed by Hicks *et al.* (1998), in which primary adhesion would be by some alternative adhesin (possibly EspA filaments) and bfp would mediate bacteria–bacteria adhesions to produce the three-dimensional microcolonies typical of intimately attached bacteria.

Although EPEC pathogenesis has provided a valuable model for the behaviour of *E. coli* O157 and other attaching–effacing VTEC, it is clear that there are fundamental differences in behaviour among such bacteria. It is, for example, notable that signal-transduction mechanisms and outcomes differ when EPEC and VTEC are compared. Notably, host proteins and/or the Tir do not appear to be phosphorylated (Ismail *et al.*, 1995, 1998). The *eae*A gene is necessary for adhesion to HEp-2 cells and colonization of the gnotobiotic piglet (McKee *et al.*, 1995). Also, a low-molecular-weight (8 kDa) outer-membrane protein (OMP) unique to O157:H7 and O26:H11 serogroups has been implicated in adherence (Zhao *et al.*, 1996). Tn*phoA*-generated mutants deficient in expression of this protein showed significantly less adherence to Henle 407 cells and they colonized chicken caeca at much lower levels than wild-type strains. The OMP was shown to have a close association with the lipid A portion of lipopolysaccharide (LPS) on the cell and was expressed in greater amounts when bile salts and acriflavin were present in the medium.

Structure and function of verotoxins

Verotoxins can be divided into two groups: VT1, which differs in sequence from shiga toxin produced by *Shigella dysenteriae* type 1 by only one amino acid and is antigenically indistinguishable; and VT2, which has only 50–60% sequence homology with VT1 and is not neutralized by antisera to shiga toxin. Verotoxins are so called because of their lethal effect on vero (green-monkey kidney) cell lines. VTs are also enterotoxic, mediating fluid accumulation in ligated ileal loops, and are lethally paralytic when injected into mice and rabbits. VT1 toxins are conserved; only one variant has been found and it differs by two amino acids (Paton *et al.*, 1993). In contrast, VT2 toxins form a diverse group with many antigenic variants. VTs are AB toxins, composed of a single A subunit (M_r 32,200) non-covalently associated with a pentamer of B subunits (M_r 7962 each). Binding of VT to mammalian cells is accomplished by interaction of B subunits with the membrane glycolipid of the globo-series G3b. This glycolipid molecule contains a terminal Galα 1–4Gal disaccharide, which appears to be the minimum determinant necessary for toxin binding. After binding, the active A subunit enters the cell by receptor-dependent endocytosis. The internalized vesicles fuse with lysosomes and are translocated, first to the Golgi apparatus, and then to the cytosol (Sandvig *et al.*, 1992). The A subunit is a ribosomal ribonucleic acid (rRNA) *N*-glycosidase, cleaving a single adenine residue near the 3′ end of eukaryotic 28S rRNA, thus preventing elongation factor-1-dependent binding of aminoacyl-transfer RNA (tRNA) (Saxena *et al.*, 1989). The resultant blockade of protein synthesis leads to cell death.

Although both VT1 and VT2 have the same mode of action, their effect *in vitro* and *in vivo* differs considerably. VT1 binds more efficiently to the G3b receptor and is more potent on vero cells (Tesh *et al.*, 1993a). However, VT2 is 400 times more lethal for mice than VT1 when injected intravenously (Tesh *et al.*, 1993b) and is 1000 times more active on human renal microvascular endothelial cells (Louie and Obrig, 1995). Lethality in streptomycin-treated mice requires colonization of the gut with an *E. coli* strain producing large amounts of VT2, and colonization with strains expressing VT1 is not lethal in such models (Waldolkowski *et al.*, 1990a). VT1 and VT2 are equivalent in their capacity to inhibit protein synthesis in cell-free assays, suggesting that differences in enzymatic activity do not contribute to differences observed in cytotoxicity *in vitro* or in mouse lethality (Tesh *et al.*, 1993a).

Human umbilical-vein endothelial cells (HUVECs) are 100 times more sensitive *in vitro* to the action of VTs in the presence of inflammatory mediators, such as LPS, or cytokines, e.g. tumour necrosis factor (TNF) or interleukin-1 (IL-1) (Louie and Obrig, 1995). Such mediators are believed to increase the amount of G3b receptor molecules on the endothelial cell surface, leading to greater susceptibility (Jackson, 1990; Fig. 1.2). Indeed, patients infected with VTEC who present with fever or have a high white blood-cell count in the early stages of infection are more likely to progress to HUS and TTP (Walters *et al.*, 1989; Pavia *et al.*, 1990).

The A subunit of VT contains a single intrachain disulphide bond, encompassing a hydrophilic loop that contains two trypsin-sensitive arginine residues (Burgess and Roberts, 1993). The VT1 A subunit is extremely sensitive to trypsin (Olsnes *et al.*, 1981) and cleavage results in the two predicted fragments, A1 and A2, required for cytotoxic effects in other toxins. When proteolysis is blocked by site-directed mutagenesis at the disulphide loop, the toxin remains effective, having a similar catalytic activity to that of the wild-type molecule and only a marginally reduced cytotoxicity towards cultured cells (Burgess and Roberts, 1993). However, processing of the toxin at alternative accessible sites has not been ruled out, and studies involving VT2 variant toxins have shown that activation can take place (Melton-Celsa *et al.*, 1996).

B2F1, an O91:H21 strain from a patient with HUS, produces two VT2 variant toxins, VT2vha and VT2vhb, but lacks the *eae*A gene and the ability to induce att/eff lesions in the intestine (Ito *et al.*, 1990). However, it is much more potent in mouse models, having a median lethal dose (LD_{50}) < 10, compared with an $LD_{50} > 10^{10}$ for EHEC strains expressing VT2 or the variant toxin VT2c (Melton-Celsa *et al.*, 1996). Culture supernatants from B2F1 grown in mouse intestinal mucous were 35- to 350-fold more toxic for vero cells than culture supernatants from B2F1 grown in LB broth. In addition, purified VT2hb from B2F1 exhibited greater toxicity when preincubated with human colonic or mouse intestinal mucus. Trypsin-nicked VT2vhb shows no increase in activity and yet still has the capacity to be activated by colonic mucus. Amino acid differences between activatable and non-activatable toxins occur in the A2 peptide, indicating this as the site for activation. Such activation, however, is not a prerequisite for lethality, since VT2 and VT2c cannot be activated but are lethal in mouse models when expressed at high levels. The activation of VT2vha and VT2vhb, but not VT2 or VT2c, thus occurs via an unknown mechanism, involving components of murine intestinal mucus that enhance potency of the toxin.

The VT1 operon consists of tandemly arranged *slt* IA and *slt* IB genes, encoding A and B units, respectively. The promoter sequence is identical to that of shiga toxin, containing a Fur-binding site, permitting the iron-dependent regulation of VT1 by the Fur–iron corepressor complex (Calderwood *et al.*, 1987). VT1a- and VT1b-encoding genes are transcribed as a single polycistronic messenger RNA (mRNA) (DeGrandis *et al.*, 1987). There is evidence for a second independent promoter for *slt* IB (Koslov *et al.*, 1988) and control of subunit expression might occur at the translational level. Differences in the ribosome binding site may result in differential translation, producing a differing ratio of A and B subunits, as is the case with cholera toxin (Sung *et al.*, 1990). The VT2 operon is similarly arranged; the genes encoding A and B subunits are in tandem, transcribed as a single polycistronic message with a gap of 14 nucleotides between them. Putative ribosomal binding sites are present immediately upstream of the A subunit coding region and within the intercistronic gap (Sung *et al.*, 1990). The promoter for the VT2 gene shows no homology to that for VT1 and transcription is not regulated by the Fur protein or iron corepressor.

VT phages containing either VT1 or VT2 operons form a generally homogeneous group of lamboid viruses, but differ dramatically in their immunity profiles. Such heterogeneity may aid in the evolution of VTEC strains with greater and more varied toxin production that confers enhanced ability to overwhelm host defences. Since both VT1 and VT2 are phage-encoded, they should be induced by substances, such as mitomycin C, that induce lysogenic λ phage to enter the lytic cycle (Al-Jumaili *et al.*, 1992). Mitomycin C activates RecA-mediated cleavage of phage immunity repressors, resulting in expression of mid to late phage genes, leading to replication of the phage genome and eventual lysis of the host cell. As the phage genome replicates in host cells, VT gene copy number increases, leading to a concomitant increase in expression of toxin. Furthermore, on cellular lysis, large amounts of free VT are released. However, most VTEC do not produce any discernible free phage particles, even after treatment with mitomycin C (Rietra *et al.*, 1989), presumably because they contain non-inducible defective prophage(s). Even so, treatment of these strains with mitomycin C greatly increases VT expression, which cannot be accounted for by phage replication alone (Yee *et al.*, 1993; Muhldorfer *et al.*, 1996). It seems likely that the VT1 genes are not integral components of the phage genomes. Indeed, regulation by iron concentration implies that the toxin-encoding sequences may have been originally acquired by phages from the *S. dysenteriae* chromosome, where the shiga-toxin gene is also iron-regulated (Calderwood *et al.*, 1987). In contrast, VT2 expression seems to be more closely phage-linked, as its regulation is common to that of other viral genes requiring RecA and phage-encoded regulatory factors. Treatment with antibiotics, such as trimethoprim–sulphamethoxazole or gentamicin, increases the chance of an infection leading to HUS (Ostroff *et al.*, 1989). At sublethal concentrations, like mitomycin C, such antibiotics markedly increase VT2 production *in vitro* (Karch *et al.*, 1995). Additionally, patients with neoplasia routinely treated with mitomycin C are more likely to develop HUS (Lesene *et al.*, 1989). Stressful conditions encountered in the gut or the open environment may also cause phage induction and subsequent increased production of VT2.

Haemolysin production by EHEC

EHEC strains produce two genetically and serologically unrelated haemolysins. Haemolysin genes are found in all O157 strains and about half of non-O157 EHEC. The 60-MDa EHEC plasmid confers a haemolytic phenotype on sheep blood cells, although only small zones of lysis are apparent (Schmidt *et al.*, 1994). The haemolytic determinant (Ehx) comprises two genes (*ehx*A and *ehx*C), which share approximately 60% homology with the *hly*A and *hly*C genes of the *E. coli* α-haemolysin operon (Schmidt *et al.*, 1995). α-Haemolysin is usually present in *E. coli* that cause extraintestinal infections and is a member of the RTX toxin family (Bauer and Welch,

1996a). The 110-kDa α-haemolysin encoded by *hly*A is activated by acylation requiring HlyC, and is secreted through a *sec*-independent pathway involving both HlyB and HlyD (Bauer and Welch, 1996a). The genes *hly*B and *hly*D are lacking in the EHEC operon, indicating that Ehx may not be secreted. This may explain the small zones of lysis observed on blood agar and lack of haemolytic activity in culture supernatants. When α-haemolysin genes *hly*BD are supplied *in trans* to wild-type EHEC or *E. coli* K-12 strains carrying plasmid-encoded *ehx*AC, zones of haemolysis become much larger and haemolytic activity can be detected in culture supernatants (Bauer and Welch, 1996b). Ehx is unique among RTX toxins in that it demonstrates both leucocyte specificity and haemolytic activity. It is active on human and sheep erythrocytes and lyses bovine lymphoma cells (which may suggest a role in maintenance of EHEC populations in cattle), but is inactive on human lymphoma cell lines (Bauer and Welch, 1996b). Of 20 serum samples from HUS patients, 19 reacted specifically with the EHEC haemolysin antigen, compared with only one out of 20 in control samples (Schmidt *et al.*, 1995).

Enterohaemolysin (Ehly), which is serologically and genetically distinct from α-haemolysin and Ehx, is closely associated with VT production in EHEC (Beutin *et al.*, 1989). Ehly is a 30-kDa protein with low activity when expressed in *E. coli* K-12, but it can form a dimer of 60 kDa with increased activity in wild-type strains (Stroeher *et al.*, 1993). It is not secreted, and is associated with the outer membrane. An Ehly-specific deoxyribonucleic acid (DNA) probe only hybridized to seven of 21 *E. coli* strains exhibiting an Ehly$^+$ phenotype, indicating that most of such strains produce a genetically distinct Ehly (Stroeher *et al.*, 1993). A second *ehly* gene cloned from one such strain and designated *ehly2*, only hybridized to 11 of 21 Ehly$^+$ strains, suggesting that a family of genetically distinct Ehly exist in VTEC. Both *ehly1* and *ehly2* are encoded on lamboid-like temperate phages (Beutin *et al.*, 1993b). Ehly1 is encoded on a temperate lamboid phage, with a genome of approximately 41 kbp, which is specific for O26 serogroups and could not be propagated in *E. coli* K-12 (Beutin *et al.*, 1990). Expression of *ehly1* proved lethal to all *E. coli* strains, apart from the strain from which the phage was isolated. Ehly is involved in phage-mediated lysis of bacteria, but acts as a haemolysin of mammalian cells (Beutin *et al.*, 1990, 1993b). Interestingly, gene products involved in invasion by *Shigella* and *Salmonella* have conserved sequence motifs in common with phage lytic transglycosylases (Mushegian *et al.*, 1996), suggesting a possible dual role for such toxins. A number of phages of 40–43 kb harbouring *ehly2* have been isolated and classified into two groups on the basis of genomic DNA restriction profiles (Beutin *et al.*, 1993b).

Bacteriophages and virulence of *E. coli* O157

EHEC readily lose their ability to produce VT when cultured on agar plates, suggesting that the encoding genes are carried on an extrachromosomal element (Karch *et al.*, 1995). Originally, a plasmid was thought to be responsible for encoding transfer of VT production, but recipients that had acquired VT from VT^+ strains became lysogenic (Smith and Lingwood, 1971). Of 519 *E. coli* strains from diseased and healthy humans or domestic animals, 68 were VT^+, of which four exhibited transfer of VT production to *E. coli* K-12 in mixed culture. In three such strains, all recipients that had become VT^+ also became lysogenic. Generally, depending on the recipient host used, lysogenization was not always associated with acquisition of VT^+, implying that some phages do not carry VT genes. It was also possible to differentiate phages from the same VTEC strain by means of their immunity patterns. For strains H19 and H28, 'mutants' (lysogens) were obtained that were phage-resistant. Phages produced by that strain were then differentiated into type A, able to lyse all of the resistant 'mutants', and type B, able to lyse only some of the mutants. Two phages isolated by O'Brien *et al.* (1984) from O157 EDL 933 were shown to encode VT1 and VT2 toxins, respectively (Strockbine *et al.*, 1986). A more extensive study of VT-encoding phages, involving characterization of eight VT phages isolated from clinical EHEC strains and VTEC strains isolated from cattle, was carried out by Rietra *et al.* (1989). Their phages could be subdivided into two groups, depending on whether they were isolated from O26 or O157 serotypes. Phages from O157 serotypes, irrespective of which VT they encoded, exhibited similar restriction fragment length polymorphisms (RFLPs) (Rietra *et al.*, 1989). All O157 phages also had similar virion morphology, with regular hexagonal heads and short tails. In contrast, the phages from O26 serotypes had elongated hexagonal heads and long tails. RFLP patterns of DNA from O26 phages were distinct from those of O157-type phages with only limited relatedness to each other. An exception was phage 933J, isolated from an O157 strain, with the same morphology as O26-type phages. However, between all of the phages there is DNA homology that is independent of the VT genes. In general, immunity patterns of the phages differed, but, interestingly, the immunity patterns of VT1 and VT2 phages from the same strain were exactly the same. Thus, for example, ϕ933-VT1 could not infect a lysogen carrying ϕ933-VT2.

The genome of the VT1 phage H-19B has been shown to have cohesive (*cos*) ends, which become covalently bound during integration (Huang *et al.*, 1987). Homologous regions with λ include the J gene (tail protein), the *int–xis* region (chromosomal integration) and the O and P genes. Unlike other toxin-converting phages, the VT1 gene is not located next to the phage *att*P site, but between O and P (DNA replication), suggesting that it was not acquired from a host chromosome by abnormal excision events (Huang *et al.*, 1987). Acquisition could have involved a transposable element associated with VT genes or the shiga-toxin gene itself in *S. dysenteriae* (Paton *et al.*, 1992). Newland and Neill (1988), using probes developed from fH-19J (VT1, O26 phage) and f933W (VT2, O157 phage) found that, in general, VT genes were associated with phage sequences. Of strains expressing VT1 and VT2, 93% were positive for both probes. Of strains carrying only VT1, 87% were positive for just the fH-19J (VT1) probe. In contrast, 77% of VT2 strains were positive for both probes. This may be explained by multiple copies of the VT2 gene encoded by both H-19J- and 933W-like phage. Alternatively, the VT2 gene may be present on a hybrid phage containing DNA sequences homologous to both fH-19J and f933W. Only 10% of EPEC and normal *E. coli* flora were positive for phage DNA, but 47% of bacteraemic isolates were positive for the fH-19J (VT1) probe. This phage may carry a gene similar to *iss*, which is involved in serum resistance (Huang *et al.*, 1987). Only 25% of 28 pig oedema strains carrying the VT2e gene reacted with the fH-19J (VT1) probe, confirming that VT2 variant genes are usually chromosomally encoded.

The P gene from a VT2 phage (Datz *et al.*, 1996) has 95.3% sequence similarity to the λ P gene. In all O157 strains tested there was close linkage between the P and VT genes (Datz *et al.*, 1996). Differences in DNA fragments hybridizing with P- and VT-specific probes were observed within individual O157 strains. *E. coli* O157 strains undergo rapid genotypic alteration in the course of an infection (Karch *et al.*, 1995), as judged by RFLP patterns when probed with λ DNA. The change in RFLP patterns and VT genotypes has been attributed to loss of VT2-encoding genes and phage sequences, accompanied by loss of bacterial DNA (Datz *et al.*, 1996). When an *E. coli* K-12 strain is infected with a single phage that only carries one copy of the VT2 gene, VT2 sequences have been shown to be located on two different-sized restriction fragments within the chromosome (Paton *et al.*, 1992). This could result from the phage integrating twice into different chromosomal locations or the VT gene being present on an invertible DNA element.

We found that nearly all VT phages we isolated formed a heterogeneous group, which differed dramatically in immunity profiles (Sergeant, 1998). Heterogeneity of immunity patterns may aid in the evolution of VTEC with enhanced pathogenicity, because superinfection could result in multiple lysogenizations of the same strain with different phages that could coreside. This would lead to strains carrying not only VT1 and VT2 genes, but also multiple variants of VT2 (Schmitt *et al.*, 1991). The resulting antigenic heterogeneity of toxin production by such strains might confer the ability to overwhelm host defences. It has also been suggested that VT2 and VT1 act synergistically to produce greater toxin effects (Tesh *et al.*, 1993a). VT1, having a greater affinity for its Gb3 receptor, should cause most damage to the colonic epithelium, perforating the gut and permitting access of VT2 into the bloodstream. Once there, VT2 would presumably target organs, such as the kidney, where Gb3 is particularly abundant (Tesh *et al.*, 1993b).

Continual acquisition of bacteriophage-associated virulence genes may group them together at chromosomal *att* sites and eventually lead to the formation of pathogenicity islands. The use of tRNA genes as integration sites is common to a wide range of bacteriophages and plasmids (Cheetham and Katz, 1995), pathogenicity islands of both EPEC and uropathogenic *E. coli* (McDaniel *et al.*, 1995) and other virulence determinants, such as the *vap* region of *Dichelobacter nodosus* (Bloomfield *et al.*, 1997). Conservation of secondary structure in tRNA genes may be important in recognition by enzymes involved in both homologous and site-specific recombination (Cheetham and Katz, 1995). Grouping of virulence genes could also be the result of homologous recombination between related phage genomes carrying different virulence genes adjacent to *att*P sites. Both the Ehly and VT phages in EHEC are λ-like and it has been shown that lambdoid phages are capable of exchanging sequences (Highton *et al.*, 1990; Campbell, 1994). Some EHEC carry at least three VT genes (VT1 and two VT2 variants) and two enterohaemolysin genes (*ehly1* and *ehly2*), all presumably imported on different lamboid bacteriophages. Multiple infection by such a family of bacteriophages could lead to increased fitness and associated virulence. Certainly, *E. coli* λ lysogens have a significant growth advantage over non-lysogens under certain conditions and such increased fitness correlates with altered outer-membrane protein profiles (Edlin *et al.*, 1977). Lysogeny can increase the survival of some *E. coli* strains in serum due to the λ *bor* gene (Barondess and Beckwith, 1990), which shows homology to the *iss* serum-resistance gene of the conjugative plasmid ColV2 (Binns *et al.*, 1979). Another λ gene, *lom*, which may affect properties of *E. coli* lysogens in animal hosts, displays significant homology to virulence loci involved in macrophage survival in *Salmonella typhimurium* and invasiveness in *Yersinia enterocolitica*. However, such advantages could be offset by the potential burden of maintaining approximately 250 kbp of additional DNA. Although the genomes of the phages would be largely silenced by immunity repressors, loss of parts of the bacteriophage genome that do not benefit the lysogenized strain might therefore be expected in the course of evolution of VTEC strains. This is consistent with the observation in clinical isolates of EHEC that phages carrying virulence determinants are generally uninducible. This would suggest loss of wild-type phage genes during their evolutionary history.

Most VTEC strains from human and animal sources that we examined failed to produce VT phages (Sergeant, 1998) and therefore presumably harboured defective prophages, a phenomenon commonly encountered among toxigenic phages. Plaques with VT phages are in any case generally smaller and burst sizes reduced when compared with wild-type or laboratory strains of phage λ. This may be because the *slt*AB operon has become inserted into a lamboid phage genome in such a way that late/lytic gene functions of the phage have been ablated or reduced in expression. Alternatively, there may be a hot spot within the phage genome, with mutations there rendering the phage more or less defective for lytic growth. The VT2 gene seems to be non-essential *in vitro*, since recombinant phages where we have inserted a marker gene such as *kan*, *lux*AB or *gus* into the VT gene are still viable and infective (Sergeant, 1998). The VT gene also seems of little obvious benefit to lysogenized bacteria. However, it could be argued that VT1, being more active on the gut epithelium (Tesh *et al.*, 1993b), could assist the host bacterium by lysing enterocytes, thus releasing limiting nutrients, such as iron. Expression of the *slt*AB1 gene increases in low-iron conditions (Calderwood *et al.*, 1987), supporting this notion. VT2 does not act primarily on the gut, but on organs where cells are expressing large amounts of the toxin receptor G3b (Tesh *et al.*, 1993a). These organs, such as the brain and kidney, are distal to the site of bacterial infection in the gut, where damage would seem to be of little benefit to the bacteria. Also, the VT gene is under the control of bacteriophage genes (Muhldorfer *et al.*, 1996), only being expressed in large quantities on phage induction. If the VT gene is not advantageous to the bacterium, why it is maintained in so many serotypes of *E. coli*, as judged by the high frequency of VTEC strains isolated from domestic animals (Beutin *et al.*, 1993a), is perhaps puzzling.

It is possible that the non-O157 VTEC sometimes found in patients infected with *E. coli* O157:H7 (Griffin, 1995), rather than being ingested from the same source, could arise by *in vivo* phage transfer to a commensal *E. coli* serotype in the gut. The only example of *in situ* phage conversion in humans is in *Corynebacterium diphtheriae*, where a healthy woman harboured three strains of *C. diphtheriae*, two toxigenic (strains A and C) and the other non-toxigenic (strain B). Strains A and B were identical, differing only in production of toxin by strain A. Strain C was morphologically different from A and B, but carried a prophage identical to the prophage in A. *E. coli* O157 requires only a low dose to cause infections (Willshaw *et al.*, 1994), but is a relatively poor competitor in the mammalian gut (Waldolkowski *et al.*, 1990a, b). These contradictory findings could be explained by transfer of the toxin gene to gut commensals *in situ*. Levels of verotoxin in faecal samples from patients infected with VTEC remain high even after the strain causing the original infection can no longer be detected (Scotland *et al.*, 1988). Also, HUS can occur after initial infection when no VTEC can be detected in the stools of patients (Griffin, 1995). This would be consistent with *in situ* lytic infection of gut commensals by a VT phage, releasing sufficient toxin to trigger the cascade of events leading to HUS. Although a commensal lysogenized with a VT phage(s) would probably not contain other virulence determinants, such as *eae*A, it would be difficult for the host to combat, as its only distinguishing feature might be production of VT2, which does not induce an antibody response (Johnson *et al.*, 1996). Therefore, such a commensal might lead to a less severe but more protracted illness, as caused typically by non-O157 VTEC (Ramotar *et al.*, 1995). Lambdoid VT phages containing analogues of *lom* and *bor* (Barondess and Beckwith, 1990) might confer sufficient selective advantage *in vivo* to allow a VT lysogen to outcompete its competitors and resulting in a second wave of disease in an infected host, which would probably remain undiagnosed.

Phages are more recalcitrant in the environment and can be spread more easily by aerosol formation than their host bacteria, which might provide selection pressure for the maintenance and development of VT phages by EHEC. However, there are problems with the hypothesis that secondary phage infections contribute to VT-induced disease. VT phages would have to be able to remain infective after passage through the human or animal stomach. Most VTEC isolated are smooth strains (Griffin, 1995), possessing intact O side-chains. Furthermore, VT phages appear to infect only rough strains of *E. coli* and *Shigella flexneri* (Smith *et al.*, 1983), suggesting that the phage receptor is masked by the O portion of LPS. This would limit the number of potential host strains in the intestine, since wild-type *E. coli* would presumably be expressing smooth LPS, unless subject to phase variation in production of LPS structure *in vivo*.

In order to begin to answer some of the questions posed, we have constructed recombinant VT phages where the toxin genes have been replaced by antibiotic-resistance markers (kanamycin resistance – Kan^r) or reporter genes, such as luciferase (*luxAB*) or green fluorescent protein (*gus*), which allow tracking and measurement of gene expression in VT phages (Sergeant, 1998). These have been used to make a putative identification and cloning of the gene for the VT phage receptor (Vpr) as an approximately 800-kDa OMP (Fig. 1.3; Sergeant, 1998).

CONCLUSIONS

Relatively little is known about the biology of VT phages and their role in the pathogenicity of *E. coli* O157 or other EHEC. For example, how the

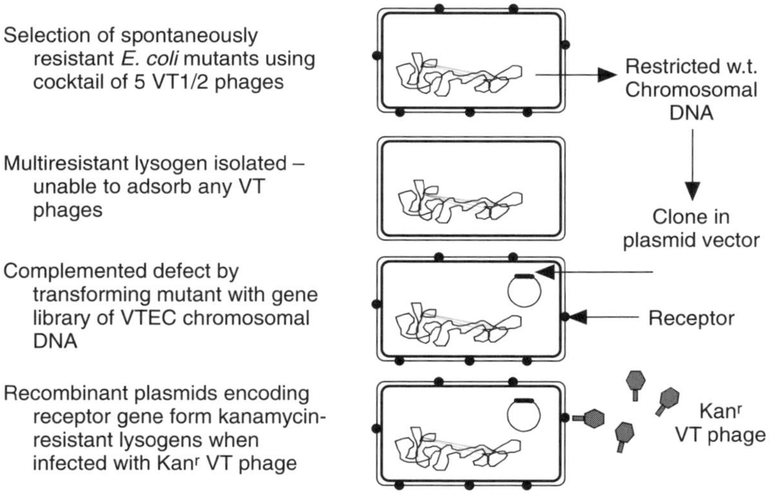

Fig. 1.3. Strategy for identification of VT phage receptor.

phage is transferred and expressed in new host strains, the nature of its receptor on the bacterial surface, sites of chromosomal attachment, immunity mechanisms and gene regulatory networks remain relatively unexplored. Differences in the pathology of *E. coli* O157 in humans and animals, notably cattle, are still enigmatic.

VT phages could in the future conceivably be responsible for the creation of novel pathogens by transfer to other *E. coli* serotypes. It is thus possible that the VT genes might find their way into a bacterium more pathogenic than O157:H7. O157:H7 is relatively rare in cattle; less than 2% carriage has been observed (Chapman *et al.*, 1993). It also proliferates in the colon, where absorption of VT is not as great as in the ileum (Waldolkowski *et al.*, 1990b), and is a poor competitor in the gut. Therefore, infection by VT phage of an *E. coli* that was a more aggressive gut competitor could potentially create a superpathogen of greater clinical significance than O157. Phages could also represent an environmental reservoir for toxin genes and allow a cycle whereby toxin genes could be maintained in a herd of cattle. Whether VT phages can contribute to the pathogenesis of VTEC strains by lysogenic or lytic infection of other gut commensals is unknown. Also, the possibility of phage-mediated toxin transfer in animal and environmental reservoirs and the role this may have in the creation and emergence of new pathogens remain to be determined.

ACKNOWLEDGEMENTS

Some of the work described in this chapter was supported by a post-graduate studentship from the Natural Environment Research Council (to MJS) and a Wellcome Trust Prize Studentship (to KJM).

REFERENCES

Acheson, D.W.K., Moore, R., De Breucker, S., Lincicome, L., Jacewicz, M., Skutelsky, E. and Keusch, G.T. (1996) Translocation of shiga toxin across polarized intestinal cells in tissue culture. *Infection and Immunity* 64, 3294–3300.

Al-Jumaili, A.R., Burke, I., Scotland, D.A., Al-Mardini, S.M. and Record, C.O. (1992) A method of enhancing verocytotoxin production by *Escherichia coli*. *FEMS Microbiology Letters* 93, 121–126.

Barondess, J.J. and Beckwith, J. (1990) A bacterial virulence determinant encoded by the lysogenic coliphage λ. *Nature* 346, 871–874.

Bauer, M.E. and Welch, R.A. (1996a) Characterisation of an RTX toxin from enterohaemorrhagic *Escherichia coli* O157:H7. *Infection and Immunity* 64, 167–175.

Bauer, M.E. and Welch, R.A. (1996b) Association of RTX toxins with erythrocytes. *Infection and Immunity* 64, 4665–4672.

Beutin, L., Montenegro, M.A., Orskov, I., Orskov, F., Prada, J., Zimmerman, S. and Stephen, R. (1989) Close association of verotoxin (shiga-like toxin) production with enterohaemolysin production in strains of *Escherichia coli*. *Journal of Clinical Microbiology* 27, 2559–2564.

Beutin, L., Bode, L., Mushin, O. and Stephan, R. (1990) Enterohaemolysin production is associated with a temperate bacteriophage in *Escherichia coli* serogroup O26 strains. *Journal of Bacteriology* 172, 6469–6475.

Beutin, L., Grier, D., Steinrueck, H., Zimmerman, S. and Schuetz, F. (1993a) Prevalence and some properties of verotoxin (shiga-like toxin) producing *Escherichia coli* in seven different species of healthy domestic animals. *Journal of Clinical Microbiology* 31, 2483–2488.

Beutin, L., Stroeher, U.H. and Manning, P.A. (1993b) Isolation of enterohaemolysin associated sequences encoded on temperate phages of *Escherichia coli*. *Gene* 132, 95–99.

Beutin, L., Geier, D., Zimmermann, S. and Karch, H. (1995) Virulence markers of shiga-like toxin-producing strains originating from healthy domestic animals of different species. *Journal of Clinical Microbiology* 33, 629–530.

Binns, M.M., Davies, D.L. and Hardy, K.G. (1979) Cloned fragments of the plasmid ColV I-K94 specifying virulence and serum resistance. *Nature* 279, 778–781.

Bloomfield, G.A., Whittle, G., McDonagh, B., Katz, M.E. and Cheetham, B.F. (1997) Analysis of sequences flanking the *vap* regions of *Dichelobacter nodosus*: evidence for multiple integration events, a killer system and a new genetic element. *Microbiology* 143, 553–562.

Burgess, B.J. and Roberts, L.M. (1993) Proteolytic cleavage at arginine residues within the hydrophilic disulphide loop of *Escherichia* shiga-like toxin I A subunit is not essential for cytotoxicity. *Molecular Microbiology* 10, 171–179.

Calderwood, S.B., Auclair, F., Donohue-Rolfe, A., Keusch, G.T. and Mekalanos, J.J. (1987) Nucleotide sequence of the shiga-like toxin genes of *Escherichia coli*. *Proceedings of the National Academy of Sciences USA* 84, 4364–4368.

Campbell, A. (1994) Comparative molecular biology of lamboid phages. *Annual Reviews in Microbiology* 48, 193–222.

Chapman, P.A., Siddons, C.A., Wright, D.J., Norman, P., Fox, J. and Crick, E. (1993) Cattle as a possible source of verocytotoxin-producing *Escherichia coli* O157 infections in man. *Epidemiology and Infection* 111, 439–444.

Cheetham, B.F. and Katz, M.E. (1995) A role for bacteriophages in the evolution and transfer of bacterial virulence determinants. *Molecular Microbiology* 18, 201–208.

Christopher-Hennings, J., Willgohs, J.A., Francis, D.H., Raman, U.A.K., Moxley, R.A. and Hurley, D.J. (1993) Immunocompromise in gnotobiotic pigs induced by verotoxin-producing *Escherichia coli* (O111:NM). *Infection and Immunity* 61, 2304–2308.

Datz, M., Janetzki-Mittman, C., Franke, S., Gunzer, F., Schmidt, H. and Karch, H. (1996) Analysis of the enterohemorrhagic *Escherichia coli* O157 DNA region containing lamboid phage gene P and Shiga-like toxin structural genes. *Applied and Environmental Microbiology* 62, 791–797.

DeGrandis, S., Ginsberg, J., Toone, M., Climie, S., Friesen, J. and Brunton, J. (1987) Nucleotide sequence and promoter mapping of the *Escherichia coli* shiga-like toxin operon of bacteriophage H-19B. *Journal of Bacteriology* 169, 4313–4319.

Donnenberg, M.S. and Kaper, J.B. (1992) Enteropathogenic *Escherichia coli*. *Infection and Immunity* 60, 3953–3961.

Donnenberg, M.S., Giron, J.A., Nataro, J.P. and Kaper, J.B. (1992) A plasmid encoded type IV fimbrial gene of enteropathogenic *Escherichia coli* associated with localised adherence. *Molecular Microbiology* 6, 3427–3437.

Dytoc, M.T., Ismaili, A., Philpot, D.J., Soni, R., Brunton, J.L. and Sherman, P.M. (1994) Distinct binding properties of *eae*A-negative verocytotoxin-producing *Escherichia coli* of serotype O113:H21. *Infection and Immunity* 62, 3494–3505.

Edlin, G., Lin, L. and Bitner, R. (1977) Reproductive fitness of P1, P2, Lambda and Mu lysogens of *Escherichia coli*. *Journal of Virology* 21, 560–564.

Griffin, P.M. (1995) *Escherichia coli* O157:H7 and other enterohaemorrhagic *Escherichia coli*. In: Blaser, M.J., Smith, J.I., Ravdin, H.B., Greenberg, H.B. and Guerrant, R.L. (eds) *Infections of the Gastrointestinal Tract*. Raven Press, New York, pp. 121–145.

Griffin, P.M. and Tauxe, R.V. (1991) The epidemiology of infections caused by *Escherichia coli* O157:H7, other enterohaemorrhagic *E. coli*, and the associated haemolytic uraemic syndrome. *Epidemiological Reviews* 13, 60–98.

Gunzer, F., Bohm, H., Russmannn, H., Bitzan, M., Aleksic, S. and Karch, H. (1992) Molecular detection of sorbitol-fermenting *Escherichia coli* O157 in patients with haemolytic uraemic syndrome. *Journal of Clinical Microbiology* 30, 1807–1810.

Hales, B., Batt, R.M., Hart, C.A. and Saunders, J.R. (1992) The large plasmids found in enterohaemorrhagic and enteropathogenic *Escherichia coli* constitute a related series of transfer-defective IncF-IIA replicons. *Plasmid* 28, 183–193.

Haque, Q.M., Sugiyama, A., Iwade, Y., Midorikawa, Y. and Yamauchi, T. (1997) Diarrheal and environmental isolates of *Aeromonas* spp. produce a toxin similar to shiga-like toxin 1. *Current Microbiology* 32, 239–245.

Hart, C.A., Batt, R.M. and Saunders, J.R. (1993) Diarrhoea caused by *Escherichia coli*. *Annals of Tropical Paediatrics* 13, 121–131.

Hicks, S., Frankel, G., Kaper, J.B., Dougan, G. and Phillips, A.D. (1998) Role of intimin and bundle-forming pili in enteropathogenic *Escherichia coli* adhesion to pediatric tissue *in vitro*. *Infection and Immunity* 66, 1570–1578.

Highton, P.J., Chang, Y. and Myers, R.J. (1990) Evidence for the exchange of segments between genomes during the evolution of lamboid bacteriophages. *Molecular Microbiology* 4, 1329–1340.

Huang, A., Friesen, J. and Brunton, J.L. (1987) Characterisation of a bacteriophage that carries the genes for production of shiga-like toxin 1 in *Escherichia coli*. *Journal of Bacteriology* 169, 4308–4312.

Ismail, A., Philpot, D.J., Dytoc, M.T. and Sherman, P.M. (1995) Signal transduction responses following adhesion of verocytotoxin-producing *Escherichia coli*. *Infection and Immunity* 63, 3316–3326.

Ismail, A., McWhirter, R., Handelsman, M.Y.C., Brunton, J.L. and Sherman, P.M. (1998) Divergent signal transduction responses to infection with attaching and effacing *Escherichia coli*. *Infection and Immunity* 66, 1688–1696.

Ito, H.A., Terai, H., Kurazono, H., Takeda, Y. and Nishibushi, M. (1990) Cloning and nucleotide sequencing of Vero Toxin 2 variant genes from the *Escherichia coli* O91:H21 isolated from a patient with hemolytic uremic syndrome. *Microbial Pathology* 8, 47–60.

Jackson, M.P. (1990) Structure–function analyses of shiga toxin and shiga-like toxins. *Microbial Pathogenesis* 8, 235–242.

Jerse, A.E. and Kaper, J.B. (1991) The *eae* gene of enteropathogenic *Escherichia coli* encodes a 94-kilodalton membrane protein, the expression of which is influenced by the EAF plasmid. *Infection and Immunity* 59, 4302–4309.

Jerse, A.E., Yu, J., Tall, B.D. and Kaper, J.B. (1990) A genetic locus of enteropathogenic *Escherichia coli* necessary for the production of attaching and effacing lesions on tissue culture cells. *Proceedings of the National Academy of Sciences USA* 87, 7839–7843.

Johnson, R.P, Cray, W.C. and Johnson, S.T. (1996) Serum antibody responses of cattle following experimental infection with *Escherichia coli* O157:H7. *Infection and Immunity* 64, 1879–1883.

Junkins, A.D. and Doyle, M.P. (1989) Comparison of adherence-properties of *Escherichia coli* O157:H7 and a 60-megadalton plasmid-cured derivative. *Current Microbiology* 19, 21–27.

Karch, H., Heesemann, J., Laufs, R., O'Brien, A.D., Tacket, C.O. and Levine, M.M. (1987) A plasmid of enterohaemorrhagic *Escherichia coli* O157:H7 is required for expression of a new fimbrial antigen for adhesion to epithelial cells. *Infection and Immunity* 55, 455–461.

Karch, H., Russmann, H., Scmidt, A., Schwarzkopf, A. and Heesemann, J. (1995) Long term shedding and clonal turnover of enterohemorrhagic *Escherichia coli* O157 in diarrheal diseases. *Journal of Clinical Microbiology* 33, 1602–1605.

Karmali, M.A., Steele, B.T., Pectric, M., and Lim, C. (1983) Sporadic cases of haemolytic uraemic syndrome associated with faecal cytotoxin and cytotoxin-producing *Escherichia coli* in stools. *Lancet* i, 619–620.

Knutton, S.T., Baldwin, P.H. and McNeish, A.S. (1989) Actin accumulation of sites of bacterial adhesion to tissue culture: basis of a new diagnostic test for enteropathogenic and enterohaemorrhagic *Escherichia coli. Infection and Immunity* 57, 1290–1298.

Knutton, S., Rosenshine, I., Pallen, M.J., Nisan, I., Neves, B.C., Bain, C., Wolff, C., Dougan, G. and Frankel, G. (1998) A novel EspA-associated surface organelle of enteropathogenic *Escherichia coli* involved in protein translocation into epithelial cells. *EMBO Journal* 17, 2166–2176.

Koslov, Y.U., Kabishev, A.A., Lukyanov, E.V. and Bayev, A.A. (1988) The primary structure of the operon coding for *Shigella dysenteriae* toxin and temperate phage H30 shiga-like toxin. *Gene* 67, 213–221.

Kurioka, T., Yunou, Y. and Kita, E. (1998) Enhancement of susceptibility to Shiga toxin-producing *Escherichia coli* O157:H7 by protein calorie malnutrition in mice. *Infection and Immunity* 66, 1726–1734.

Lesene, J.B., Rothschild, N., Erikson, B., Korec, S., Sisk, R. and Keller, J. (1989) Cancer associated haemolytic-uraemic syndrome: an analysis of 85 cases from the national registry. *Journal of Clinical Oncology* 7, 781–789.

Levine, M.M., Bergquist, E.J., Nalin, D.R., Waterman, D.H., Hornwick, R.B., Young, C.R., Sotman, S. and Rowe, B. (1985) The diarrheal response of humans to some classic serotypes of enteropathogenic *E. coli* is dependent on plasmid encoding an enteroinvasiveness factor. *Journal of Infectious Diseases* 152, 550–557.

Louie, C.B. and Obrig, T.G. (1995) Specific interaction of *Escherichia coli* O157:H7-derived shiga-toxin II with human renal endothelial cells. *Journal of Infectious Diseases* 172, 1397–1401.

McDaniel, T.K., Jarvis, K.G., Donnenberg, M.S. and Kaper, J.B. (1995) A genetic locus of enterocyte effeacement conserved among diverse enterobacterial pathogens. *Proceedings of the National Academy of Sciences USA* 92, 1664–1668.

McKee, M.L. and O'Brien, A.D. (1995) Investigation of enterohaemorrhagic *Escherichia coli* O157:H7 adherence characteristics and invasion potential reveals a new attachment pattern shared by intestinal *E. coli*. *Infection and Immunity* 63, 2070–2074.

McKee, M.L., Melton-Celsa, A.R., Moxely, R.A., Francis, D.H. and O'Brien, A.D. (1995) Enterohemorrhagic *Escherichia coli* O157:H7 requires intimin to colonize the gnotobiotic pig intestine and to adhere to HEp-2 cells. *Infection and Immunity* 63, 3739–3744.

Maloney, M.D. and Lingwood, C.A. (1994) CD19 has a potential CD77 (globotriaosyl ceramide)-binding site with sequence similarity to verotoxin B-subunits: implications in molecular mimicry for B cell adhesion and enterohemorrhagic *Escherichia coli* infections. *Journal of Experimental Medicine* 180, 191–201.

Melton-Celsa, A.R., Darnell, S.C. and O'Brien, A.D. (1996) Activation of shiga-like toxins by mouse and human intestinal mucus correlates with virulence of enterohaemorrhagic *Escherichia coli* O91:H21 isolates in orally infected, streptomycin-treated mice. *Infection and Immunity* 64, 1569–1576.

Mobbs, K.J. (1997) Molecular, phenotypic, and ecological studies of verotoxigenic and enterohaemorrhagic *Escherichia coli*. PhD thesis, University of Liverpool.

Muhldorfer, I., Hacker, J., Keusch, G.T., Acheson, D.W., Tschape, H., Kane, A.V., Ritter, A., Olschlager, T. and Donohue-Rolfe, A. (1996) Regulation of the shiga-like toxin II operon in *Escherichia coli*. *Infection and Immunity* 64, 495–502.

Mushegian, A.R., Fullner, K.J., Koonin, E.V. and Nester, E.W. (1996) A family of lysozyme-like virulence factors in bacterial pathogens of plants and animals. *Proceedings of the National Academy of Sciences USA* 93, 7321–7326.

Nataro, J.P., Sclalesky, L.C.A., Kaper, J.B., Levine, M.M. and Trabulsi, L.R. (1985) Plasmid mediated factors conferring diffuse and localised adherence of enteropathogenic *Escherichia coli*. *Infection and Immunity* 48, 378–383.

Newland, J.W. and Neill, R.J. (1988) DNA probes for shiga-like toxins I and II and for toxin-converting bacteriophages. *Journal of Clinical Microbiology* 21, 1292–1297.

O'Brien, A.D., Newland, J.W., Miller, S.F., Holmes, R.K., Smith, H.W. and Formal, S.B. (1984) Shiga-like toxin-converting phages from *Escherichia coli* strains that cause hemorrhagic colitis or infantile diarrhea. *Science* 226, 694–696.

Olsnes, S., Reisbig, R. and Eiklid, K. (1981) Subunit structure of *Shigella* cytotoxin. *Journal of Biological Chemistry* 256, 8732–8738.

Ostroff, S.M., Kobayashi, J.M. and Lewis, J.H. (1989) Infections with *Escherichia coli* O157:H7 in Washington State: the first year of state wide disease surveillence. *Journal of the American Medical Association* 262, 355–359.

Paton, A.W. and Paton, J.C. (1996) *Enterobacter cloacae* producing a shiga-like toxin II related cytotoxin associated with a case of haemolytic uraemic syndrome. *Journal of Clinical Microbiology* 34, 463–465.

Paton, A.W., Paton, J.C., Heuzenroeder, M.W., Goldwater, P.N. and Manning, P.A. (1992) Cloning and nucleotide sequence of a variant shiga-like toxin II gene from *Escherichia coli* OX3:H21 isolated from a case of sudden infant death syndrome. *Microbial Pathogenesis* 13, 225–236.

Paton, A.W., Paton, J.C., Goldwater, P.N., Heuzenroeder, M.W. and Manning, P.A. (1993) Sequence of a variant Shiga-like toxin type-1 operon of *Escherichia coli* O111:H-. *Gene* 129, 87–92.

Paton, A.W., Ratcliff, R., Doyle, R.M., Seymour-Murray, J., Davos, D., Lanser, J.A. and Patton, J.C. (1996) Molecular microbiology investigation of an outbreak of haemolytic uraemic syndrome caused by dry fermented sausage contaminated with shiga-like toxin producing *Escherichia coli*. *Journal of Clinical Microbiology* 34, 1622–1627.

Paton, A.W., Voss, E., Manning, P.A. and Paton, J.C. (1997) Shiga toxin-producing *Escherichia coli* isolates from cases of human disease show enhanced adherence to intestinal epithelial (Henle 407) cells. *Infection and Immunity* 65, 3799–3805.

Pavia, A.T., Nichols, C.R. and Green, D.P. (1990) Hemolytic uremic syndrome during an outbreak of *Escherichia coli* O157:H7 infections in institutions for mentally retarded persons: clinical and epidemiological observations. *Journal of Pediatrics* 116, 544–551.

Porter, J., Mobbs, K., Hart, C.A., Saunders, J.R., Pickup, R.W. and Edwards, C. (1997) Detection, distribution and probable fate of *Escherichia coli* O157 around an asymptomatic dairy farm. *Journal of Applied Microbiology* 83, 297–306.

Ramotar, K., Henderson, E., Szumski, R. and Louie, T.J. (1995) Impact of free verotoxin testing on the epidemiology of diarrhoea caused by verotoxin-producing *Escherichia coli*. *Journal of Clinical Microbiology* 33, 1114–1120.

Rietra, P.J.G.M., Willshaw, G.A., Smith, H.R., Field, A.M., Scotland, S.M. and Rowe, B. (1989) Comparison of Vero-cytotoxin encoding phages from *Escherichia coli* of human and bovine origin. *Journal of General Microbiology* 135, 2307–2318.

Rosenshine, I., Donnenberg, M.S., Kaper, J.B. and Finlay, B.B. (1992) Signal transduction between enteropathogenic *E. coli* and epithelial cells: EPEC induces tyrosine phosphorylation of host cell proteins to initiate cytoskeletal rearrangement and bacterial uptake. *EMBO Journal* 11, 3551–3560.

Sandvig, K., Garred, O., Prydz, K., Koslar, J.V., Hansen, S.H. and Van Deurs, B. (1992) Retrograde transport of endocytised shiga toxin to the endoplasmic reticulum. *Nature* 358, 510–512.

Saxena, S.F., O'Brien, A.D. and Alderman, E.J. (1989) Shiga toxin, shiga-like toxin II variant, and ricin are all single site RNA N-glycosidases of 28S RNA when micro-injected into *Xenopus* oocytes. *Journal of Biological Chemistry* 264, 596–601.

Schmidt, H., Montag, M., Bockemuhl, J., Heeseman, J. and Karch, H. (1993) Shiga like toxin II related cytotoxins in *Citrobacter freundii* strains from humans and beef samples. *Infection and Immunity* 61, 534–543.

Schmidt, H., Karch, H. and Beutin, L. (1994) The large-sized plasmids of enterohaemorrhagic *Escherichia coli* O157 strains encode haemolysins which are presumably members of the *E. coli* α-haemolysin family. *FEMS Microbiology Letters* 117, 189–196.

Schmidt, H., Beutin, L. and Karch, H. (1995) Molecular analysis of the plasmid-encoded haemolysin of *Escherichia coli* O157:H7 strain EDL 933. *Infection and Immunity* 63, 1055–1061.

Schmitt, C.K., McKee, M.L. and O'Brien, A.D. (1991) Two copies of Shiga-like toxin II-related genes common in enterohemorrhagic *Escherichia coli* strains are responsible for the antigenic heterogeneity of the O157:H- strain E32511. *Infection and Immunity* 59, 1065–1073.

Scotland, S.M., Rowe, B., Smith, H.R., Willshaw, G.A. and Gross, R.J. (1988) Vero cytotoxin-producing strains of *Escherichia coli* from children with haemolytic uraemic syndrome and their detection by specific DNA probes. *Journal of Medical Microbiology* 25, 237–243.

Sergeant, M.J. (1998) Molecular biological characterisation of verotoxigenic bacteriophages in *Escherichia coli*. PhD thesis, University of Liverpool.

Sherman, P., Soni, R., Petric, M. and Karmali, M. (1987) Surface properties of the vero cytotoxin-producing *Escherichia coli* O157:H7. *Infection and Immunity* 55, 1824–1829.

Smith, H.W. and Lingwood, M.A. (1971) The transmissable nature of enterotoxin production in a human enteropathogenic strain of *Escherichia coli*. *Journal of Medical Microbiology* 4, 301–305.

Smith, H.W., Green, P. and Parsell, S. (1983) Vero cell toxins in *Escherichia coli* and related bacteria: transfer by phage conjugation and toxic action in laboratory animals, chickens and pigs. *Journal of General Microbiology* 129, 3121–3137.

Strockbine, N.A., Marques, L.R.M., Newland, J.W., Smith, H.W., Holmes, R.K. and O'Brien, A.D. (1986) Two toxin-converting phages from *Escherichia coli* O157:H7 strain 933 encode antigenically distinct toxins with similar boiological activities. *Infection and Immunity* 53, 135–140.

Stroeher, U.H., Bode, L., Beutin, L. and Manning, P.A. (1993) Characterisation and sequence of a 33 kDa enterohaemolysin (Ehly1) associated protein in *Escherichia coli*. *Gene* 132, 89–94.

Sung, L.M., Jackson, M.P., O'Brien, A.D. and Holmes, R.K. (1990) Transcription of the shiga-like toxin type II and shiga-like toxin type II variant operons of *Escherichia coli*. *Journal of Bacteriology* 172, 6386–6395.

Taylor, C.M., Milford, D.V. and Rose, P.E. (1990) The expression of blood group P1 in post-enteropathic haemolytic uraemic syndrome. *Pediatric Nephrology* 4, 59–61.

Tesh, V.L., Samuel, J.E., Perera, L.P., Sharefkin, J.B. and O'Brien, A.D. (1993a) Evaluation of the role of shiga and shiga-like toxins in mediating direct damage to human vascular endothelial cells. *Journal of Infectious Diseaeses* 164, 344–352.

Tesh, V.L., Burris, J.A., Owens, J.E., Gordon, V.M., Waldolkowski, E.A., O'Brien, A.D. and Samuel, J.E. (1993b) Comparison of relative toxicities of shiga-like toxins typeI and typeII for mice. *Infection and Immunity* 61, 3392–3402.

Toth, I., Cohen, M.L., Rumschlag, H.S., Riley, L.W., White, E.H., Carr, J.H., Nond, W.W. and Wachsmuth, I.K. (1990) Influence of the 60-megadalton plasmid on adherence of *Escherichia coli* O157:H7 and genetic derivatives. *Infection and Immunity* 58, 1223–1231.

Tzipori, S., Gibson, R. and Montanaro, J. (1989) Nature and distribution of mucosal lesions with enteropathogenic and enterohaemorrhagic *Escherichia coli* in piglets and the role of plasmid mediated factors. *Infection and Immunity* 57, 1142–1150.

Tzipori, S., Gunzer, F., Donnenberg, M.S., Montigny, L., Kaper, J.B. and Donohue-Rolfe, A. (1995) The role of the *eae*A gene in diarrhoea and neurological complications in a gnotobiotic piglet model of enterohaemorrhagic *Escherichia coli* infection. *Infection and Immunity* 63, 3621–3627.

Waldolkowski, E.A., Burris, J.A. and O'Brien, A.D. (1990a) Mouse model for colonization and disease caused by enterohaemorrhagic *Escherichia coli* O157:H7. *Infection and Immunity* 58, 2438–2445.

Waldolkowski, E.A., Sung, J.A., Burris, J.E., Samuel, J.E. and O'Brien, A.D. (1990b) Acute renal tubular necrosis and death of mice orally infected with *Escherichia coli* strains that produce shiga-like toxin type II. *Infection and Immunity* 58, 3959–3965.

Walters, M.D.S., Matthei, U., Kay, R., Dillon, M.J. and Barret, T.M. (1989) The polymorphonuclear leucocyte count in childhood haemolytic uraemic syndrome. *Paediatric Nephrology* 10, 130–134.

Whittam, T.S. (1995) Genetic population structure and pathogenicity in enteric bacteria. In: Baumberg, S., Young, J.P.W., Wellington, E.M.H. and Saunders, J.R. (eds) *Population Genetics of Bacteria.* Society for General Microbiology, Cambridge University Press, Cambridge, pp. 217–246.

Willshaw, G.A., Smith, H.R., Scotland, S.M. and Rowe, B. (1985) Cloning of genes determining the production of vero cytotoxin by *Escherichia coli. Journal of General Microbiology* 131, 3047–3053.

Willshaw, G.A., Smith, H.R., Scotland, S.M., Field, A.M. and Rowe, B. (1987) Heterogeneity of *Escherichia coli* phages encoding vero cytotoxins: comparison of cloned sequences determining VT1 and VT2 and development of specific gene probes. *Journal of General Microbiology* 133, 1309–1317.

Willshaw, G.A., Thirlwell, J., Jones, A.P., Parry, S., Salmon, R.L. and Hickey, M. (1994) Verocytotoxin-producing *Escherichia coli* O157:H7 in beefburgers linked to an outbreak of diarrhoea, haemorrhagic colitis and haemolytic uraemic syndrome in Britain. *Letters in Applied Microbiology* 19, 404–407.

Wolff, C., Nisan, I., Hanski, E., Frankel, G. and Rosenshine, I. (1998) Protein translocation into host epithelial cells by infecting enteropathogenic *Escherichia coli. Molecular Microbiology* 28, 143–155.

Yee, A.J., De Grandis, S. and Gyles, L.G. (1993) Mitomycin-induced synthesis of a shiga-like toxin from enteropathogenic *Escherichia coli* H.I.8. *Infection and Immunity* 61, 4510–4513.

Yu, J. and Kaper, J.B. (1992) Cloning and characterisation of the *eae*A gene of enterohaemorrhagic *Escherichia coli* O157:H7. *Molecular Microbiology* 6, 411–417.

Zhao, S., Meng, J., Doyle, M.P., Meinersman, R., Wang, G. and Zhao, P. (1996) A low molecular weight outer-membrane protein of *Escherichia coli* O157:H7 associated with adherence to INT407 cells and chicken caeca. *Journal of Medical Microbiology* 45, 90–96.

2

Acid Tolerance of *Escherichia coli* – the Sting in the Tail?

I.R. Booth,[1] F. Thomson-Carter,[2] P. Carter,[3] S. Jordan,[4] S. Park,[4] L. Malcolm[1] and J. Glover[1]

[1] *Department of Molecular and Cell Biology, Institute of Medical Sciences, University of Aberdeen, UK;* [2] *Scottish Reference Laboratory for* E. coli *O157 and* Campylobacter, *Department of Medical Microbiology, University of Aberdeen, UK;* [3] *Department of Medical Microbiology, Institute of Medical Sciences, University of Aberdeen, UK;* [4] *Department of Microbiology, Institute of Food Research, Reading, UK*

> ... however secure and well-regulated civilized life may become bacteria, Protozoa, viruses, infected fleas, lice, ticks, mosquitoes, and bedbugs will always lurk in the shadows ready to pounce when neglect, poverty, famine, or war lets down the defenses. And even in normal times they prey on the weak, the very young and the very old, living along with us in mysterious obscurity awaiting their opportunities.
>
> (Zinsser, 1934)

INTRODUCTION

Analysis of the molecular origin of *Escherichia coli* O157:H7 has shown considerable similarity between strains at the molecular level, despite diverse geographical origins, and indicates that the organism started on its path to its current genetic state some 5 million years ago (Armstrong *et al.*, 1996). There is a great diversity of pathogenic *E. coli* and *Shigella* pathogenic strains, which appear to have arisen by the acquisition by 'commensal' organisms of gene clusters that enable them to cause disease (Pupo *et al.*, 1997). In contrast, it is thought that *E. coli* O157:H7 strains arose from a single stock despite their current diversity (Whittam *et al.*, 1988). However, *E. coli* O157:H7 has become recognized as a major cause of food poisoning only in the last 15 years (Armstrong *et al.*, 1996). Infections have serious sequelae for the very young and the elderly and are considered to be one of the primary causes of the haemolytic uraemic syndrome, which often leads to serious kidney damage. Thus, there is no doubting the serious nature of the persistence of this organism in foods.

The organism is usually transmitted through contaminated food or drink, with a wide range of processed and minimally processed foods implicated in disease outbreaks (Armstrong *et al.*, 1996; Tilden *et al.*, 1996). For those routes of infection that have been resolved, the cause seems to be equally distributed between failures in establishment of good preservation barriers and poor hygiene in the preparation of food and its distribution (Armstrong *et al.*, 1996). It is clear that the infective dose of *E. coli* O157:H7 is very low. Estimates derived from an outbreak due to dry-cured salami suggested that doses between five and 50 organisms were effective in causing bloody diarrhoea (Armstrong *et al.*, 1996; Tilden *et al.*, 1996). Such a low infective dose has given rise to the view that this organism is unusually tolerant of the stresses that are used by the body as defence mechanisms. However, as will be documented below, an equally plausible model is that the surviving cells are themselves physiologically adapted to the niche through which they are transmitted. In this review, we focus on acid tolerance in particular, which has been highlighted as an important physiological characteristic of this organism (Small *et al.*, 1994; Wang and Doyle, 1998). The last 10 years have seen considerable growth in the understanding of the mechanisms that enable bacteria to withstand acid stress, largely, but not exclusively, through the work of John Foster with *Salmonella typhimurium* and *E. coli* O157:H7 (Bearson *et al.*, 1997; see also Rowbury, 1995). This chapter will briefly review the current understanding of pH homoeostasis and acid tolerance and how this aids our understanding of *E. coli* O157:H7 transmission.

pH HOMOEOSTASIS

It is generally held that bacteria maintain their cytoplasmic pH relatively constant, despite variations in the pH of the environment (Booth, 1985). This observation is true for the enteric bacteria, where respiratory metabolism appears to enable a finer degree of pH homoeostasis than may be observed in organisms that are fermenting. Thus, it follows that, as the lifestyle of *E. coli* O157:H7 changes from aerobic to anaerobic, there may be changes in the capacity for pH homoeostasis. It is not our purpose here to review extensively what is understood about mechanisms by which the pH of the cell is sensed and adjustments made. Recent reviews (Booth, 1985, 1999; Booth and Stratford, 1999) have noted the developments in this field. Suffice it to say that the mechanisms are complex and still relatively poorly understood, even in *E. coli*. Critical to an understanding of the physiology of *E. coli* O157:H7 is that the conditions that induce acid tolerance do not make profound changes in the capacity for pH homoeostasis. The absence of good probes of cytoplasmic pH for use at pH 3 has not made understanding this problem easy and there remains a paucity of good data that would enable precise conclusions to be drawn. In our own studies, we have found that the cytoplasmic pH of *E. coli* O157:H7 does not change over the range pH 4–7 when the cells are rendered acid-tolerant by growth at mildly acidic conditions (Jordan, S.L. *et al.*, 1999). At lower pH values, it is possible that there is a slightly higher cytoplasmic pH in habituated cells, similar to the observations made with *S. typhimurium* (Foster and Hall, 1991). Stationary-phase cells of *E. coli* O157:H7 exhibit a lower cytoplasmic pH across the range studied (pH 4–7) than either exponential phase or habituated cells, and this may be due to the energy-limited status of these cells. The addition of 50 mM lactate at pH 4–5 caused an almost identical final pH in cells derived from exponential phase, habituated cells or stationary-phase cells (Table 2.1). These data suggest that there is no significant difference between these three types of cells in their ability to buffer perturbation of the cytoplasm. Despite this, both habituated and stationary-phase cells were 3–4 logs more resistant to the effects of lactate than were exponential-phase cells (Jordan, S.L. *et al.*, 1999). Below pH 4, we found that low concentrations of ethanol (5%) could also perturb pH homoeostasis and this was a contributory factor in cell death at extreme acid pH in the presence of the alcohol (Jordan, S.L. *et al.*, 1999). Again, habituated and stationary-phase cells were more resistant to the effects of perturbation of cytoplasmic pH by ethanol than were exponential-phase cells. The capacity to maintain the cytoplasmic pH at a value where enzyme systems can function to maintain cell integrity is important. The cytoplasmic pH must be maintained in a range that is compatible with enzyme activity and with protein and DNA stability. However, it is more probably the level of expression of systems that function to repair macromolecules (such as those induced during habituation or during the stationary phase (Raja *et al.*, 1991; also see below)) that determine life or death.

Table 2.1. Effect of ethanol and lactate on cytoplasmic pH in *E. coli* O157:H7. Cells of *E. coli* O157:H7 (strain 30-2C4) were grown as described in the text and the cytoplasmic pH measured as described previously (Jordan, S.L. *et al.*, 1999). The pH of the incubation was pH 4.

	Additions		
Growth phase	None	Lactate (50 mM)	Ethanol (5% v/v)
Exponential pH 7	6.58 ± 0.01	5.07 ± 0.06	5.53 ± 0.07
Exponential pH 5.8	6.42 ± 0.09	5.13 ± 0.06	5.46 ± 0.08
Stationary	5.77 ± 0.18	4.83 ± 0.11	5.52 ± 0.14

ACID TOLERANCE

The transfer of a wide range of bacteria from neutral to extreme acid pH (< pH 3.3) leads to rapid cell death and frequently greater than 5-logs killing can be achieved in a few minutes (Fig. 2.1). However, if the organism is cultured at a moderately acidic pH (pH 5–6), it acquires increased tolerance of extreme acid as a consequence of the expression of a number of gene products (Goodson and Rowbury, 1989; Foster and Hall, 1990, 1991; Rowbury, 1995; Bearson *et al.*, 1997; Wang and Doyle, 1998). Induction of the heat-shock response has been reported to render *E. coli* O157:H7 acid-tolerant (Wang and Doyle, 1998), although cells that had survived mild acid in Lebanon Bologna were not subsequently heat-resistant (Ellajosyula *et al.*, 1998). Cells that are growing slowly ($\mu < 1\ h^{-1}$) (Ferguson *et al.*, 1998; see below) or have ceased growth upon entry into the stationary phase induce the expression of a further subset of genes that confer stress tolerance, including resistance to acid stress (Hengge-Aronis, 1993; Small *et al.*, 1994; Cheville *et al.*, 1996). In addition, there are acid-resistance mechanisms that depend upon the presence of amino acid and the induction of specific decarboxylases (Bearson *et al.*, 1997). These systems are subject to complex regulation and may be particularly important if the recent history of the organism is a rich 'medium' at moderately acid pH and possibly low oxygen (Bearson *et al.*, 1997). Thus, acid stress poses a serious threat only to those organisms that have entered acidic environments immediately following rapid growth at neutral pH. For organisms that are expressing one or more of the acid-tolerance systems, survival for many hours or days at pH 3 is a reality, since the rate of death is frequently very small (Jordan, K.N. *et al.*, 1999). The risk of food-borne disease arising from contaminated food then becomes dependent upon the size of the infective dose, the susceptibility of individual cells to acid (see below) and the population size. It is often said that bacteria in their natural environment are most likely to be growing slowly and therefore possess a high degree of acid tolerance. However, in foods that either lack or have diminished preservatives, bacteria may attain higher growth rates and consequently be more susceptible to very low pH. In contrast, however, mild preservative conditions that inhibit growth but do not kill may potentiate long-term survival by the induction of protective mechanisms (Leyer *et al.*, 1995).

The studies in our laboratory were undertaken to assess the acid tolerance of *E. coli* O157:H7, relative to other *E. coli* organisms isolated from human faeces, and the relationship to pH homoeostasis. Acid tolerance has been assessed in 12 *E. coli* O157:H7 isolates obtained either from Scottish outbreaks or from international sources. Five *E. coli* isolates (J1, J2, J4–J6) were obtained from the faeces of healthy volunteers and other isolates have been obtained from cattle. All of the organisms were grown under the same regime (glucose-based McIlvaine's medium at either pH 7 or pH 5.8) into mid-exponential phase before transfer to McIlvaine's buffer at pH 3.

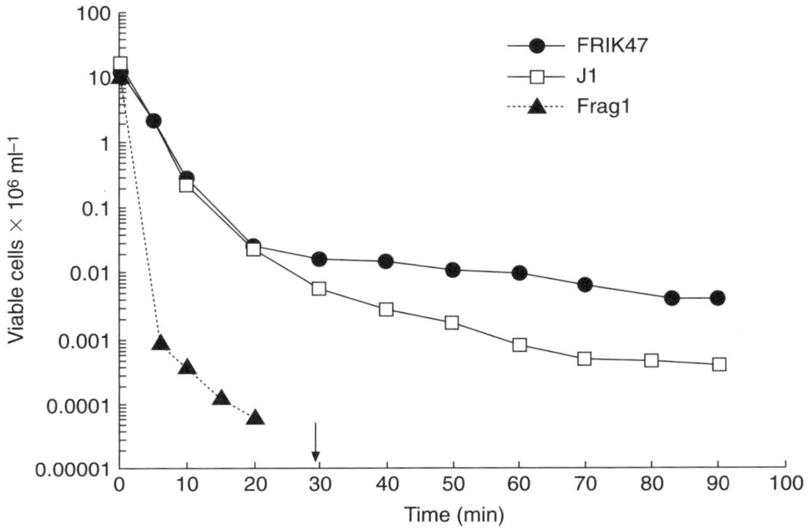

Fig. 2.1. Survival of incubation at pH 3 vs time for Frag1, J1 and an O157:H7 strain, FRIK47. The three strains were grown to mid-exponential phase in McIlvaine's minimal medium (Jordan, S.L. *et al.*, 1999) at pH 7 and then diluted 20-fold into McIlvaine's buffer pH 3 at zero time. All three strains exhibited similar growth rates prior to transfer to buffer at pH 3. Samples were taken and serially diluted into McIlvaine's buffer pH 7 and colonies recovered on LB plates. Arrow indicates no viable cells detected after the indicated time point.

Stationary-phase cells were grown for 18 h in the same medium. Survival was analysed by sampling at intervals and analysis of the numbers of colony-forming units recovered on complex medium. Consistent patterns of survival were seen for all the isolates investigated. There was an initial exponential loss of viability for approximately 20 min, followed by the survival of a more acid-resistant population (the 'tail' population), which persisted for up to 4 h, at which time monitoring ceased (Fig. 2.1). In other studies, the persistence of a 'tail' of O157:H7 cells for several days has been seen in broth cultures acidified to pH 2 (Jordan, K.N. *et al.*, 1999). When cells were grown into exponential phase at pH 5.8, they underwent habituation – the specific acquisition of tolerance to extreme acid conditions (Glover *et al.*, 1999; Jordan, K.N. *et al.*, 1999; Jordan, S.L. *et al.*, 1999). The only significant difference between the isolates was that the habituation was incomplete for the O157:H7 isolates compared with all other *E. coli* strains investigated (Glover *et al.*, 1999). All stationary-phase cells were very tolerant of acid conditions. However, Jordan and colleagues (Jordan, K.N. *et al.*, 1999) noted that stationary-phase cultures incubated in broth lost their acid tolerance more rapidly than habituated cells. These detailed analyses of intrinsic acid tolerance and of stationary-phase resistance reveal considerable variability between O157:H7 isolates and commensal organisms, such that it cannot be stated that these organisms have greater acid resistance.

Several surveys of acid tolerance have now been completed and are published or in press. Although initial studies suggested that O157:H7 strains were more acid-tolerant than other *E. coli* strains (Small *et al.*, 1994; Benjamin and Datta, 1995; Wang and Doyle, 1998), there is an emerging consensus that this is not the case. Firstly, laboratory K-12 strains provide no guide to the level of intrinsic acid tolerance to be expected in either commensal or pathogenic *E. coli.* We define intrinsic acid tolerance as that expressed by cells when growing exponentially at a defined growth rate (close to $\mu = 0.9\ h^{-1}$) in minimal medium at pH 7, since, under these conditions, no specific attempt has been made to induce the known acid-resistance mechanisms (see below however). In general, laboratory K-12 strains are tenfold, or greater, more sensitive to acid conditions than are commensal organisms (Glover *et al.*, 1999). Laboratory strains show the expected increased resistance associated with the stationary phase and growth at mildly acidic pH, but they are generally more sensitive to acid than commensal and pathogenic organisms. Secondly, there is very significant diversity in the level of intrinsic acid tolerance between different isolates of commensal and pathogenic organisms (Lin *et al.*, 1996; Glover *et al.*, 1999; Jordan, S.L. *et al.*, 1999). There are examples of very resistant commensal organisms and very acid-sensitive O157:H7 isolates and therefore it is unwise to consider either group to be especially well adapted to facing pH stress. Thirdly, although the RpoS regulon is an important determinant of survival of acid stress, a significant number of O157:H7 isolates from patients were acid-sensitive and could be rendered acid-resistant by transformation with the cloned wild-type *rpoS* gene (Waterman and Small, 1996). This suggests that, while the RpoS regulon is important for survival, it is not the sole determinant of survival of either acid stress or other stresses in the natural environment. The ability of cells to acquire acid tolerance during growth at mildly acidic pH is independent of RpoS, the stationary phase sigma factor, (Fig. 2.2; Glover *et al.*, 1999; see below). However, the regulation of accumulation and activity of the RpoS sigma factor is complex and variations in intrinsic acid tolerance in $RpoS^+$ strains may relate to different balances in the regulation.

In one respect, the O157:H7 isolates did differ from commensal organisms. In these investigations (Glover *et al.*, 1999), we noted that, although cell death started immediately upon transfer to acid pH, after 20–30 min there was no further decline in the viable counts and the acid-resistant survivors persisted for many hours (Fig. 2.1). This population was variable in size between different *E. coli* isolates, but in general was consistent for any given isolate in repeat experiments. As a rule, this population was ten- to 100-fold greater for the O157:H7 isolates than for commensal isolates. Similar heterogeneity in response to the applied stress

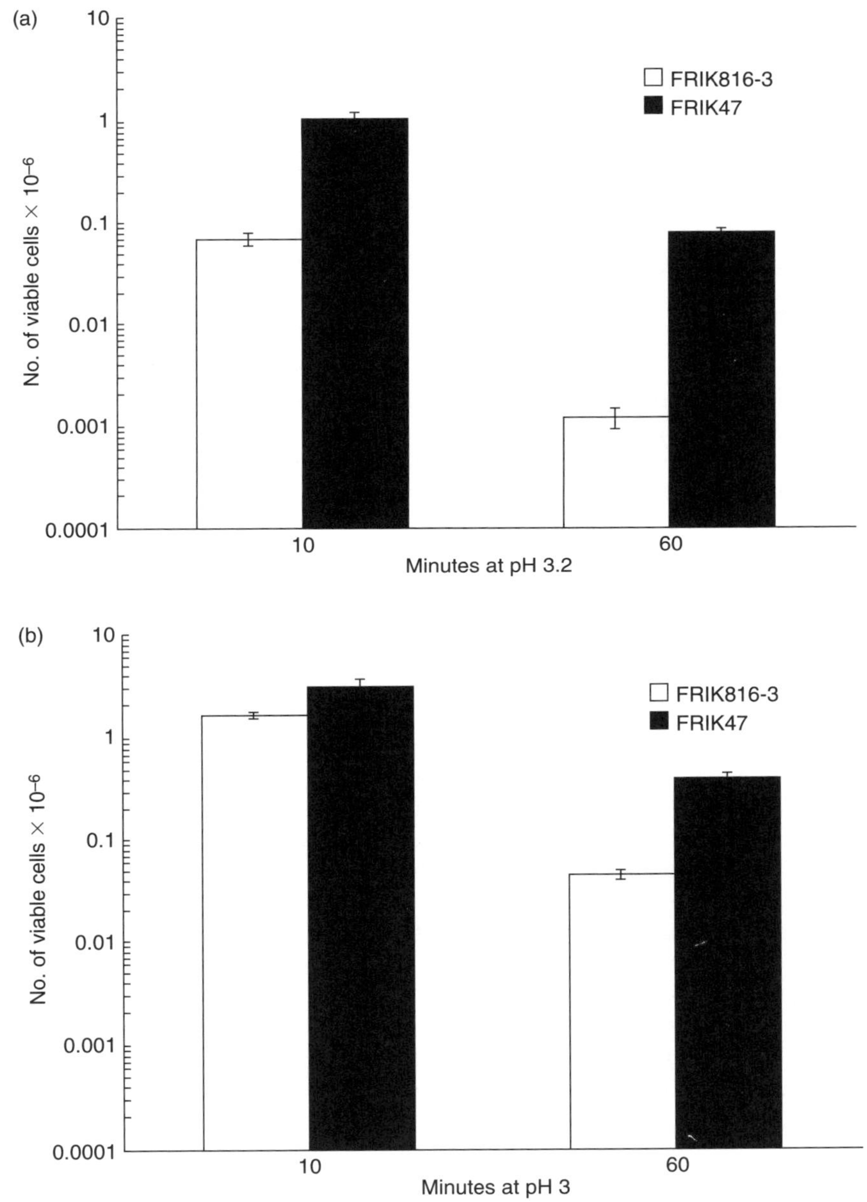

Fig. 2.2. Survival at acid pH for an *rpoS* mutant of O157:H7. Cells were prepared as described in Fig. 2.1 and were grown at either (a) pH 7 or (b) pH 5.8 habituated. The data show a comparison of survival at 10 min and 60 min after transfer to (a) pH 3.2 or (b) pH 3.0. Strain FRIK47 ($RpoS^+$) (closed bar) and FRIK816-3 ($RpoS^-$) (open bar) were isolated and created, respectively, by Cheville and colleagues (Cheville *et al.*, 1996).

has been noted in heat-treated *S. typhimurium*, in *Shigella* and in *E. coli* O157:H7 frozen in chicken-breast meat in the presence of NaCl and in defined media (Benjamin and Datta, 1995; Connor and Hall, 1996; Brown *et al.*, 1997; Humpheson *et al.*, 1998).

It is clear that the organisms that survive stress are those most likely to colonize a new environment upon release from the stress and hence are those that might generate food poisoning. The basis of the acid tolerance of the 'tail' population is the subject of our current investigations. Possible explanations for the presence of the acid-resistant population of cells are as follows.

1. A few cells manage to induce proteins that confer acid tolerance during incubation at pH 3.
2. A small number of cells retain stationary-phase gene products into exponential-phase growth.
3. The population contains genetic and non-genetic variants that survive the acid conditions.

Induction of acid-tolerance genes

Studies with inhibitors of protein and RNA synthesis showed that the presence of the survivors was not dependent upon new protein synthesis (Glover *et al.*, 1999). Although, under some conditions, there was a slight reduction in the size of the acid-tolerant population (Glover *et al.*, 1999; Jordan, K.N. *et al.*, 1999), this may be due to direct toxicity of the antibiotics themselves, since it was not evident with all the antibiotics tested. However, the heat-resistant 'tail' of *Salmonella enteridis* PT4 was shown to be eliminated if chloramphenicol was included during heating (Humpheson *et al.*, 1998). This suggested that induction of heat-shock genes during the heating treatment was the cause of the heat-tolerant 'tail'. At lower temperatures, which might be expected to allow more gene expression, the tailing effect was not as significant, despite a similar degree of killing. This suggests the possibility that chloramphenicol eliminates the 'tail', due to synergy between the antibiotic (or the solvent) and heat, rather than primarily through prevention of induction of heat-shock genes.

The role of the RpoS regulon

A mutant strain of *E. coli* O157:H7 lacking RpoS, created by Kaspar and colleagues (Cheville *et al.*, 1996), also continued to show the two populations of cells (Glover *et al.*, 1999). However, the demonstration of this required some modification of the experimental conditions. When exponentially growing cells of the mutant were transferred from pH 7 to pH 3, cell death was so extensive that no surviving population was observed. The rate of death of the cells in the RpoS mutant was faster than the equivalent culture of the RpoS$^+$ parent (Fig. 2.2) and therefore the RpoS regulon has a significant role in setting the background level of acid tolerance, even in rapidly growing exponential-phase cultures (μ = 0.8–1.0 h^{-1}). However, raising the pH to 3.2 allowed greater survival of the *rpoS* mutant and then two populations of cells were observed (Glover *et al.*, 1999). In addition, culture of the *rpoS* mutant at pH 5.8 for three generations induced the acid-tolerance regulon and increased the overall tolerance of the strain to acid, which incidentally demonstrates the independence of the acid habituation response from RpoS (Fig. 2.2). In such cultures, two populations of cells were also evident: those that were killed at pH 3 and those that survived. Thus, the generation of heterogeneity does not require the presence of the RpoS regulon and cannot be ascribed to the persistence of genes under the control of this sigma factor. We recently demonstrated that lactate and ethanol can be combined with low pH to effect high rates of killing of *E. coli* O157:H7 (Jordan, S.L. *et al.*, 1999; see also Leyer *et al.*, 1995). As described above, the addition of either lactate or ethanol at pH 3 causes a lowering of the cytoplasmic pH and this is probably one of the factors that determine the rate of death, particularly in exponential-phase cells (Jordan, S.L. *et al.*, 1999). All the *E. coli* isolates investigated could be killed at acid pH by incubation with either ethanol or lactate, even those that possessed very high levels of intrinsic acid tolerance. When ethanol (5%) was added to the acid-treated culture after 40 min incubation at pH 3, there was a rapid decline in the viable population (Glover *et al.*, 1999). These data suggest that the surviving 'tail' population is not generally stress-tolerant and this again is consistent with this phenomenon not arising from the persistence of the products of the RpoS regulon in some cells in the exponential phase.

Physiological and unstable genetic variation

All of the data available point to the survivors arising as a result of either unstable genetic variation or physiological variation. Cultures generated by recovery of the population of survivors at pH 3 exhibited similar acid sensitivity to the initial inoculum. The kinetics of killing during the initial phase of cell death in the recultured survivors was frequently heterogeneous, suggesting that there had been some enrichment for stable mutants (Glover *et al.*, 1999). These data suggest that the acid-resistance properties possessed by the majority of the survivors are readily lost on transfer to fresh growth medium (Glover *et al.*, 1999; Jordan, K.N. *et al.*, 1999). This is not the place for detailed theoretical treatment of the origins of variation within growing populations of cells. Such heterogeneity phenomena are well established in the literature (Novick and Weiner, 1957; Spudich and Koshland, 1976; Russo-Marie *et al.*, 1993; Lupski *et al.*, 1996; Whiteley *et al.*, 1996; Tolker-

Neilsen *et al.*, 1998). In the context of survival of acid conditions, a number of possibilities are obvious: variation in pools of cell metabolites, differences in cell-cycle stage, heterogeneous protein composition, transient gene amplification, transient variations in cell envelope composition, variation in individual cell growth rate. Each of these has the potential to contribute to intrinsic acid tolerance through alterations in the capacity for pH homoeostasis and for either recovery from or protection against acid damage to cytoplasmic and membrane components of the cell.

CONCLUSIONS

There is no doubt that *E. coli* O157:H7 represents a persistent threat as a food-poisoning agent. It has been speculated that the two major factors that have given rise to the increased prevalence of this form of food poisoning are changes in agriculture and changes in food preparation (both domestic and commercial). In the context of acid tolerance, the organism does not appear to be greatly different from commensal *E. coli.* However, O157:H7 may have the ability to generate a higher 'tail' population and this, coupled with the low infective dose and changes in our lifestyle, has allowed the organism to become a major pathogen. From our own studies and those of others, it is evident that the organism can be killed by appropriate hygiene, food preservation and cooking regimes. Thus truly, in the sense that Zinsser (1934) meant it, this may be an organism 'living along with us in mysterious obscurity awaiting their opportunities'. Those opportunities are created by human complacency, not by biological advances by the organism.

ACKNOWLEDGEMENTS

This work was funded by the Department of Health and the Ministry of Agriculture, Fisheries and Food. Special thanks are due to Conor O'Byrne, John Foster, Charles Kaspar and Hugh Pennington.

REFERENCES

Armstrong, G.L., Hollingsworth, J. and Morris, J.G. (1996) Emerging foodborne pathogens: *Escherichia coli* O157:H7 as a model of entry of a new pathogen into the food supply of the developed world. *Epidemiological Reviews* 18, 29–51.

Bearson, S., Bearson, B. and Foster, J.W. (1997) Acid stress in enterobacteria. *FEMS Microbiology Letters* 147, 173–180.

Benjamin, M.M. and Datta, A.R. (1995) Acid tolerance of enterohemorrhagic *Escherichia coli. Applied and Environmental Microbiology* 61, 1669–1672.

Booth I.R. (1985) Regulation of cytoplasmic pH in bacteria. *Microbiological Reviews* 49, 59–78.

Booth, I.R. (1999) Regulation of cytoplasmic pH in bacteria. In: *Novartis Foundation Symposium* 221, 28–37.

Booth, I.R. and Stratford, M. (1998) Acidulants and low pH. In: Gould, G.W. and Russell, N.J. (eds) *The Molecular Basis of Food Preservative Action.* Blackie, London (in press).

Brown, J.L., Ross, T., McMeekin, T. and Nichols, P.D. (1997) Acid habituation of *Escherichia coli* and the potential role of cyclopropane fatty acids in low pH tolerance. *International Journal of Food Microbiology* 37, 163–173.

Cheville, A.M., Arnold, K.W., Buchrieser, C., Cheng, C.-M. and Kaspar, C.W. (1996) *rpoS* Regulation of acid, heat, and salt tolerance in *Escherichia coli* O157:H7. *Applied and Environmental Microbiology* 62, 1822–1824.

Connor, D.E. and Hall, G.S. (1996) Temperature and food additives affect the growth and survival of *Escherichia coli* O157:H7 in poultry meat. *Dairy, Food and Environmental Sanitation* 16, 150–153.

Ellajosyula, K.R., Doores, S., Mills, E.W., Wilson, R.A., Anantheswaran, R.C. and Knabel, S.J. (1998) Destruction of *Escherichia coli* O157:H7 and *Salmonella typhimurium* in Lebanon Bologna by interaction of fermentation pH, heating temperature, and time. *Journal of Food Protection* 61, 152–157.

Ferguson, G.P., Creighton, R.I., Nikolaev, Y. and Booth, I.R. (1998) The importance of RpoS and Dps in the survival of exposure of both exponential and stationary phase cells to the electrophile, *N*-ethylmaleimide. *Journal of Bacteriology* 180, 1030–1036.

Foster, J.W. and Hall, H.K. (1990) Adaptive acidification tolerance response of *Salmonella typhimurium. Journal of Bacteriology* 172, 771–778.

Foster, J.W. and Hall, H.K. (1991) Inducible pH homeostasis and the acid tolerance response of *Salmonella typhimurium. Journal of Bacteriology* 173, 5129–5135.

Glover, J., Malcolm, L., Thomson-Carter, F.M., Carter, P., Jordan, S., Park, S.J. and Booth, I.R. (1999) Non-genetic variation as a mechanism of survival of acid stress in *E. coli* O157:H7. *Molecular Microbiology* (in press).

Goodson, M. and Rowbury, R.J. (1989) Habituation to normal lethal acidity by prior growth of *Escherichia coli* at a sub-lethal pH value. *Letters in Applied Microbiology* 8, 77–79.

Hengge-Aronis, R. (1993) Survival of hunger and stress – the role of rpoS in early stationary phase gene regulation in *E. coli. Cell* 72, 165–168.

Humpheson, L., Adams, M.R., Anderson, W.A. and Cole, M.B. (1998) Biphasic thermal inactivation kinetics in *Salmonella enteridis* PT4. *Applied and Environmental Microbiology* 64, 459–464.

Jordan, K.N., Oxford, L. and O'Byrne, C.P. (1999) Survival of low pH stress by *Escherichia coli* O157:H7: a correlation between alterations in the cell envelope and increased acid tolerance. *Applied and Environmental Microbiology* (in press).

Jordan, S.L., Glover, J., Malcolm, L., Thomson-Carter, F.M., Booth, I.R. and Park, S.F. (1999) Augmentation of killing of *Escherichia coli* O157:H7 by combinations of low pH, lactate and ethanol. *Applied and Environmental Microbiology* 65, 1308–1311.

Leyer, G.J., Wang, L.L. and Johnson, E.A. (1995) Acid adaptation of *Escherichia coli* O157:H7 increases survival in acidic foods. *Applied and Environmental Microbiology* 61, 3752–3755.

Lin, J., Smith, M.P., Chapin, K.C., Baik, H.S., Bennett, G.N. and Foster, J.W. (1996) Mechanisms of acid resistance in enterohemorrhagic *Escherichia coli*. *Journal of Applied and Environmental Microbiology* 62, 3094–3100.

Lupski, J.R., Roth, J.R. and Weinstock, G.M. (1996) Chromosomal duplications in bacteria, fruit flies, and humans. *American Journal of Human Genetics* 58, 21–27.

Novick, A. and Weiner, M. (1957) Enzyme induction is an all or none phenomenon. *Proceedings of the National Academy of Sciences USA* 43, 553–566.

Pupo, G.M., Karaolis, D.K.R., Lan, R. and Reeves, P.R. (1997) Evolutionary relationships among pathogenic and nonpathogenic *Escherichia coli* strains inferred from multilocus enzyme electrophoresis and *mdh* sequence studies. *Infection and Immunity* 65, 2685–2692.

Raja, N., Goodson, M., Smith, D.G. and Rowbury, R.J. (1991) Decreased DNA damage and increased repair of acid-damaged DNA in acid-habituated *Escherichia coli*. *Journal of Applied Bacteriology* 70, 507–511.

Rowbury, R.J. (1995) An assessment of environmental factors influencing acid tolerance and sensitivity in *Escherichia coli*, *Salmonella* spp. and other enterobacteria. *Letters in Applied Microbiology* 20, 333–337.

Russo-Marie, F., Roederer, M., Sager, B., Herzenberg, L.A. and Kaiser, D. (1993) β-Galactosidase activity in single differentiating bacterial cells. *Proceedings of the National Academy of Sciences USA* 90, 8194–8198.

Small, P., Blankenhorn, P., Welty, D., Zinser, E. and Slonczewski, J.L. (1994) Acid and base resistance in *Escherichia coli* and *Shigella flexneri*: role of *rpoS* and growth pH. *Journal of Bacteriology* 176, 1729–1737.

Spudich, J.L. and Koshland, D.E., Jr (1976) Non-genetic individuality: chance in the single cell. *Nature (London)* 262, 467–471.

Tilden, J., Jr, Young, W., McNamara, A., Custer, C., Boesel, B., Lambert-Fair, M.A., Majkowski, J., Vugia, D., Werner, S.B., Hollingsworth, J. and Morris, J.G., Jr (1996) A new route of transmission for *Escherichia coli*: infection from dry fermented salami. *American Journal of Public Health* 86, 1142–1145.

Tolker-Neilsen, T., Homstrom, K., Boe, L. and Molin, S. (1998) Non-genetic population heterogeneity studied by *in situ* polymerase chain reaction. *Molecular Microbiology* 27, 1099–1105.

Wang, G. and Doyle, M.P. (1998) Heat shock response enhances acid tolerance of *Escherichia coli* O157:H7. *Letters in Applied Microbiology* 26, 31–34.

Waterman, S.R. and Small, P.L.C. (1996) Characterization of the acid resistance phenotype and *rpoS* alleles of shiga-like toxin-producing *Escherichia coli*. *Infection and Immunity* 64, 2808–2811.

Whiteley, A.S., O'Donnell, A.G., Macnaughton, S.J. and Barer, M.R. (1996) Cytochemical colocalization of phenotypic and genotypic characteristics in individual bacterial cells. *Applied and Environmental Microbiology* 62, 1873–1879.

Whittam, T.S., Wachsmuth, I.K. and Wilson, R.A. (1988) Genetic evidence for clonal descent of *Escherichia coli* O157:H7 associated with hemorrhagic colitis and hemolytic uremic syndrome. *Journal of Infectious Diseases* 157, 1124–1133.

Zinsser, H. (1934) *Rats, Lice and History*. Little, Brown, Boston, Massachusetts.

Escherichia coli O157:H7 and the Rumen Environment

3

M.A. Rasmussen, T.L. Wickman, W.C. Cray, Jr and T.A. Casey

National Animal Disease Center, ARS–USDA, Ames, Iowa, USA

INTRODUCTION

The occurrence of facultative anaerobes, such as *Escherichia coli*, in an anaerobic environment like the rumen has, in the past, been dismissed as unimportant. These microbes were considered poor competitors in relation to the predominant population of strict anaerobes found in this environment. Microbial interactions within the rumen are complex, intensely competitive and known to inhibit the growth of enterobacteria. Although facultatively anaerobic enterobacteria are present in the rumen, they usually occur at relatively low population densities and are generally regarded to be transient and non-growing. In recent years, the human pathogen *E. coli* O157:H7 has forced microbiologists to re-evaluate long-held beliefs concerning the ecology of facultative anaerobes like *E. coli* in the rumen and other gastrointestinal (GI) tract compartments.

COMPETITIVE FITNESS OF *E. COLI* IN THE RUMEN

Rumen microbiologists have long considered *E. coli* to be an unimportant member of the rumen microbiota. This general conclusion was based upon extensive population surveys showing the predominance of strict anaerobes and upon the early work of Wolin (1969), which demonstrated the inhibitory relationship between pH and the volatile fatty acids (VFA) produced during rumen fermentation. Media with low pH and high VFA concentrations were most inhibitory. In more recent work, intracellular anion accumulation has been proposed as a mechanism of action for the

VFA's effects upon facultative anaerobes like *E. coli* (Russell, 1992). Inoculation studies have demonstrated the inhospitable nature of the rumen with respect to *E. coli*. Under *in vivo* conditions, inoculated strains have failed to establish permanent populations when introduced into the rumen (Wallace *et al.*, 1989; Cray and Moon, 1995).

RUMINANTS, FASTING STRESS AND *ESCHERICHIA COLI*

A diurnal variation exists in the GI tract for the fermentation parameters, pH and VFA. These parameters are related to the feeding frequency of the animal. In animals fed only once a day, rumen pH and VFA levels will fluctuate widely, whereas these values will remain somewhat constant in animals with constant or semicontinuous access to feed. In animals that are fasted for 24–48 h, rumen pH can rise above 7.5, while VFA concentrations will decline below 50 mM (Brownlie and Grau, 1967; Rasmussen *et al.*, 1993). Classic studies have borne out the relationship between fasting and fermentation parameters and their effect upon microbial populations like *Salmonella* and *E. coli* (Grau *et al.*, 1969). In other studies, a variety of *E. coli* strains, including strains of O157:H7, were inhibited by the prevailing pH and VFA concentrations of the rumen of well-fed cattle (Rasmussen *et al.*, 1993). Strains of *E. coli* O157:H7 did not display superior tolerance to normal rumen parameters, as compared with other strains of *E. coli*. Furthermore, all strains of *E. coli* showed unrestricted growth in rumen fluid collected from fasted cattle, thus indicating a role for fasting in the ecology of *E. coli* in cattle.

Based upon this evidence, a fasting protocol was devised in order to test the relationship between fasting and faecal shedding of *E. coli* (Fig. 3.1). This protocol was designed to mimic the sporadic periods of feedings and fasting that occur when animals are transported long distances over several days (Knowles, 1998). Using this protocol, fasting routinely increased total coliform counts by 4–6 log colony-forming units (CFU) in both rumen and faecal samples (Fig. 3.2). The peak in coliform population corresponded closely with the single feeding given to the test animals during the middle of the fasting period (day 2). It was concluded that a combination of fasting and sporadic feeding perturbed normal gut microflora to such an extent that minor population members like *E. coli* could temporarily predominate in this environment.

In further studies, a nalidixic acid resistant strain of *E. coli* was used to monitor the effects of fasting in sheep (Fig. 3.3). When this strain was inoculated into sheep which were then subjected to fasting, the usual pattern of increased coliform populations was observed from both rumen and faecal samples. When normal feeding was resumed, the marked strain of *E. coli* became undetectable. However, further fasting caused this microbe to repopulate the gut without further inoculation. In one animal, this pattern of repopulation was repeated in each of three subsequent fasting cycles over a period of 70 days.

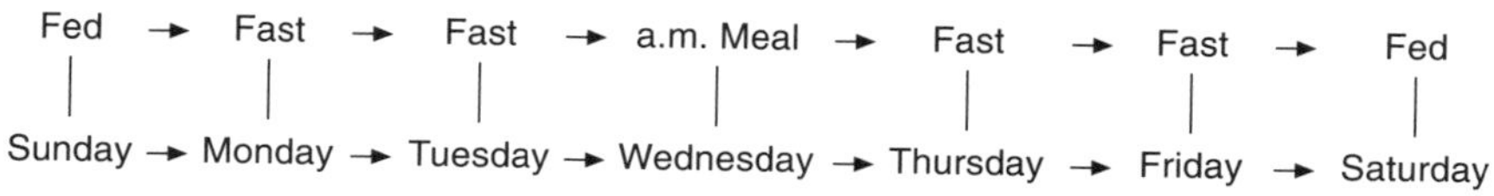

Fig. 3.1. Fasting protocol time line (Cray *et al.*, 1998).

In cattle, fasting's effects upon the population dynamics of *E. coli* O157:H7 have not been as pronounced as that observed for other strains of the microbe. Cray *et al.* (1998) found no significant increase in faecal shedding of strain O157:H7 as a result of fasting. However, fasting did make calves more susceptible to a given inoculation dose. A dose of 10^7 CFU combined with fasting resulted in faecal shedding patterns that were similar to those obtained when using a dose of 10^{10} CFU without fasting.

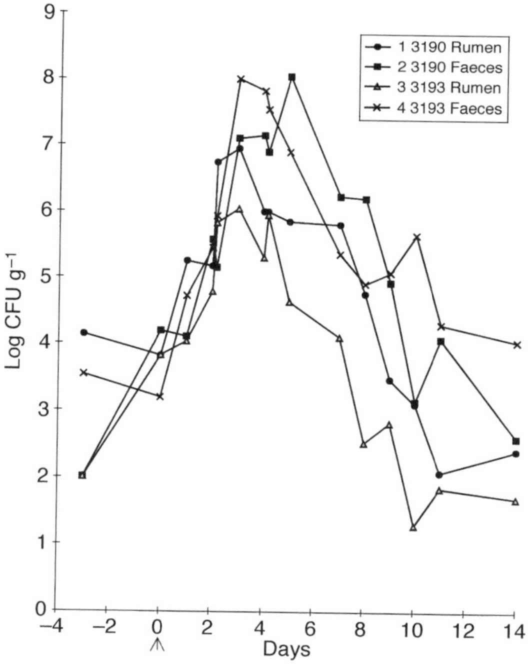

Fig. 3.2. The effect of fasting upon coliform populations in the rumen and faeces of sheep. Total coliform CFU (MacConkey agar) from sheep nos 3190 and 3193. Animals were subjected to the fasting protocol of Cray *et al.* (1998) (see Fig. 3.1), with arrow symbolizing initiation of fasting period. Meals were given to sheep only on days −1, 2 and 4. On days thereafter, the sheep were given regular twice-daily meals.

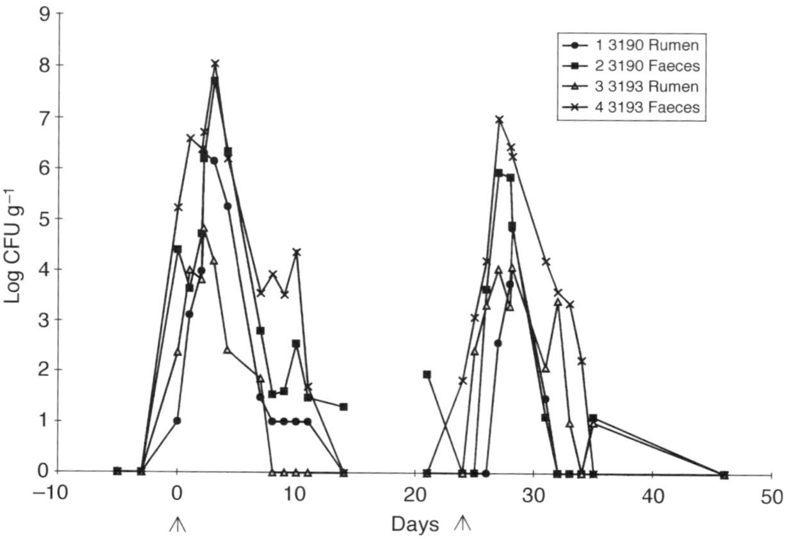

Fig. 3.3. Repeated recovery of a nalidixic acid-resistant *E. coli* from the rumen and faeces of sheep. Bacterial strain (6 × 10^{10} CFU) orally inoculated into sheep at day −1. Animals were subjected to the fasting protocol of Cray *et al.* (1998) (see Fig. 3.1), with initiation of each fasting period indicated by arrow. Meals were given to sheep only on days −1, 2 and 4. On days thereafter, the sheep were given regular twice-daily meals. In the period between fasts, animals were given regular twice-daily meals.

TRANSPORT STRESS AND *SALMONELLA*: THE AUSTRALIAN EXPERIENCE

Australian workers have provided a good example of the effect that fasting can have upon the microbial ecology of the rumen. Their research was undertaken in response to a very practical problem. During the early 1980s, the Australian sheep industry developed a market for live sheep in the Middle East. This market required sheep to be transported by sea on large 'stockyard ships' from ports in Western Australia to Middle Eastern slaughter facilities. Early voyages encountered high death losses, which prompted concerns about animal welfare and management (Norris *et al.*, 1989). Further investigations demonstrated that many of the afflicted sheep were suffering from *Salmonella* infections and that inappetence was a contributing factor to the high death losses. The poor feed and water consumption was attributed to the abrupt change in diet, as well as to the unfamiliar feed and watering equipment used on the transport ships. This information was combined with the earlier *Salmonella* research of Grau *et al.* (1969), Chambers and Lysons (1979) and Mattila *et al.* (1988) to arrive at a solution. These earlier works had all demonstrated a basic relationship between fasting, transport and *Salmonella* infections. The work can best be summarized by a passage from Mattila *et al.* (1988): 'to maintain the inhibitory capacity of the rumen for *Salmonella*, minimize the time in transport and feed animals often'. Using this information, new management practices were implemented. Prior to boarding, sheep were gradually introduced to the types of feeding facilities and pelleted feeds that they would encounter once on board. These changes improved feed intake during the voyages and reduced the deaths.

UBIQUITOUS POPULATIONS OF FAECAL COLIFORMS?

That *E. coli* and other coliform bacteria are present in animal faeces at high population levels is a widely held belief. Each new generation of microbiologists has accepted this belief without question and has assumed that this 'fact' applies to all individuals, animal species and circumstances. This concept has also formed the basis of the standard methods for examination of water purity and meat carcass cleanliness. However, evidence exists that calls this concept into question. Smith and Crabb (1961) reported that they found little or no evidence of *E. coli* in the faeces of rabbits and guinea-pigs and wide population differences in cattle. Later work substantiated these unusual observations in respect of guinea-pigs (McLean and Boquest, 1977). In recent work with cattle, we have also found wide variations in faecal coliform counts from cattle (from 0 to 10^8 CFU (authors' unpublished data)). These results raise many questions with regard to faecal coliform populations. One of those questions pertains to the current practice of using generic *E. coli* (biotype 1) as a marker for faecal contamination in US livestock-processing plants (Food Safety and Inspection Service, 1996).

The variability of specific *E. coli* populations in the gut is also reflected in other literature. Epidemiological data support the concept that *E. coli* O157:H7 'infections' in cattle are relatively transient events, on an individual animal basis (Garber *et al.*, 1995; Besser *et al.*, 1997; Hancock *et al.*, 1997) and on a herd basis (Rahn *et al.*, 1997). This transient behaviour brings into question the widely held belief that cattle serve as a reservoir for *E. coli* O157:H7. An objective reappraisal of this concept does not fully support this belief but instead suggests that cattle are transient 'incubators' for this strain, as they are for other strains of *E. coli*.

DIETARY FACTORS AND *ESCHERICHIA COLI* O157

Epidemiological studies have investigated a wide variety of factors in an attempt to identify those factors that may influence the presence of *E. coli* in cattle (Hancock *et al.*, 1994; Herriott *et al.*, 1998). These studies have considered management, facility and dietary factors that are currently used for beef- and dairy-cattle production. Diet has been considered a potentially important area, given the biological plausibility that it influences gut microbial populations. Most of the factors investigated have shown little or no statistical relationship to *E. coli* O157:H7. However, some dietary factors have shown enough of a pattern for further investigation to be warranted. These include factors that indicate a negative relationship to *E. coli* (cottonseed and clover feeding) and others with a positive relationship (ionophore feeding).

The use of ionophores has attracted interest, given the apparent temporal relationship between initial ionophore use in the US cattle industry (1970s) and the increase in *E. coli* O157:H7 cases. However, experimentation in cattle has not been able to establish a direct cause-and-effect relationship between ionophore use and *E. coli* O157:H7 shedding. In spite of this, it is still possible that these compounds do alter the gut microbiota in ways that give *E. coli* a selective advantage, but the effects may be indirect and subtle. Further research in this area is needed.

The other dietary factors that have been identified by epidemiology include the feeding of cottonseed and clover hay. Although complete experimental data are lacking, it is interesting to speculate that chemical constituents within these plants may play a role in suppressing *E. coli* in the gut. For example, gossypol, a compound that is found in cottonseed, is known to inhibit the growth of a wide variety of Gram-positive bacteria. However, in our experiments, gossypol had little effect upon the growth of *E. coli* (authors' unpublished data). In spite of these data, it is possible that other compounds are present (e.g. other terpenoids in cotton and saponins in clover) which show activity against *E. coli* and thus explain the epidemiological evidence.

The feeding of grain to cattle is another dietary factor, the impact of which is currently undergoing a vigorous debate. Some authors (Diez-Gonzalez *et al.*, 1998) have suggested, on very preliminary data, that grain feeding creates an acidic environment in the gut of cattle and this in turn leads to the selection of acid-tolerant *E. coli*, including O157 strains, which are then heavily shed in the faeces. The authors propose that cattle producers could solve the *E. coli* problem by feeding hay to cattle before slaughter. Earlier studies by Allison *et al.* (1975) partially support these claims, because they found increased caecal coliform populations in cattle and sheep fed high-grain diets. However, these earlier studies were on animals suffering from experimentally induced grain overload and, as such, these results may not be directly applicable to healthy grain-fed ruminants. The majority of the other literature available contradicts the claims of Diez-Gonzalez *et al.* (1998). The epidemiological data of Hancock *et al.* (1994) demonstrated no difference in O157:H7 prevalence between grain-fed and hay-fed cattle. Others have shown no difference in faecal *E. coli* shedding patterns when cattle were fed a grain- or forage-based diet (Jordan and McEwen, 1998). Still others have found exactly the opposite effect, observing that forage feeding resulted in the highest levels of *E. coli* O157:H7 (Kudva *et al.*, 1995; Robert Elder, personal communication). It is also worthwhile to note that Argentina has a very high prevalence rate of *E. coli* O157:H7, but its cattle industry is almost entirely based upon forage and grassland agriculture (Reilly, 1998).

For researchers investigating the possible causes of an increased incidence of *E. coli* O157:H7 in cattle, it may be useful to consider other cattle-management practices which, unlike grain feeding, were actually initiated in the 1970s, when human cases of *E. coli* O157:H7 began to be reported. One dietary factor from the 1970s to consider is the feeding of protein supplements with high rumen-bypass potential. An extensive literature on this feeding practice exists with regard to animal performance but essentially none with regard to their microbiological effects post-ruminally. Although experimental evidence is lacking to support this speculation, it is possible that increased protein flow into the lower gut may alter the environment and provide selective advantages for some strains of *E. coli.*

Another dietary change implemented in the 1970s is the supplementation of livestock diets with selenium. In the USA, it became legal to add selenium to the diets of lambs and ewes at a level of 0.1 p.p.m. in 1978 (Ullrey, 1992). This authority was extended to all classes of sheep and cattle in 1979. Still later, in 1987, the level of selenium supplementation was increased to 0.3 p.p.m. For purposes of discussion, we propose a relationship between selenium and *E. coli*, including the strain O157:H7. We propose that this relationship is due in part to this element's chemical similarity to other oxyanions of periodic groups 5a and 6a, most notably tellurite, nitrite and nitrate, for which some substantiating microbiological literature exists. Zadik *et al.* (1993) found that adding tellurite (2.5 mg l^{-1}) to MacConkey medium markedly increased the rate of isolation of *E. coli* O157:H7 from rectal swabs of cattle. Although these researchers were primarily interested in method development, their work offers a useful clue with regard to the ecology of *E. coli* O157 in cattle. Similarly, Chernyaeva *et al.* (1993) reported *in vitro* data which indicated that nitrates stimulated the development of 'pathogenic' strains of enterobacteria.

The toxicity of the oxyanions nitrate, nitrite, tellurite, selenite and selenate to microorganisms, especially Gram-negative bacteria, is well known, as are some of the resistance mechanisms that microbes use to overcome the effects of these compounds. Some microbes can obtain energy for growth from the reduction of the compounds. Others reduce them to less toxic forms, such as elemental tellurium, only as a means of preventing cell damage. In *E. coli*, resistance is believed to be a consequence of nitrate-reductase activity (Lloyd-Jones *et al.*, 1994; Avazeri *et al.*, 1997). Tellurite- and selenate-reductase activities from membrane-protein extracts were also found to reduce nitrate (Avazeri *et al.*, 1997). These workers found that mutants lacking nitrate-reductase activity were hypersensitive to tellurite. It was also noted that anaerobic conditions like those encountered in the gut stimulated additional reductase activity, which increased the bacteria's resistance to tellurium. These authors concluded that nitrate reductases conferred resistance to oxyanions like tellurite.

We have attempted to relate these findings to the ecology of *E. coli* in cattle. In preliminary experiments, a rumen-fistulated goat was fed increasing levels of supplemental selenium (sodium selenate). Populations of enterobacteria in the rumen were monitored through the use of a 27-base oligonucleotide probe for *E. coli* and other enterobacteria (5′ TCAGCAAAGCAGCA–AGCTGCTTCCTGT 3′). We found that selenium supplementation, up to 3 p.p.m., resulted in a corresponding increase in probe hybridization signal (Table 3.1). By inference, it was concluded that populations of *E. coli* in the rumen had increased in size. Although these are very preliminary data, it is worthwhile speculating that selenium may be an environmental selection factor for *E. coli* in the gut of cattle. A reanalysis of previously conducted epidemiological surveys should be undertaken if selenium-feeding practices were recorded as part of these surveys. These and other more direct studies could then be used to determine whether this selenium hypothesis is valid.

CONCLUDING SUMMARY

In this chapter, we introduce several factors that may influence the relationship between *E. coli* O157:H7 and ruminants. These include the following.

1. The inhibitory effects of the rumen on *E. coli*. In our experiments, all strains of *E. coli* tested, including strains of *E. coli* O157:H7, grew poorly in media designed to mimic the well-fed rumen. Rumen fluid from fasted animals which was depleted of VFA supported rapid growth of *E. coli*.
2. Faecal shedding patterns of *E. coli* after oral inoculation. Adult cattle that were orally inoculated with *E. coli* O157:H7 (10^{10} CFU) usually eliminated

Table 3.1. The effect of dietary selenium supplementation upon a population of enterobacteria in the goat rumen.

Day of treatment	Supplemented selenium (p.p.m.)	Hybridization intensity*
0	0	500
10	0.3	600
20	0.3	1000
30	0.6	9100
35	1.0	8500
40	2.0	8000

* Relative intensity determined by hybridization of extracted rRNA to a ^{32}P-radiolabelled probe and quantitated with a Packard Imager (Packard Instrument Co., Meriden, Connecticut, USA).

this microbe within a few weeks. Calves carried the organism for a longer period of time, in some cases for several months, but most animals eventually eliminated the microbe from the gut. Calves subjected to a dietary fast had patterns of *E. coli* O157:H7 shedding that were not different from those of well-fed animals. In contrast to *E. coli* O157:H7 shedding, total faecal coliforms routinely increased when calves were fasted. Fasted calves were more susceptible to lower inoculation doses (10^7 CFU) and shed significantly more *E. coli* O157:H7 than calves maintained on a normal diet.

3. Cattle as a reservoir for *E. coli* O157:H7. Rumen inhibition and the variability in faecal shedding raise questions concerning the nature of the bovine reservoir and whether a 'true carrier state' exists. The data indicate that individuals can carry and clear *E. coli* O157:H7 within a relatively brief period of time. Similarly, herds can remain culture-positive indefinitely only if the environment is favourable for interanimal transmission. Such factors may explain the observed seasonality of herd infection rates.

4. Differences between the rumen and hind-gut. In contrast with the rumen, little is known about the physiology and microbiology of the hind-gut in relation to *E. coli* O157:H7 persistence. Rumen fermentation, with its abundance of substrate, usually restricts the growth of *E. coli*, but the more distal compartments of the digestive tract (colon and caecum) are often substrate-limited. These sites may play a very different role in the growth and excretion of pathogenic *E. coli*.

5. Hind-gut microbiology of animals that do not contain *E. coli*. Some individuals and animal species, such as the guinea-pig, do not shed *E. coli* in their faeces. Such animals may yield important clues concerning the microbial ecology of the gut and the exclusion of *E. coli*.

6. Emergence of *E. coli* O157:H7 and the role of feed ingredients and additives. There has been much speculation on the factors that have led to the 'emergence' of *E. coli* O157:H7 in cattle. This issue requires a critical reappraisal. However, in the absence of extensive pre-1980 baseline data, it is difficult to determine if *E. coli* O157:H7 truly emerged or was always present in the cattle population. A variety of dietary and management factors have been proposed as factors contributing to the increased prevalence of this microbe. Evidence that supports a role for these factors remains inconclusive and, in some cases, controversial. As a consequence, producers have been given little useful guidance on management practices that they can implement in order to reduce the incidence of *E. coli* O157:H7 in their herds.

REFERENCES

Allison, M.J., Robinson, I.M., Dougherty, R.W. and Bucklin, J.A. (1975) Grain overload in cattle and sheep: changes in microbial populations in the caecum and rumen. *American Journal of Veterinary Research* 36, 181–185.

Avazeri, C., Turner, R.J., Pommier, J., Weiner, J.H., Giordono, G. and Vermeglio, A. (1997) Tellurite reductase activity of nitrate reductase is responsible for the basal resistance of *Escherichia coli* to tellurite. *Microbiology* 143, 1181–1189.

Besser, T.E., Hancock, D.D., Pritchett, L.C., McRae, E.M., Rice, D.H. and Tarr, P.I. (1997) Duration of detection of fecal excretion of *Escherichia coli* O157:H7 in cattle. *Journal of Infectious Diseases* 175, 726–729.

Brownlie, L.E. and Grau, F.H. (1967) Effect of food intake on growth and survival of *Salmonella* and *Escherichia coli* in the bovine rumen. *Journal of General Microbiology* 46, 125–134.

Chambers, P.G. and Lysons, R.J. (1979) The inhibitory effect of bovine rumen fluid on *Salmonella typhimurium*. *Research in Veterinary Science* 26, 273–276.

Chernyaeva, I.I., Pishchik, V.N., Timopheeva, S.V., Glavin, A.A., Tiktin, L.A. and Rubenchik, B.L. (1993) The influence of nitrates, nitrites and *n*-nitrosodimethylamine on the metabolism of enterobacteriaceae family of bacteria. *Eksperimentalnaya Onkologiya* 15, 34–38.

Cray, W.C., Jr and Moon, H.W. (1995) Experimental infection of calves and adult cattle with *Escherichia coli* O157:H7. *Applied and Environmental Microbiology* 61, 1586–1590.

Cray, W.C., Jr, Casey, T.A., Bosworth, B.T. and Rasmussen, M.A. (1998) Effect of dietary stress on fecal shedding of *Escherichia coli* O157 in calves. *Applied and Environmental Microbiology* 64, 1975–1979.

Diez-Gonzalez, F., Callaway, T.R., Kizoulis, M.G. and Russell, J.B. (1998) Grain feeding and the dissemination of acid-resistant *Escherichia coli* from cattle. *Science* 281, 1666–1668.

Food Safety and Inspection Service, USDA (1996) Pathogen reduction: hazard analysis and critical control point (HACCP) systems. *Federal Register* 61, 38806–38989.

Garber, L.P., Wells, S.J., Hancock, D.D., Doyle, M.P., Tuttle, J., Shere, J.A. and Zhao, T. (1995) Risk factors for fecal shedding of *Escherichia coli* O157:H7 in dairy calves. *Journal of the American Veterinary Medical Association* 207, 46–49.

Grau, F.H., Brownlie, L.E. and Smith, M.G. (1969) Effects of food intake on numbers of *Salmonella* and *Escherichia coli* in rumen and faeces of sheep. *Journal of Applied Bacteriology* 32, 112–117.

Hancock, D.D., Besser, T.E., Kinsel, M.L., Tarr, P.I., Rice, D.H. and Paros, M.G. (1994) The prevalence of *Escherichia coli* O157:H7 in dairy and beef cattle in Washington state. *Epidemiology and Infection* 113, 199–207.

Hancock, D.D., Besser, T.E., Rice, D.H., Herriott, D.E. and Tarr, P.I. (1997) A longitudinal study of *Escherichia coli* O157 in fourteen cattle herds. *Epidemiology and Infection* 118, 193–195.

Herriott, D.E., Hancock, D.D., Ebel, E.D., Carpenter, L.V., Rice, D.H. and Besser, T.E. (1998) Association of herd management factors with colonization of dairy cattle by Shiga toxin-positive *Escherichia coli* O157. *Journal of Food Protection* 61, 802–807.

Jordan, D. and McEwen, S.A. (1998) Effect of duration of fasting and a short-term, high-roughage ration on the concentration of *Escherichia coli* Biotype I in cattle faeces. *Journal of Food Protection* 67, 531–534.

Knowles, T.G. (1998) A review of the road transport of slaughter sheep. *Veterinary* 143, 212–219.

Kudva, I.T., Hatfield, P.G. and Hovde, C.J. (1995) Effect of diet on the shedding of *Escherichia coli* O157:H7 in a sheep model. *Applied and Environmental Microbiology* 61, 1363–1370.

Lloyd-Jones, G., Osburn, A.M., Ritchie, D.A., Strike, P., Hobman, J.L., Brown, N.L. and Rouch, D.A. (1994) Accumulation and intracellular fate of tellurite in tellurite-resistant *Escherichia coli*: a model for the mechanism of resistance. *FEMS Microbiology Letters* 118, 113–120.

McLean, A.J. and Boquest, A. (1977) Enteric flora of normal laboratory guinea pigs. *British Journal of Experimental Pathology* 58, 251–254.

Mattila, T., Frost, A.J. and O'Boyle, D. (1988) The growth of *Salmonella* in rumen fluid from cattle at slaughter. *Epidemiology and Infection* 101, 337–345.

Norris, R.T., Richards, R.B. and Dunlop, R.H. (1989) An epidemiological study of sheep deaths before and during export by sea from Western Australia. *Australian Veterinary Journal* 66, 276–279.

Rahn, K., Renwick, S.A., Johnson, R.P., Wilson, J.B., Clarke, R.C., Alves, D., McEwen, S., Lion, H. and Spika, J. (1997) Persistence of *Escherichia coli* O157:H7 in dairy cattle and the dairy farm environment. *Epidemiology and Infection* 119, 251–259.

Rasmussen, M.A., Cray, W.C., Jr, Casey, T.A. and Whipp, S.C. (1993) Rumen contents as a reservoir of enterohemorrhagic *Escherichia coli*. *FEMS Microbiology Letters* 114, 79–84.

Reilly, A. (1998) Prevention and control of enterohaemorrhagic *Escherichia coli* (EHEC) infections: memorandum from a WHO meeting. *Bulletin of the World Health Organization* 76, 245–255.

Russell, J.B. (1992) Another explanation for the toxicity of fermentation acid at low pH: anion accumulation versus uncoupling. *Journal of Applied Bacteriology* 73, 363–370.

Smith, H.W. and Crabb, W.E. (1961) The faecal bacterial flora of animals and man: its development in the young. *Journal of Pathology and Bacteriology* 82, 53–66.

Ullrey, D.E. (1992) Basis for regulation of selenium supplements in animal diets. *Journal of Animal Science* 70, 3922–3927.

Wallace, R.J., Falconer, M.L. and Bhargava, P.K. (1989) Toxicity of volatile fatty acids at rumen pH prevents enrichment of *Escherichia coli* by sorbitol in rumen contents. *Current Microbiology* 19, 277–281.

Wolin, M.J. (1969) Volatile fatty acids and the inhibition of *Escherichia coli* growth by rumen fluid. *Applied and Environmental Microbiology* 17, 83–87.

Zadik, P.M., Chapman, P.A. and Siddons, C.A. (1993) Use of tellurite for the selection of verocytotoxigenic *Escherichia coli* O157. *Journal of Medical Microbiology* 39, 155–158.

4

Bovine Infection with *Escherichia coli* O157:H7

E.A. Dean-Nystrom,[1] B.T. Bosworth,[1] A.D. O'Brien[2] and H.W. Moon[3]

[1] *Enteric Diseases and Food Safety Research Unit, National Animal Disease Center, ARS–USDA, Ames, Iowa, USA;* [2] *Department of Microbiology and Immunology, F. Edward Hebert School of Medicine, Uniformed Services University of the Health Sciences, Bethesda, Maryland, USA;* [3] *Veterinary Medical Research Institute, College of Veterinary Medicine, Iowa State University, Ames, Iowa, USA*

INTRODUCTION

Cattle are a major reservoir of enterohaemorrhagic *Escherichia coli* (EHEC) O157:H7 and non-O157 shiga toxin-producing *E. coli* (STEC) strains that cause disease in humans. The majority of human EHEC outbreaks for which a source has been identified have been associated with consumption of cattle products, especially improperly cooked ground hamburger and raw milk.

STEC are commonly isolated from the intestines of healthy cattle (Whipp *et al.*, 1994). However, EHEC strains are pathogenic for multiple species, including humans, piglets, rabbits, chickens, monkeys and mice (Whipp *et al.*, 1994; Karpman *et al.*, 1997). EHEC serotypes that are associated with human disease are not usually associated with disease in cattle and are not considered to be bovine pathogens. However, many STEC isolates from healthy cattle share common virulence factors (e.g. shiga toxin and intimin) with attaching and effacing (att/eff) *E. coli* (AEEC), enteric pathogens that cause diarrhoea in young calves.

EXPERIMENTS WITH CALVES

We have shown that EHEC O157:H7 bacteria are pathogenic for neonatal calves (Dean-Nystrom *et al.*, 1997, 1998). As early as 18 h postinoculation with EHEC O157:H7, colostrum-deprived neonatal (< 12 h old) calves develop severe, sometimes fatal, diarrhoea, accompanied by the presence of att/eff lesions in the large and small intestines (Table 4.1; Figs 4.1 and 4.2; Dean-Nystrom *et al.*, 1997). Att/eff lesions can be detected by histological staining only in tissues that contain ≥ 10^6 colony-forming units (CFU) of O157:H7 bacteria per gram of tissue. As shown in Table 4.1, an EHEC O157:H7 strain (strain 3081) that was isolated from a healthy calf (Cray and Moon, 1995) is as pathogenic for neonatal calves as are EHEC O157:H7 strains 933 and 86-24 that were isolated from human food-borne outbreaks (Tarr *et al.*, 1989; O'Brien *et al.*, 1993).

Earlier studies showed that weaned calves remain clinically healthy following experimental infection with EHEC O157:H7, but are colonized and shed variable numbers of EHEC O157:H7 for variable periods (Cray and Moon, 1995). Thus, a weaned-calf model of asymptomatic EHEC O157:H7 infection may be more suitable than the symptomatic neonatal-calf model for identifying specific virulence factors that promote intestinal colonization

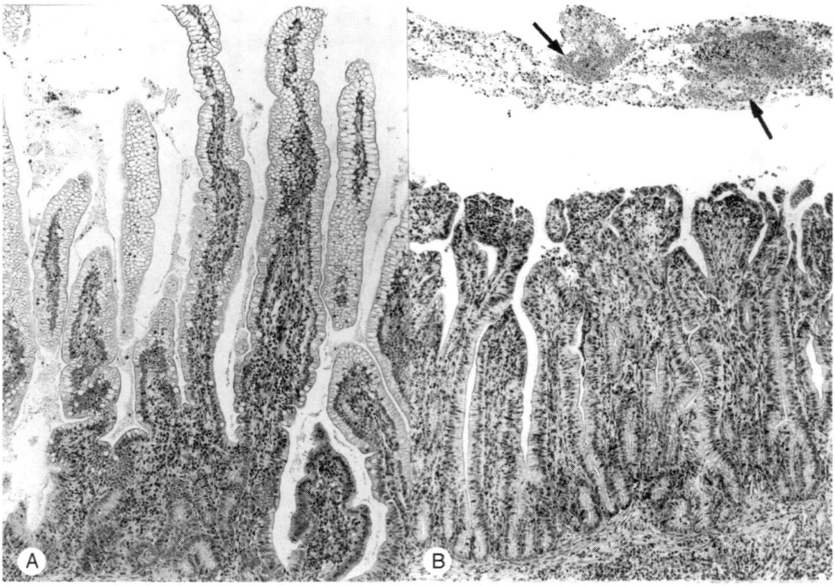

Fig. 4.1. H&E-stained sections of neonatal calf ileum (from Dean-Nystrom *et al.*, 1997, with permission). A. 18 h postinoculation with control *E. coli* strain 123. The long villi and vacuolated, tall columnar epithelium characteristic of normal neonatal calves are preserved. B. 3 days postinoculation with EHEC O157:H7 stain 3081. There is diffuse atrophy of villi. Atrophic villi have irregular, disrupted epithelium at their tips and cellular infiltrates (determined at higher magnification to be neutrophils) in distal lamina propria. Haemorrhage (plugs of erythrocytes at arrows) and fibrinocellular exudate have formed a pseudomembrane in the lumen.

Table 4.1. Findings in neonatal calves after inoculation with EHEC O157:H7 bacteria.

EHEC O157:H7 strain	*stx* gene[a]	*eae* gene[b]	Source	Hours after inoculation	Number of calves positive/number of calves tested: Diarrhoea	Death	AEB[c]	Reference
3081	1, 2	+	Healthy cow	18	2/3	0/3	3/3	Dean-Nystrom *et al.*, 1997
933	1, 2	+	Hamburger	18	0/4	0/4	4/4	Dean-Nystrom *et al.*, 1997
86-24	2	+	Human	18	2/2	0/2	2/2	Dean-Nystrom *et al.*, 1998
				42	3/3	1/3	3/3	
ATCC 43888	–	+	Human	42	2/3	0/3	3/3	Dean-Nystrom *et al.*, not published
86-24*eae*Δ10	2	–	Laboratory	42	0/3	0/3	0/3	Dean-Nystrom *et al.*, 1998
86-24*eae*Δ10(pEB310)	2	+	Laboratory	42	3/4	1/4	3/4	Dean-Nystrom *et al.*, 1998

[a] Presence or absence of *stx* gene.
[b] Presence or absence of *eae* gene.
[c] Att/eff bacteria detected by haematoxylin-and-eosin (H&E) staining or immunohistochemical staining with goat anti-O157:H7.

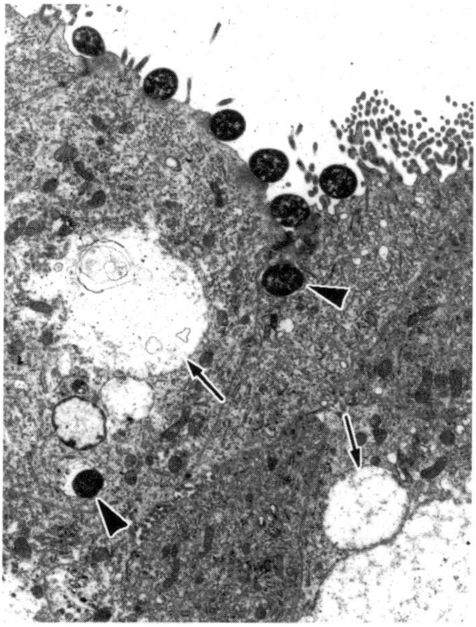

Fig. 4.2. Electron micrograph of absorptive cells from the ileum of a neonatal calf 18 h postinoculation with EHEC O157:H7 strain 3081 (from Dean-Nystrom *et al.*, 1997, with permission). Bacteria are intimately attached to absorptive cell membranes. Absorptive cell microvilli have been effaced to the left, but remain in the uncolonized area to the right. There are electron-dense filaments (presumably polymerized actin) in host cytoplasm subjacent to attached bacteria. Vacuolation of absorptive cells (arrows) is normal at this age. Two bacteria appear to be intracellular in vacuoles (arrowheads).

and faecal shedding in older cattle. We hypothesized that O157:H7 cause att/eff lesions in weaned calves, as they do in neonatal calves, but the lesions caused by the att/eff bacteria were not identified in earlier studies because the bacterial counts were too low (i.e. $< 10^6$ CFU g^{-1} of tissue). Since fasted ruminants shed higher numbers of *E. coli* and other enteric pathogens than do well-fed animals (Rasmussen *et al.*, 1993), we fasted weaned calves for 48 h prior to inoculation to increase the likelihood of recovering $\geq 10^6$ CFU of the inoculated bacteria per gram of tissue. Weaned 3–4-month-old calves were inoculated via stomach tube with 10^{10} CFU of EHEC O157:H7 or with a non-pathogenic *E. coli* control strain. All calves remained clinically healthy, but calves inoculated with EHEC O157:H7 had higher intestinal and faecal levels of inoculated *E. coli* than did the control animals. Att/eff bacteria were found by histopathological examination in three of nine O157-infected calves, but not in any of the control calves. Att/eff bacteria were found only in the rectum and caecum and only in tissues that contained $> 10^{5.5}$ CFU of O157:H7 g^{-1} of tissue (Fig. 4.3). These

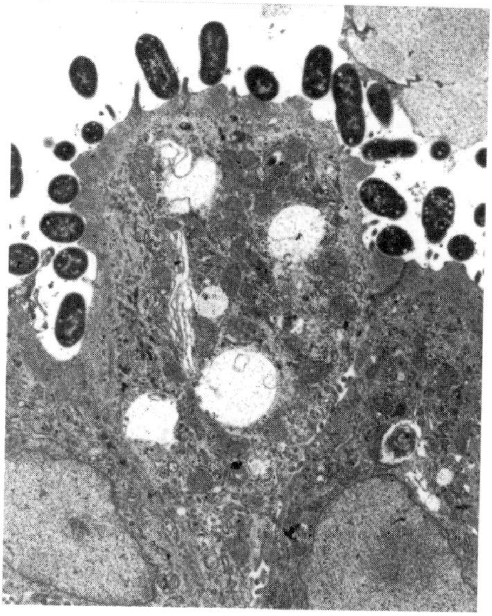

Fig. 4.3. Electron micrograph of enterocytes from the rectum of a 3-month-old weaned calf 4 days postinoculation with EHEC O157:H7 strain 86-24. Bacteria are intimately attached to epithelial cell membranes and most of the microvilli have been effaced.

results demonstrate that weaned calves, like neonatal calves, are susceptible to intestinal damage induced by *E. coli* O157:H7, but there is less EHEC-induced damage in weaned calves than in neonatal calves.

We are using the neonatal and weaned calf O157:H7 infection models to identify virulence factors that are involved in EHEC O157:H7 infections, colonization and bacterial shedding in cattle. EHEC O157:H7 bacteria require intimin, an adhesin encoded by the EHEC *eae* gene, to colonize, induce intestinal damage and cause disease in neonatal calves. As shown in Table 4.1, unlike the intimin-positive wild-type strain 86-24, an intimin-negative mutant of EHEC O157:H7 strain 86-24 (86-24*eae*Δ10) does not cause diarrhoea or induce att/eff lesions in neonatal calves. However, pathogenicity is fully restored in strain 86-24*eae*Δ10(pEB310) in which the *eae* deletion is complemented *in trans*. In weaned calves, intimin increases EHEC O157:H7 colonization in the intestines and shedding in the faeces. The intimin-positive strain 86-24 is present in higher numbers in the large intestines and shed longer in the faeces of weaned calves than is the intimin-negative strain 86-24*eae*Δ10 (Table 4.2). Att/eff bacteria were found in three of nine calves inoculated with 86-24, but not in any of the four calves inoculated with the intimin-negative mutant.

Table 4.2. Findings in weaned calves after inoculation with EHEC O157:H7 bacteria.

Inoculum strain		*n*	Average $\log_{10}$ CFU of inoculated bacteria per gram of tissue				
			Ileum	Caecum	Spiral colon	Rectum	Faeces
86-24	(*stx*$^+$ intimin$^+$)						
	All calves	9	< 3.0	4.5	4.6	4.7	5.6
	Calves with AEB[a]	3	3.4	5.0	4.6	6.6	6.3
	Calves with no AEB	6	< 3.0	4.2	4.7	3.8	5.3
86-24*eae*Δ10	(*stx*$^+$ intimin$^-$)	4	< 3.0	< 3.0	< 3.0	< 3.0	< 3.0
ATCC 43888	(*stx*$^-$ intimin$^+$)	2	< 3.0	< 3.0	< 3.0	< 3.0	< 3.0

[a] Attached and effacing bacteria, found only in the caecum and rectum.

Production of shiga toxin does not appear to be essential for EHEC O157:H7 pathogenicity in neonatal calves, but it may play a role in promoting intestinal colonization and shedding in older calves. As shown in Table 4.1, a shiga toxin-negative *E. coli* O157:H7 strain (American Type Culture Collection (ATCC) strain 43888) produced clinical symptoms and att/eff lesions in neonatal calves that were similar to those caused by shiga toxin-positive strains 86-24 (shiga toxin 2 only) and strains 3081 and 933 (shiga toxins 1 and 2). However, greater numbers of inoculated bacteria were recovered from the large intestines and faeces of weaned calves inoculated with the shiga toxin-producing strain 86-24 than from weaned calves inoculated with the shiga toxin-negative strain 43888 (Table 4.2).

These results show that both intimin and shiga toxin play a role in the pathogenesis of EHEC O157:H7 infections in cattle. Therefore, vaccines directed against intimin or shiga toxin have the potential to interfere with EHEC infections and block transmission in bovines. This would help reduce the level of EHEC in cattle and reduce the number of EHEC infections in humans.

ACKNOWLEDGEMENTS

This work was partly supported by grants from the National Institutes of Health (AI20148-15) and the United States Department of Agriculture (97-35201-4578) to Alison D. O'Brien.

REFERENCES

Cray, W.C., Jr and Moon, H.W. (1995) Experimental infection of calves and adult cattle with *Escherichia coli* O157:H7. *Applied and Environmental Microbiology* 61, 1586–1590.

Dean-Nystrom, E.A., Bosworth, B.T., Cray, W.C., Jr and Moon, H.W. (1997) Pathogenicity of *Escherichia coli* O157:H7 in the intestines of neonatal calves. *Infection and Immunity* 65, 1842–1848.

Dean-Nystrom, E.A., Bosworth, B.T., Moon, H.W. and O'Brien, A.D. (1998) *Escherichia coli* O157:H7 requires intimin for enteropathogenicity in calves. *Infection and Immunity* 66, 4560–4563.

Karpman, D., Connell, H., Svensson, M., Scheutz, F., Alm, P. and Svandborg, C. (1997) The role of lipopolysaccharide and shiga-like toxin in a mouse model of *Escherichia coli* O157:H7 infection. *Journal of Infectious Diseases* 175, 611–620.

O'Brien, A.D., Melton, A.R., Schmitt, C.K., McKee, M.L., Batts, M.L and Griffin, D.E. (1993) Profile of *Escherichia coli* O157:H7 pathogen responsible for hamburger-borne outbreak of hemorrhagic colitis and hemolytic uremic syndrome in Washington. *Journal of Clinical Microbiology* 31, 2799–2801.

Rasmussen, M.A., Cray, W.C., Jr, Casey, T.A. and Whipp, S.C. (1993) Rumen contents as a reservoir of enterohemorrhagic *Escherichia coli*. *FEMS Microbiology Letters* 114, 79–84.

Tarr, P.I., Neill, M.A., Clausen, C.R., Newland, J.W., Neill, R.J. and Moseley, S.L. (1989) Genotypic variation in pathogenic *Escherichia coli* O157H7 isolated from patients in Washington, 1984–1987. *Journal of Infectious Diseases* 159, 344–347.

Whipp, S.C., Rasmussen, M.A. and Cray, W.C., Jr (1994) Animals as a source of *Escherichia coli* pathogenic for human beings. *Journal of the American Veterinary Medical Association* 204, 1168–1175.

5

Faecal Shedding and Rumen Proliferation of *Escherichia coli* O157:H7 in Calves: an Experimental Model

B.G. Harmon,[1] M.P. Doyle,[2] C.A. Brown,[1] T. Zhao,[2] S. Tkalcic,[1] E. Mueller,[1] A.H. Parks[1] and K. Jacobsen[1]

[1]*College of Veterinary Medicine, The University of Georgia, Athens, Georgia, USA;* [2]*Centre for Food Safety and Quality Enhancement, College of Agricultural and Environmental Sciences, Griffin, Georgia, USA*

INTRODUCTION

Escherichia coli O157:H7 is an important food-borne human pathogen that causes haemorrhagic colitis and haemolytic uraemic syndrome in humans (Doyle, 1991; Griffin and Tauxe, 1991; Bell *et al.*, 1994). Cattle serve as an important reservoir for contamination of meat and dairy products with *E. coli* O157:H7 (Griffin and Tauxe, 1991; Wells *et al.*, 1991). The herd prevalence for *E. coli* O157:H7 can be quite high, up to 75% in some dairy herds in the Pacific Northwest (Hancock *et al.*, 1997a) and 63% in US feedlots (Hancock *et al.*, 1997b). The prevalence for individual cattle within herds is relatively low and ranges from 0 to 5.5% (Hancock *et al.*, 1997a). The prevalence in weaned dairy calves may be as high as 5% (Garber *et al.*, 1995; Zhao *et al.*, 1995). In a survey of cattle at a large abattoir in The Netherlands, 10.6% of cattle tested were positive for *E. coli* O157:H7 (Heuvelink *et al.*, 1998).

Experimental evidence in sheep (Kudva *et al.*, 1995) and evidence from epidemiological studies in cattle indicate that horizontal transmission of *E. coli* O157:H7 occurs in groups of animals and contaminated water may serve as a vehicle in the spread and persistence of *E. coli* O157:H7 within herds (Faith *et al.*, 1996). Also, these surveys suggest that faecal shedding is intermittent and variable in cattle (Zhao *et al.*, 1995; Faith *et al.*, 1996). The concentration of *E. coli* O157:H7 populations shed in faeces ranges from 10^5

colony-forming units (CFU) g^{-1} of faeces to detectable only by enrichment procedures (Zhao *et al.*, 1995).

To study carriage and faecal shedding of *E. coli* O157:H7 in cattle, we (Brown *et al.*, 1997) and others (Cray and Moon, 1995) have inoculated weaned calves with *E. coli* O157:H7 under experimental conditions. We have used this same model to investigate the effects of fasting on carriage and faecal shedding of *E. coli* O157:H7 (Harmon *et al.*, 1999). Preliminary studies to determine the effects of roughage and concentrate diets on faecal shedding and rumen proliferation of *E. coli* O157:H7 in calves have been conducted (Tkalcic *et al.*, 1998). Finally, this model has been used to evaluate the use of probiotic bacteria to reduce faecal shedding of *E. coli* O157:H7 in weaned calves (Zhao *et al.*, 1998).

In our studies (for details, see Brown *et al.*, 1997), 8–12-week-old weaned Holstein calves were tested for enteric pathogens and adjusted to a diet of grain and lucerne pellets or Bermuda hay and given water *ad libitum*. Some calves were fitted with rumen cannulas. Calves were inoculated by nasogastric tube or rumen cannula with a five-strain mixture of nalidixic acid-resistant *E. coli* O157:H7 (10^{10} total bacteria). Faeces (and rumen contents in some experiments) were collected daily for enumeration of *E. coli* O157:H7. Calves were necropsied sequentially or at the end of the study, 27–32 days postinoculation. At necropsy, sections from each part of the gastrointestinal (GI) tract were taken for culture and histopathology was performed on these same sections, as well as on sections from all visceral tissues (Brown *et al.*, 1997).

CARRIAGE OF *E. COLI* O157:H7 IN CALVES

Field surveys have indicated that calves and adult cattle shed *E. coli* O157:H7 intermittently in the faeces, with populations that range from 10^5 g^{-1} of faeces to detectable only by enrichment procedures (Zhao *et al.*, 1995). In addition, there is no evidence from the field studies that *E. coli* O157:H7 causes clinical disease in adult or weaned calves (Garber *et al.*, 1995). Following experimental inoculation of calves and adults with 10^{10} *E. coli* O157:H7, there is a sharp decline in populations shed in the faeces for the first 2 weeks, followed by intermittent shedding of populations ranging from approximately 5×10^4 g^{-1} of faeces to detectable only by enrichment (Brown *et al.*, 1997; Fig. 5.1). *E. coli* O157:H7 populations as a percentage of total faecal coliforms decrease dramatically after the first few days (Table 5.1). Calves shed larger populations of *E. coli* O157:H7 and for longer periods (up to 189 days) compared with adult cattle (up to 100 days) (Cray and Moon, 1995). The size of populations shed by individual calves is highly variable after the first 2 weeks and, in some calves, populations varied considerably from day to day (Fig. 5.1).

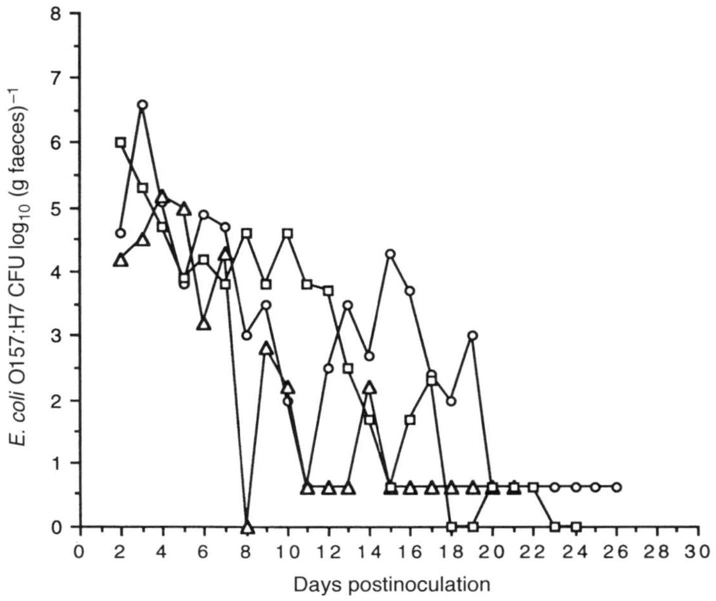

Fig. 5.1. Temporal faecal shedding of *E. coli* O157:H7 in three calves following inoculation of calves with a five-strain mixture of 10^{10} *E. coli* O157:H7 on day 0. Each symbol represents $\log_{10}$ CFU g^{-1} of faeces for an individual calf.

In our studies (Brown *et al.*, 1997), the only clinical signs observed were mild transient diarrhoea shortly after inoculation and a few calves were febrile at the same time. Calves remained bright and alert and

Table 5.1. *E. coli* O157:H7 expressed as a percentage of the total coliform populations isolated from faeces following oral inoculation of calves with 10^{10} of a five-strain mixture of *E. coli* O157:H7 (data from Brown *et al.*, 1997).

	Calf number				
Day postinoculation	2	3	4	5	6
0	0	0	0	0	0
1	99	79	ND	80	50
3	99	0.31	5.1	50	10
4	79	0.50	0.03	0.79	1.2
5	40	0.10	0.31	0.03	0.03
6	ND	1.6	0.40	0.63	0.31
15	0.02	ND	2.0	0.01	0.001
20	0.02	ND	0.02	0.001	0.001

ND, not done.

continued to eat. At necropsy, we could detect no attaching and effacing lesions in small or large intestines of calves necropsied between 13 and 27 days postinoculation (Brown *et al.*, 1997). In fact, there was no microscopic evidence of attachment to the mucosa. No gross or microscopic intestinal lesions were detected in calves necropsied between 3 and 18 days postinoculation or in adult cattle necropsied between 2 and 4 days postinoculation (Cray and Moon, 1995). Much larger populations of *E. coli* O157:H7 were detected in GI contents than in simultaneously cultured mucosal samples (Table 5.2; Brown *et al.*, 1997). Therefore, sites of mucosal colonization in weaned calves and adults have yet to be determined and it is unclear if mucosal colonization is necessary for cattle to serve as a reservoir host for *E. coli* O157:H7.

At necropsy, the largest populations of *E. coli* O157:H7 were most consistently detected in rumen, reticulum, omasum, proximal and distal caecum, ascending colon, spiral colon, transverse colon and descending colon. Populations in these sites ranged from detectable only by enrichment to 3200 CFU g^{-1} of contents. Small populations were detected in the duodenum in two of nine calves and in the ileum in four of nine calves (Brown *et al.*, 1997). Persistence in the rumen may serve as a source of *E. coli* O157:H7 for continued reintroduction into the colon, where more substantial proliferation may occur. *E. coli* O157:H7 was not isolated from any tissues outside the GI tract, including kidney, spleen, liver, gall-bladder, jejunal lymph node, ileal lymph node and caecal lymph node (Brown *et al.*, 1997).

In summary, *E. coli* O157:H7 does not appear to be pathogenic in weaned calves or adult cattle. *E. coli* O157:H7 does not appear to displace the resident flora, as it comprises only a very small percentage of the total faecal coliforms only a few days following inoculation. Calves are capable

Table 5.2. Isolation of *E. coli* O157:H7 from calves at necropsy 14 and 26 days following oral inoculation with 10^{10} of a five-strain mixture of *E. coli* O157:H7. *E. coli* O157:H7 populations are expressed as CFU g^{-1} of tissue or g^{-1} of contents (data from Brown *et al.*, 1997).

	Calf no. 1, 14 days PI (CFU g^{-1})		Calf no. 2, 26 days PI (CFU g^{-1})	
Organ	Contents	Mucosa	Contents	Mucosa
Rumen	3160	63	32	(−)
Omasum	2510	80	125	4
Ileum	(−)	(−)	20	(−)
Caecum	400	(+)	63	(−)
Colon	630	10	25	(−)

PI, postinoculation; (−), negative culture results with enrichment procedure; (+), positive results with enrichment procedure, but negative on direct plating.

of shedding *E. coli* O157:H7 for extended periods following experimental inoculation with a large dose of 10^{10} *E. coli* O157:H7; however, the size of the populations shed is highly variable among calves and fluctuates over time for individual animals for unknown reasons. A definitive site for mucosal colonization has not been demonstrated for weaned calves or adult cattle. Even so, *E. coli* O157:H7 persists in the rumen, recticulum, omasum and all parts of the large colon during the period of faecal shedding. Control of this type of subclinical carriage in ruminants is a daunting task. Control measures such as traditional vaccination procedures and/or detection and culling would be impractical. New knowledge about the epidemiology of *E. coli* O157:H7 on the farm and novel control measures at several stages in the production cycle are needed.

EFFECTS OF DIFFERENT FEEDING PRACTICES ON RUMEN PROLIFERATION AND FAECAL SHEDDING OF *ESCHERICHIA COLI* O157:H7 IN WEANED CALVES

Little is known about the effects of different feeding practices on rumen growth and faecal shedding of *E. coli* O157:H7 in cattle. Fasting cattle results in proliferation of coliforms in the bovine rumen and subsequent increases in faecal shedding. Feed withdrawal can result in 3×10^4- and 10^7-fold increases in ruminal *Salmonella* sp. and *E. coli* populations, respectively (Brownlie and Grau, 1967). Also, withholding feed from rams has resulted in increased shedding of *E. coli* O157:H7 (Kudva *et al.*, 1995). In *in vitro* fermentation systems, *E. coli* O157:H7 growth is restricted in rumen fluid collected from well-fed cattle, but grows normally in rumen fluid collected from fasted cattle (Rasmussen *et al.*, 1993). In well-fed animals, a combination of increased volatile fatty acid (VFA) concentration and low pH are responsible for the relatively poor growth of coliforms in the rumen (Wolin, 1969; Wallace *et al.*, 1989; Rasmussen *et al.*, 1993). High concentrations of VFA uncouple the proton electrochemical gradient across the cell membrane of acid-sensitive bacteria as the pH falls (Kell *et al.*, 1981). Therefore, it is expected that fasted calves might experience an increase in proliferation of *E. coli* O157:H7 in the rumen and increased faecal shedding, resulting in a greater probability of spreading the bacteria to other calves and contaminating the farm environment. At abattoirs, cattle held for longer periods without feed tend to have larger populations of *E. coli* and *Salmonella* sp. in the rumen when slaughtered (Grau and Brownlie, 1968). Cattle examined at the abattoir were found to have larger populations of verotoxigenic *E. coli* in their faeces than was found on previous examination at the farm of origin (Suthienkul *et al.*, 1990).

The effect of feed composition and feed additives on rumen proliferation and faecal shedding of *E. coli* O157:H7 is largely unknown. An epidemiological study of the prevalence of *E. coli* O157:H7 in feedlot cattle demonstrated a threefold higher prevalence in cattle that had been on feed for the shortest time (Hancock *et al.*, 1997b). However, it is unknown if this finding was due to dietary stress or some other stress factors. In another survey, feeding of cottonseed or clover hay was negatively associated with faecal shedding of *E. coli* O157:H7 in cattle (Garber *et al.*, 1995). There was no epidemiological association between feeding ionophores and faecal shedding of *E. coli* O157:H7 (Garber *et al.*, 1995). Faecal shedding of *E. coli* O157:H7 increased when sheep fed lucerne-pelleted feed were turned out on sagebrush–bunch grass range (Kudva *et al.*, 1995).

We compared faecal shedding of *E. coli* O157:H7, in calves before, during and after fasting periods. Six calves were fasted for two 48-h periods 15 or 16 and 22 or 23 days after inoculation with 10^{10} *E. coli* O157:H7 (Harmon *et al.*, 1999). We monitored rumen VFA concentrations, rumen pH and rumen and faecal populations of *E. coli* O157:H7 the day before fasting, 2 days during the fast and the day after the resumption of feeding. Fasting resulted in a dramatic decrease in rumen VFA concentration and a corresponding increase in rumen pH (Table 5.3). However, there was no consistent change in the size of the populations of *E. coli* O157:H7 shed on fasting days or on days following the resumption of feeding (Table 5.3). In addition, there was no correlation between VFA concentration or pH and the populations of *E. coli* O157:H7 in the rumen or shed in the faeces. Rumen populations of *E. coli* O157:H7 were below 50 CFU g^{-1} of rumen contents at the beginning of the fasting periods and remained at or below this concentration throughout the study, including fasting and non-fasting periods.

Table 5.3. Rumen pH, rumen VFA concentration (mM) and *E. coli* O157:H7 (CFU g^{-1} of rumen contents or faeces) for a typical calf inoculated with *E. coli* O157:H7 and fasted on days 15–16 and days 22–23 postinoculation (PI). Feeding was resumed on days 17 and 24, respectively (data from Harmon *et al.*, 1999).

Day PI	pH	Acetic acid (mM)	Propionic acid (mM)	Butyric acid (mM)	Total VFA acids (mM)	*E. coli* O157:H7 (CFU g^{-1})	
						Rumen	Faeces
14	6.10	101.4	30.1	17.8	149.3	25	3980
15 (F)	6.75	52.9	11.9	4.1	68.9	8	630
16 (F)	7.92	21.9	3.4	1.7	27.0	(+)	2510
17	6.31	62.6	20.3	12.8	95.7	(−)	795
21	5.76	104.4	25.0	19.8	149.2	(+)	25
22 (F)	6.82	59.5	15.3	13.5	88.3	(+)	(+)
23 (F)	7.73	25.9	4.4	2.5	32.8	8	(+)
24	5.72	84.3	38.1	24.0	146.4	(−)	63

(F), fasting day; (+), positive results with enrichment procedure, but negative or direct plating; (−), negative culture results with enrichment procedure.

In preliminary studies, we compared faecal shedding and rumen proliferation of *E. coli* O157:H7 in calves fed two different diets (Tkalcic *et al.*, 1998). One group of five calves was fed a diet high in roughage (Bermuda hay) and six calves were fed a diet composed primarily of grain. Both diets were balanced to meet the minimum nutrient requirements. The calves were adjusted to the diets 2 weeks before inoculation with 10^{10} *E. coli* O157:H7. The average rumen pH and the total VFA concentration were slightly higher and lower, respectively, in calves fed the high-roughage diet compared with calves fed the high-grain diet. Faecal shedding was highly variable in both groups; however, two calves in the grain-fed group shed approximately tenfold higher average populations of *E. coli* O157:H7 in the faeces compared with other calves in both groups. Rumen populations of *E. coli* O157:H7 were not different for the two groups. However, there was a positive correlation between average rumen propionate concentration and average *E. coli* O157:H7 populations shed in the faeces of the 11 calves.

The results of these two experiments are contrary to those expected. Fasting might have been expected to cause proliferation of *E. coli* O157:H7 in the rumen or colon, because rumen pH was increased and total VFA concentrations decreased. Similarly, animals fed roughage might be expected to shed higher populations of *E. coli* O157:H7, due to consistently lower VFA concentrations when compared with grain-fed calves. However, other unknown factors may have more important influences on the proliferation of *E. coli* O157:H7 in the rumen and colon. Also, some strains of *E. coli* O157:H7 are known to be acid-tolerant (Arnold and Kaspar, 1995; Benjamin and Datta, 1995). Acid-tolerant *E. coli* O157:H7 may not be sensitive to the fluctuations in VFA concentrations of the rumen and colon, as are other coliforms. *E. coli* O157:H7 may actually survive preferentially in the rumen and colon under certain acidic conditions. Acid-tolerance mechanisms could be triggered by the ruminal environment, allowing *E. coli* O157:H7 to survive passage through the abomasum and then recolonize the colon. It is also possible that higher propionate-to-acetate ratios may give a competitive advantage to *E. coli* O157:H7. Further studies are needed to address the effects of specific changes in the rumen microenvironment on survival of *E. coli* O157:H7 in the rumen and colon. If faecal shedding can be reduced by feeding practices or use of feed additives just prior to slaughter, the probability of contamination of beef products could be greatly reduced.

FAECAL SHEDDING OF *ESCHERICHIA COLI* O157:H7 IN CALVES ADMINISTERED PROBIOTIC BACTERIA

One possible approach to reducing faecal shedding of *E. coli* O157:H7 in cattle is the use of probiotic bacteria. Probiotic bacteria are bacteria that beneficially affect the host by improving its microbial balance, including eliminating or reducing microorganisms that are carried by the host and that are harmful to humans. Probiotic bacteria have not been used extensively in cattle. Undefined bacterial preparations have been used successfully to reduce *Salmonella* sp. colonization in young chickens (Rantala and Nurmi, 1973). Introduction of bovine commensal *E. coli* that colonize the same anatomic locations as *E. coli* O157:H7 and produce toxic metabolites, such as colicins, may reduce the carriage of *E. coli* O157:H7 in the bovine digestive tract.

Bacteria (1200 isolates) were obtained from bovine GI tract or faeces and screened for inhibitory activity against *E. coli* O157:H7 *in vitro* (Zhao *et al.*, 1998). Seventeen bovine *E. coli* isolates and one *Proteus mirabilis* isolate were found to inhibit the growth of *E. coli* O157:H7 *in vitro*. An approximately equal mixture of these isolates (10^{10} total bacteria) were given to nine cannulated calves 48 h prior to inoculation with 10^{10} *E. coli* O157:H7 (Zhao *et al.*, 1998). We compared faecal shedding and rumen proliferation of *E. coli* O157:H7 in calves fed probiotic bacteria with control calves fed only *E. coli* O157:H7 (Zhao *et al.*, 1998). Five of six calves treated with the probiotic bacteria stopped shedding *E. coli* O157:H7 before the nine control calves (Table 5.4). Both rumen and faecal cultures from these five probiotic-treated calves became *E. coli* O157:H7-negative within 18 days, whereas only one of the probiotic-treated calves and all of the control calves continued to shed *E. coli* O157:H7 until the study was terminated. At necropsy, all nine untreated calves were culture-positive for *E. coli* O157:H7 and only one of six probiotic-treated calves was positive. However, this

Table 5.4. Carriage of *E. coli* O157:H7 in calves treated with probiotic bacteria (P) 48 h prior to inoculation with 10^{10} *E. coli* O157:H7, compared with control calves (C) that received no treatment. The last postinoculation (PI) day that a positive culture was obtained is listed in the table (data from Zhao *et al.*, 1998).

Control calves			Probiotic-treated calves		
Calf no.	Rumen (days PI)	Faeces (days PI)	Calf no.	Rumen (days PI)	Faeces (days PI)
1C	35*	35*	1P	9	11
2C	29*	29*	2P	9	15
3C	35*	35*	3P	17	18
4C	28*	28*	4P	17	17
5C	28*	25	5P	16	18
6C	24	29*	6P	30*	30*
7C	25	29*			
8C	28*	28*			
9C	28*	28*			

* Indicates that the last positive isolation was made at the end of the study from necropsy samples.

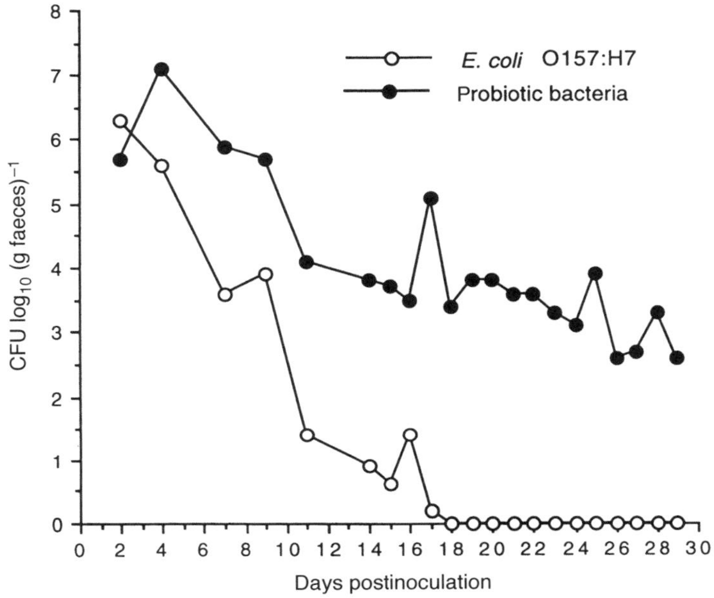

Fig. 5.2. Faecal shedding of *E. coli* O157:H7 and probiotic bacteria by a probiotic-treated calf. Calves were inoculated with 10^{10} probiotic bacteria 48 h before inoculation with a five-strain mixture of 10^{10} *E. coli* O157:H7 on day 0. Each symbol represents $\log_{10}$ CFU g^{-1} of faeces.

probiotic-treated calf failed to continue to harbour the probiotic bacteria. All other probiotic-treated calves were culture-positive for the probiotic bacteria throughout the 27–35-day study (Fig. 5.2) and the probiotic bacteria were isolated from the GI tract at necropsy (Zhao *et al.*, 1998). The probiotic bacteria were isolated from the same GI sites, as was *E. coli* O157:H7, suggesting that they reside in the same locations.

Further studies are needed to determine the duration of carriage of these probiotic bacteria in cattle, along with studies of larger populations of animals in field settings. These preliminary data suggest that a probiotic strategy could be useful for reducing carriage of *E. coli* O157:H7 in cattle. Also, feeding these competing bacteria to cattle may result in them competing with *E. coli* O157:H7 in other locations within the farm environment, such as in feedlot manure.

REFERENCES

Arnold, K.W. and Kaspar, C.W. (1995) Starvation- and stationary-phase-induced acid tolerance in *Escherichia coli* O157:H7. *Applied and Environmental Microbiology* 61, 2037–2039.

Bell, P.B., Goldoft, M., Griffin, P.M., Davis, M.A., Gordon, D.C., Tarr, P.I., Bartleson, C.A., Lewis, J.H., Barrett, T.J., Wells, J.G., Baron, R. and Kobayashi, J. (1994) A multistate outbreak of *Escherichia coli* O157:H7-associated bloody diarrhea and hemolytic uremic syndrome from hamburgers. *Journal of the American Medical Association* 272, 1349–1353.

Benjamin, M.M. and Datta, A.R. (1995) Acid tolerance of enterohemorrhagic *Escherichia coli. Applied and Environmental Microbiology* 61, 1669–1672.

Brown, C.A., Harmon, B.G., Zhao, T. and Doyle, M.P. (1997) Experimental *Escherichia coli* O157:H7 carriage in calves. *Applied and Environmental Microbiology* 63, 27–32.

Brownlie, L.E. and Grau, F.H. (1967) Effects of food intake on growth and survival of Salmonellas and *Escherichia coli* in the bovine rumen. *Journal of General Microbiology* 46, 125–134.

Cray, C.W. and Moon, H.W. (1995) Experimental infection of calves and adult cattle with *Escherichia coli* O157:H7. *Applied and Environmental Microbiology* 61, 1585–1590.

Doyle, M.P. (1991) *Escherichia coli* O157:H7 and its significance in foods. *International Journal of Food Microbiology* 12, 289–302.

Faith, N.G., Shere, J.A., Brosch, R., Arnold, K.W., Ansay, S.E., Lee, M.S., Luchansky, J.B. and Kaspar, C.W. (1996) Prevalence and clonal nature of *Escherichia coli* O157:H7 on dairy farms in Wisconsin. *Applied and Environmental Microbiology* 62, 1519–1525.

Garber, L.P., Wells, J.S., Hancock, D.D., Doyle, M.P., Tuttle, J., Shere, J.A. and Zhao, T. (1995) Risk factors for fecal shedding of *Escherichia coli* O157:H7 in dairy calves. *Journal of the American Veterinary Medical Association* 207, 46–49.

Grau, F.H. and Brownlie, L.E. (1968) Effect of some preslaughter treatments on the *Salmonella* population in the bovine rumen and faeces. *Journal of Applied Bacteriology* 31, 157–163.

Griffin, P.M. and Tauxe, R.V. (1991) The epidemiology of infections caused by *Escherichia coli* O157:H7, other enterohemorrhagic *E. coli*, and the associated hemolytic uremic syndrome. *Epidemiology Review* 13, 60–98.

Hancock, D.D., Rice, D.H., Herriott, D.E., Besser, T.E., Ebel, E.D. and Carpenter, L.V. (1997a) Effects of farm manure-handling practices on *Escherichia coli* O157:H7 prevalence in cattle. *Journal of Food Protection* 60, 363–366.

Hancock, D.D., Rice, D.H., Thomas, L.A., Dargatz, D.A. and Besser, T.E. (1997b) Epidemiology of *Escherichia coli* O157:H7 in feedlot cattle. *Journal of Food Protection* 60, 462–465.

Harmon, B.G., Brown, C.A., Tkalcic, S., Mueller, P.O.E., Parks, A., Jain, A.V., Zhao, T. and Doyle, M.P. (1999) Faecal shedding and rumen growth of *Escherichia coli* O157:H7 in fasted calves. *Journal of Food Protection* 62, 574–579.

Heuvelink, A.E., van den Biggelaar, F.A.L.M., de Boer, E., Herbes, R.G., Melchers, W.J.G., Huis In't Veld, J.H.J. and Monnens, L.A.H. (1998) Isolation and characterization of verocytotoxin-producing *Escherichia coli* O157 strains from Dutch cattle and sheep. *Journal of Clinical Microbiology* 36, 878–882.

Kell, D.B., Peck, M.W., Rodger, G. and Morris, J.G. (1981) On the permeability to weak acids and bases of the cytoplasmic membrane of *Clostridium pasteurianum*. *Biochemistry and Biophysics Research Communications* 99, 81–88.

Kudva, I.T., Hatfield, P.G. and Hovde, C.J. (1995) Effect of diet on the shedding of *Escherichia coli* O157:H7 in a sheep model. *Applied and Environmental Microbiology* 61, 1363–1370.

Rantala, M. and Nurmi, E. (1973) Prevention of the growth of *Salmonella infantis* in the intestines of broiler chicks by flora of the alimentary tract of chickens. *British Poultry Science* 14, 627–630.

Rasmussen, M.A., Cray, W.C., Casey, T.A. and Whipp, S.C. (1993) Rumen contents as a reservoir of enterohemorrhagic *Escherichia coli*. *FEMS Microbiology Letters* 114, 79–84.

Suthienkul, O., Brown, J.E., Seriwatana, J., Tienthongdee, S., Sastravaha, S. and Echeverria, P. (1990) Shiga-like toxin producing *Escherichia coli* in retail meats and cattle in Thailand. *Applied and Environmental Microbiology* 56, 1135–1139.

Tkalcic, S., Harmon, B.G., Brown, C.A., Mueller, E., Parks, A., Zhao, T. and Doyle, M.P. (1998) Dietary effects on rumen proliferation and fecal shedding of *Escherichia coli* O157:H7 in calves. In: *International Conference on Emerging and Infectious Diseases*, 8–11 March, Atlanta, Georgia, p. 82 (abstract).

Wallace, J.R., Falconer, M.L. and Bhargava, K. (1989) Toxicity of volatile fatty acids at rumen pH prevents enrichment of *Escherichia coli* by sorbitol in rumen contents. *Current Microbiology* 19, 277–281.

Wells, J.G., Shipman, L.D., Greene, K.D., Sowers, E.G., Green, J.H., Cameron D.N., Downes, F.P., Martin, M.L., Griffin, P.M., Ostroff, S.M., Potter, M.E., Tauxe, R.V. and Wachsmuth, I.K. (1991) Isolation of *Escherichia coli* serotype O157:H7 and other shiga-like-toxin-producing *E. coli* from dairy cattle. *Journal of Clinical Microbiology* 29, 985–989.

Wolin, M.J. (1969) Volatile fatty acids and the inhibition of *Escherichia coli* growth by rumen fluid. *Applied Microbiology* 17, 83–87.

Zhao, T., Doyle, M.P., Shere, J.A. and Garber, L. (1995) Prevalence of enterohemorrhagic *Escherichia coli* O157:H7 in a survey of dairy herds. *Applied and Environmental Microbiology* 61, 1290–1293.

Zhao, T., Doyle, M.P., Harmon, B.G., Brown, C.A., Mueller, P.O.E. and Parks, A.H. (1998) Reduction of carriage of enterohemorrhagic *Escherichia coli* O157:H7 in cattle by inoculation with probiotic bacteria. *Journal of Clinical Microbiology* 36, 641–647.

6

Commensal–Pathogen Interactions Involving *Escherichia coli* O157 and the Prospects for Control

S.H. Duncan, K.P. Scott, H.J. Flint and C.S. Stewart

Rowett Research Institute, Aberdeen, UK

INTRODUCTION

Ruminants are considered to act as reservoirs for enterohaemorrhagic *Escherichia coli* (EHEC). Reducing carriage and shedding of this bacterium by ruminants would be expected to decrease the incidence of zoonotic infections and the incidence of contaminated meat, vegetables, fruit, milk and water entering the human food-chain (Synge, 1997). It is relevant, therefore, to consider the many microbial, dietary and physiological factors which may influence the survival of *E. coli* in the ruminant gut and the shedding of this bacterium in ruminant faeces. The ruminant gut plays host to a very wide range of commensal and symbiotic microbial species, and understanding the interactions that occur between these microorganisms and *E. coli* is likely to be crucial in our attempts to control the spread of this pathogen.

THE RUMINANT GUT ECOSYSTEM

Ruminants, such as sheep, cattle and deer, and their close relatives the camelids (camels, llamas) are pregastric fermenters, with an enlarged non-secretory anterior section of the stomach, the reticulorumen, in which the passage of dietary plant material is delayed sufficiently to allow extensive hydrolysis of cellulose, arabinoxylans and other plant polymers (Van Soest, 1994). In cattle and sheep, the reticulorumen forms around 65–70% of the gut volume and the large bowel provides around 10–13%. Although oxygen diffuses from the bloodstream into the rumen, a specialized bacterial population forms a biofilm on the rumen wall (Fig. 6.1) and the facultative species within this biofilm scavenge oxygen, contributing to anaerobic conditions in the bulk phase of the rumen contents (Rasmussen *et al.*, Chapter 3, this volume). The predominant microbes in the rumen are anaerobic bacteria, protozoa and fungi (Fig. 6.2). Facultative bacteria, including commensal *E. coli*, normally provide 1% or less of the cultivable microbiota. The anaerobes present are predominantly fermentative, the volatile fatty acids (VFA) being formed by the dissimilation of pyruvate formed in the Embden–Meyerhof–Parnas pathway (Hungate, 1966; Russell and Wallace, 1997). Up to 75% of the anaerobic bacteria are thought to occur in biofilms which coat the digesta particles (Cheng *et al.*, 1984). The concentrations and relative proportions of VFA present vary according to the diet and the pattern of feeding, but typically may be a combined total of acetate, propionate and butyrate of between 50 and 150 mM (Hungate, 1966).

Conditions in the large intestine of ruminants are rarely reported, but, as in the rumen, the predominant anaerobic bacteria outnumber aerobes by 100-fold or more (Fig. 6.2). Protozoa and some of the species of large bacteria characteristic of the rumen, such as *Oscillospira* and large ovals, were not observed in the large intestine by Ulyatt *et al.* (1975); in contrast, anaerobic fungi are present in the ruminant large intestine (Trinci *et al.*, 1993). The substrates fermented in the hind-gut are limited to those that escape fermentation in the rumen, together with secreted mucins (Van Soest, 1994). The number of goblet cells in the large intestine of sheep exceeds that in the small intestine, the secreted mucus enabling rapid passage of the digesta (Ulyatt *et al.*, 1975). Depending on the composition and particle size of the diet, up to 30% of the total amount disappearing from the rumen may be digested in the large intestine and the caecum (Demeyer, 1981). The hind-gut fermentation of sheep has been shown to generate methane (Murray *et al.*, 1978), and the nutritional interactions involved are presumed to be similar to those known to occur in the rumen (Wolin *et al.*, 1997). Cellulolytic anaerobes were detected in the caecum of sheep by Mann and Orskov (1973). The predominant caecal anaerobes present in these animals were described as *Bacteroides* species.

Rumen microorganisms pass down the digestive tract either attached to feed particles, suspended in the liquid phase of the digesta or attached to sloughed epithelial cells. The bacteria that survive the digestive process provide an inoculum for the hind-gut compartments. The dynamics of the faecal shedding of bacteria will be influenced by the phase location of the relevant species. The digesta passes more rapidly through the hind-gut than through the rumen, but in both gut compartments the liquid phase of the digesta passes more rapidly than the solid phase (Hungate, 1966; Van Soest, 1994).

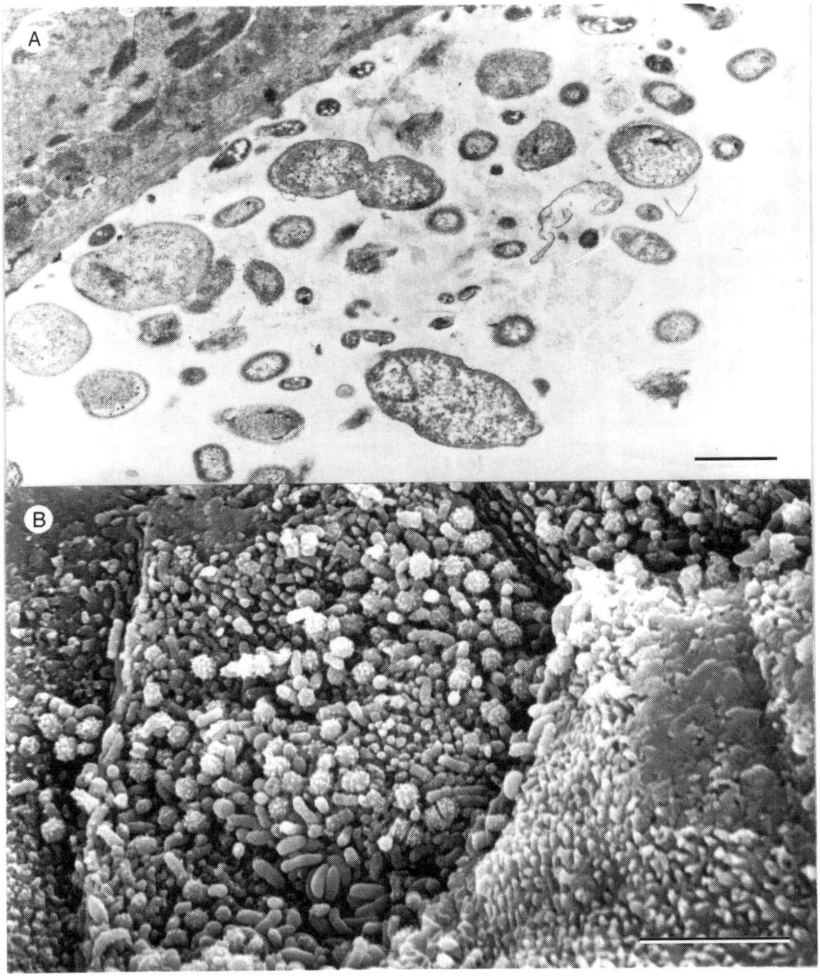

Fig. 6.1. Transmission (A) and scanning (B) electron micrographs showing the bacterial biofilm adherent to the rumen epithelium of reindeer (Cheng *et al.*, 1993, reprinted with permission from *Canadian Journal of Microbiology*). Bars, A = 1 µm, B = 5 µm.

ESCHERICHIA COLI IN RUMINANTS

Occurrence

Typically, rumen contents possesses up to around 10^5 colony-forming units (CFU) ml^{-1} of *E. coli*, depending on the diet and the feeding regime (Mann *et al.*, 1954; Grau and Brownlie, 1965). The numbers of *E. coli* in the rumen

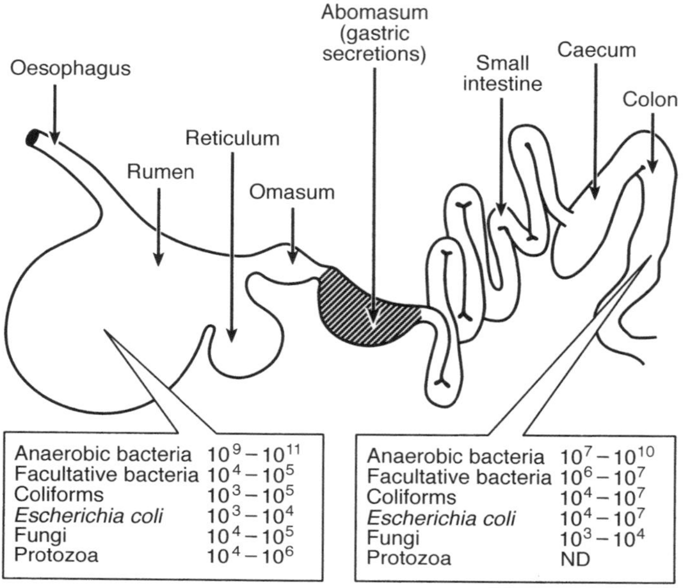

Fig. 6.2. Distribution of microorganisms in the digestive tract of ruminants. Numbers = approx. colony-forming units per ml of gut contents. (Data from Ulyatt *et al.*, 1975; Davies *et al.*, 1993; Van Soest, 1994; Diez-Gonzalez *et al.*, 1998.) ND, not detected.

of sheep fed lucerne hay have been shown to vary according to the frequency of feeding and the amount fed. During periods without feed, the concentration of VFA in the rumen fell and the numbers of *E. coli* rose (Brownlie and Grau, 1967). Howe *et al.* (1976) showed that *E. coli* was not always present in the faeces of adult cows and, when detected, was present in low numbers; in contrast, calves regularly excreted high numbers of *E. coli.* Fifty per cent of the cows studied possessed only one O-type of *E. coli* and, in total, only six O-types were found. In contrast, 37 different O-types were isolated from the calves. Generally, it is non-O157:H7 serotypes of *E. coli* strains that cause infections, such as mastitis, in ruminants (Verheijden *et al.*, 1983). Such infections are routinely treated with antibiotics. Antibiotics have also been used for several decades as growth promoters for farm animals and poultry (Gustafson and Bowen, 1997). Drug-resistant *E. coli* have been isolated from adult ruminants (Flint *et al.*, 1987) and from calves between 1 and 6 weeks of age (Fliegerova, 1993). Resistant strains isolated from adult sheep were of two types. One group of ten isolates that included the strain F38 carried two large plasmids, one of which was responsible for cotransmission of resistance to tetracycline, ampicillin and streptomycin. A second group of five isolates, exemplified by F318, lacked plasmids and carried non-transmissible resistances to tetracycline and streptomycin (Flint *et al.*, 1987). Remarkably, the two rumen strains were shown to be capable of exchanging a native plasmid carrying an ampicillin-resistance determinant at detectable rates when added to whole-rumen contents (Scott and Flint, 1995). Caprioli *et al.* (1991) detected multiply drug-resistant *E. coli* isolates in almost one-third of red-deer faecal samples screened. These wild deer in the central Alps had not been treated with antibiotics but may have shared grazing land with domesticated animals.

Since 1982, there have been numerous reports of the occurrence of *E. coli* O157 in ruminants, including cows, sheep and wild animals, such as deer. Links to human infection have been described, and it is clear that they may be the result of direct contact with animals or their faeces or of contamination of the human food-chain. These and related findings are reviewed in the companion chapters of this volume. Despite the severity of disease that can occur in humans, EHEC is not considered to cause disease in animals, except experimentally infected neonates less than 36 h old (Dean-Nystrom *et al.*, 1998; Dean-Nystrom *et al.*, Chapter 4, this volume).

Localization

Although *E. coli* is not among the predominant organisms so far isolated from the gut epithelial biofilm, tests with cultured rumen epithelium cells *in vitro* show that strains of *E. coli* that express F1 fimbriae bind to rumen epithelium cells (Galfi *et al.*, 1998). It is possible that this bacterium may have been present but missed upon cultivation of the predominant members of this microbial community (McCowan *et al.*, 1978; Cheng *et al.*, 1979; Dehority and Grubb, 1981; Mead and Jones, 1981; Mueller *et al.*, 1984). Thus, a molecular study of the gut-wall biofilm in ruminants using polymerase chain reaction (PCR)-amplified 16S rDNA genes (Wood *et al.*, 1998) would be valuable. Although preliminary *in vitro* studies using cultured epithelial cells have not so far demonstrated attachment of *E. coli* O157 (S.H. Duncan, P. Galfi and S. Neogrady, unpublished data), it is possible that the expression of receptors is affected by growth *in vitro*. Also, whether or not some O157 reference strains, such as National Collection of Type Cultures (NCTC) 12900, possess intimin is not known (Saunders *et al.*, Chapter 1, this volume; Dean-Nystrom *et al.*, Chapter 4, this volume). In calves, EHEC are mainly found in the rumen and colon (Brown *et al.*, 1997). The rumen may be an important site for long-term carriage, because it provides a heavy 'inoculum' of bacteria for the posterior digestive tract.

A potentially valuable approach to studying the localization of *E. coli* strains in the ruminant gut is to tag cells with a visible marker, such as the green fluorescent protein (*gfp*) gene from the jellyfish *Aequorea victoria*. We have recently used a red-shifted mutant of *gfp* (Heim *et al.*, 1994) to track the persistence of marked lactic acid bacteria in fermentor simulations of the human colonic flora (Scott *et al.*, 1998). The advantages of this mutant over wild-type GFP are that it has longer optimal excitation and emission wavelengths and increased fluorescence, leading to improved detectability. A potential problem in the application of this marker to gut ecosystems lay in the requirement of oxygen for maturation of the GFP protein, but we have shown that GFP synthesized under anaerobic conditions in *E. coli* or other bacterial hosts can be activated upon subsequent exposure to oxygen (Scott *et al.*, 1998; Fig. 6.3).

E. coli O157 was initially tagged with GFP by introducing a plasmid construct originally designed for expression in lactococci, in which expression is driven by a constitutive lactococcal P32 promoter. Although strong fluorescence was observed, not surprisingly this construct proved relatively unstable in *E. coli* hosts in the absence of antibiotic selection. This instability is believed to be related to the plasmid vector rather than to GFP toxicity. A stable GFP-expressing O157 strain was therefore constructed by insertion of a Tn5-*gfp* cassette contained in plasmid pUT*gfp* (Tombolini *et al.*, 1997) into the chromosome. Chromosomally integrated *gfp* was confirmed by fluorescence and PCR, and such constructs proved stable in the absence of antibiotic selection. However, the intensity of fluorescence was diminished in the chromosomally marked strains, but studies using a fluorescence-activated cell sorter (FACS) may circumvent this problem.

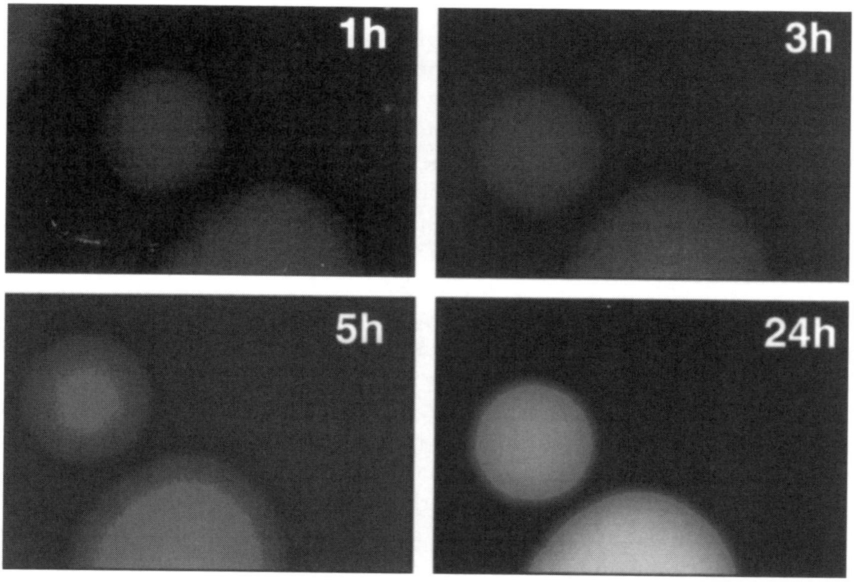

Fig. 6.3. Development of fluorescence by anaerobically grown *E. coli* carrying the plasmid pKPSP*gfp*, following exposure to air for from 1 to 24 h.

INTERACTIONS BETWEEN *E. COLI* O157 AND OTHER MICROORGANISMS

Effects of acids released by fermentation

All of the fermentative bacteria, protozoa and fungi form VFA from the carbon (C) sources present in dietary material. These VFA exert relatively small effects on anaerobes (Stewart, 1975); however, Wolin (1969) showed that the rumen concentrations of VFA were markedly inhibitory to growth of *E. coli* strains. Wallace *et al.* (1989) considered that the adverse effects of VFA would prevent the establishment of *E. coli* strains at high population levels in the ovine rumen. Further, Diez-Gonzalez and Russell (1997) found that a strain of *E.coli* O157 was more tolerant of high concentrations of acetate at pH 5.9 than was *E. coli* strain K-12. However, these studies were all performed with laboratory-conditioned strains. Rasmussen *et al.* (1993) found no evidence that strains of *E. coli* O157 were more tolerant of VFA than were commensal *E. coli* strains from ruminants. It was demonstrated that, when rumen contents was supplemented with glucose and trypticase, *E. coli* O157 grew poorly in rumen contents from well-fed animals, in which the concentration of VFA would be high, but grew rather better in rumen contents from fasted animals, in which the concentration of VFA would be low (Rasmussen *et al.*, 1993). Scott and Flint (1995) also found that the two ovine rumen commensal *E. coli* strains F38 and F318 were able to grow at normal rates in anaerobic media at pH 7 in the presence of 50 mM concentrations of VFA, whereas growth of a laboratory K-12 strain was completely inhibited under these conditions (Table 6.1). A VFA concentration of 100 mM was inhibitory to growth of the rumen strains, particularly at pH 6, and tolerance of VFA was greater under aerobic than under anaerobic growth conditions. The relative tolerance of VFA did not appear to be a unique attribute of rumen-derived strains, since it was shared by four recent random isolates of *E. coli* from porcine faeces (Scott and Flint, 1995).

The data in Table 6.1 comparing the growth rates of one O157 strain (12900) with a non-O157 rumen isolate (F318) show that there was essentially no difference in the acid tolerance of the two strains under both aerobic and anaerobic conditions. The rumen isolate (F318) and the O157 isolate were more tolerant of the higher levels of VFA likely be found in the rumen, particularly at pH 6, when compared with data obtained with laboratory strains. It appears that many laboratory strains have lost tolerance to VFA and gut conditions.

The two strains (12900 and F318) were also relatively tolerant of the acids tested singly. At 100 mM, propionate was the most inhibitory of the acids under anaerobic conditions. This is of particular interest in the light of some findings with human colonic isolates. Hinton and Hume (1995) showed that a *Veillonella* strain grown with a strain of *Bacteroides fragilis*

Table 6.1. Growth rates (h^{-1}) of an *E. coli* O157 strain (12900), a sheep rumen strain (F318) and a laboratory strain (UB281) under aerobic and anaerobic conditions in the presence of VFA (acetate:propionate:butyrate ratio 10:2:1).

	VFA conc. (mM)	pH	Strain 12900	Strain F318	Strain UB281
Aerobic	0	7	1.49	2.08	1.02
	50	7	0.87	1.32	0.49
	100	7	0.51	1.11	0.40
	0	6	0.98	ND	ND
	50	6	0.45	0.63	*
	100	6	0.24	0.59	*
Anaerobic	0	7	1.27	0.94	0.9
	50	7	0.84	1.02	*
	100	7	0.51	0.19	*
	0	6	0.53	ND	ND
	50	6	0.21	0.8	*
	100	6	*	*	*

* Little or no growth.
ND, not determined.

possessed the ability to inhibit *E. coli* O157 and some other pathogenic bacteria. The inhibitory activity of the mixed culture correlated with the concentration of acids (acetate and succinate) formed from glucose by *B. fragilis*. The succinate produced by *B. fragilis* was decarboxylated to propionate by *Veillonella* species. The combined action of acetate and propionate was thought to result in inhibition of the growth of *E. coli*.

Competition for nutrients between *E. coli* and the commensal microflora

Little is known about the nutrition of *E. coli* in the rumen. *E. coli* cannot use native proteins, but can grow on protein digests. Brecher *et al.* (1991) showed that *E. coli* can use peptides as a C or nitrogen (N) source, although, when a peptide is used as the C source under C-limited conditions, the bacteria transform the C skeleton of the amino acids to glucose. In the human large intestine, the extracellular protease activity of some of the most numerous bacteria is complemented by the activity of the pancreatic enzymes (Gibson *et al.*, 1989). In contrast, the rumen is non-secretory and *E. coli* strains may have to compete for access to peptides provided by the proteolytic microorganisms (Wallace and Brammall, 1985).

When pure cultures of rumen bacteria were grown on filter-sterilized rumen fluid supplemented with glucose, bicarbonate and reducing agents, the species most abundant in the rumen grew more rapidly than strains of the less abundant species (Van Gylswyk *et al.*, 1992). Ammonia, amino acids and peptides increased growth rates to some extent, but the greatest stimulatory effect on the growth of the less abundant bacteria was provided by factors present in yeast extract. It was concluded that competition for unidentified factors present in yeast extract may limit the population sizes of some bacteria in the rumen.

Duncan *et al.* (1997a) examined the ability of *E. coli* O157 and a rumen strain to grow on filter-sterilized rumen contents with and without various additions. Rumen contents contain amino acids and ammonia (Hungate, 1966), so nitrogenous growth factors would not be expected to be limiting. To obtain rapid growth of *E. coli*, it was necessary to add either an additional carbon source or a peptide source. It may be that the low numbers of *E. coli* in the ruminant gut are not always the result of the effects of VFA, but may also reflect the success of the commensal anaerobes in competing for nutrients.

Interactions involving commensal *E. coli* and other Gram-negative facultative bacteria

Colicins produced by some strains of *E. coli* inhibit growth of closely related strains (Riley and Gordon, 1996). They are proteins with a narrow spectrum of inhibitory activity which attach to specific receptors. Their modes of action vary and include pore formation in the membrane of sensitive cells or DNase or RNase activity, while some inhibit peptidoglycan synthesis. They are usually extrachromosomally encoded determinants and the host-cell immunity genes are also plasmid-borne.

Colicin-sensitive cells have specific receptors located in the outer membrane. These may also serve as the attachment sites for bacteriophages. There are large numbers of bacteriophages in the rumen and they are commonly present at between 3×10^9 and 1.6×10^{10} virions ml^{-1} rumen contents (Klieve and Swain, 1993). They are largely maintained in high numbers by lysis of rumen bacteria, but their role in the ecology of *E. coli* and other bacteria in this ecosystem is unclear. Insensitivity to colicins can result from shielding of the protein receptors by O-antigenic lipopolysaccharide side-chains in some cases and through unknown mechanisms in others (Pugsley, 1985).

Bradley and Howard (1991) screened 20 *E. coli* O157 strains for their sensitivity to colicins. Col G and H inhibited all 20 strains, while Col E2 and V inhibited 12 and 18 strains, respectively. Colicins A, B, D and Ia had no inhibitory effect. Murinda *et al.* (1996) compared the inhibitory activity of colicins with and without a known inducer of colicins, mitomycin C, and screened other diarrhoeagenic serotypes for sensitivity to colicins. Even without the addition of the inducer, they found that all of the O157 strains were sensitive to Col G and H and to the microcin Mcc B17. The addition of mitomycin C resulted in *E. coli* strains becoming sensitive to a wider range of colicins, particularly within the A group. Bradley and Howard (1991) reported that EHEC strains are often colicinogenic, and predominantly produce Col D. We have shown that *E. coli* O157 strain NCTC 12900 is sensitive to fewer colicins than other *E. coli* strains (Duncan *et al.*, 1997a and unpublished data) and that, although many of the *E. coli* strains isolated from a range of animal samples are colicinogenic, none of the isolates tested were inhibitory to *E. coli* O157 (12900). The finding that so many of the gut *E. coli* isolates are colicinogenic would suggest that maintaining a niche within the rumen is a fiercely competitive task, particularly for the minor components of the rumen microflora, so that strains with high competitive ability establish at the expense of less competitively endowed strains (Tan and Riley, 1996).

Exploitation of antagonistic microbial interactions has led some workers to develop probiotic mixes of bacteria known to have inhibitory activity against EHEC. Zhao *et al.* (1998) screened 1200 bacterial isolates from cattle samples and, from these, selected 18 that possessed the ability to inhibit EHEC. These isolates were 17 strains of *E. coli* and one strain of *Proteus mirabilis*. When six calves received a probiotic mixture of the 18 strains administered prior to exposure to EHEC, Zhao *et al.* (1998) subsequently failed to find the pathogen in all of the six necropsied calves. In comparison, EHEC was detected in seven out of nine of the control animals in this study. Further experiments from this group are described in Harmon *et al.* (Chapter 5, this volume).

Duncan *et al.* (1997b) screened isolates from MacConkey agar (Oxoid) plates for inhibitory activity against EHEC, and in three out of the six ovine rumen samples studied the predominant inhibitory isolates identified, on the basis of biochemical tests, were strains of *Pseudomonas aeruginosa*. The mechanism of inhibition is twofold and it seems that under aerobic growth conditions, the major inhibitory factor is the pigment pyocyanin, which is frequently produced by this organism. Pyocyanin had little effect on the growth of some of the more numerous anaerobic bacteria found in ruminants. Under anaerobic conditions, another pigment, fluorescein, may be largely responsible for the inhibitory activity. Fluorescein can sequester iron which is required in trace amounts by *E. coli* for protein synthesis. Although both these pigments are likely to have deleterious effects in the host, structurally related model compounds with less harmful side-effects might be designed from these compounds for use as treatments to eradicate EHEC from ruminants.

Interactions involving lactic acid-producing bacteria (LAB)

Interactions between *E. coli* and LAB have been extensively studied in relation to food preservation (reviewed in Wood, 1992). Lactic acid accumulates in the ruminant gut only under conditions of dietary imbalance, so under normal conditions it is unlikely to have an important ecological role in adult animals, although it could be important in developing ruminants. Antimicrobial substances from LAB active against *E. coli* have also been reported, but it is not clear whether they have an important or potential role in the gut (Gibson and Wang, 1994).

THE EFFECT OF PLANT METABOLITES AND OTHER DIETARY FACTORS

It has been shown that *E. coli* O157 strain 12900 was inhibited by coumarin aglycones, such as aesculetin, umbelliferone, coumarin and scopoletin, under both aerobic and anaerobic conditions *in vitro* (Duncan *et al.*, 1998).

Some of the most numerous bacterial species (Stewart *et al.*, 1997) present in the colon and rumen, such as *Bacteroides* spp. and *Prevotella* spp., possess the ability to hydrolyse aesculin to the aglycone aesculetin. This ability appears to be a common feature of bacteria that possess β-1–4-glucosidase activity. Several isolates of some of the most numerous bacterial species from human and porcine gut samples also possess the ability to hydrolyse aesculin to aesculetin and, in turn, inhibit the growth of *E. coli* O157 (Maxwell *et al.*, 1998).

The effects of the simultaneous presence of aesculetin and VFA at the levels likely to be encountered in the rumen (50–100 mM) were additive (Fig. 6.4). The addition of aesculin to batch cultures of ovine rumen contents inoculated with *E. coli* O157 at around 10^6 CFU ml^{-1} resulted in a greater than 2000-fold drop in the number of the *E. coli* O157 cells surviving over a 24 h incubation period at 38°C, while in the control incubation with no added aesculin there was no change in the *E. coli* O157 numbers on selective media. The total number of anaerobes dropped from 1.2×10^8 ml^{-1} to 7.3×10^6 ml^{-1} and 6.5×10^6 ml^{-1}, respectively, with and without the addition of aesculin over the 24 h incubation period. These results suggest that the biotransformation of aesculin by the mixed rumen microflora markedly reduced the survival of *E. coli* O157. Work is in progress to elucidate the inhibitory mechanism of aesculetin and the possible value of this and other metabolites in controlling EHEC in ruminants.

One of the major effects of dietary change in ruminants is to influence the concentrations of VFA in the rumen and the colon. A reduction in numbers of *E. coli* in the sheep gut following a switch from feeding grain to hay was ascribed by Diez-Gonzalez *et al.* (1998) to the selection of strains with reduced tolerance of acidic gastric secretions.

Brownlie and Grau (1967) showed that when cattle received a regular daily ration of 6.8 kg of lucerne hay, *E. coli* was rapidly eliminated from the rumen. Decreasing the food intake or an interruption of feeding for one or more days permitted the growth of *E. coli* in the rumen. Although the

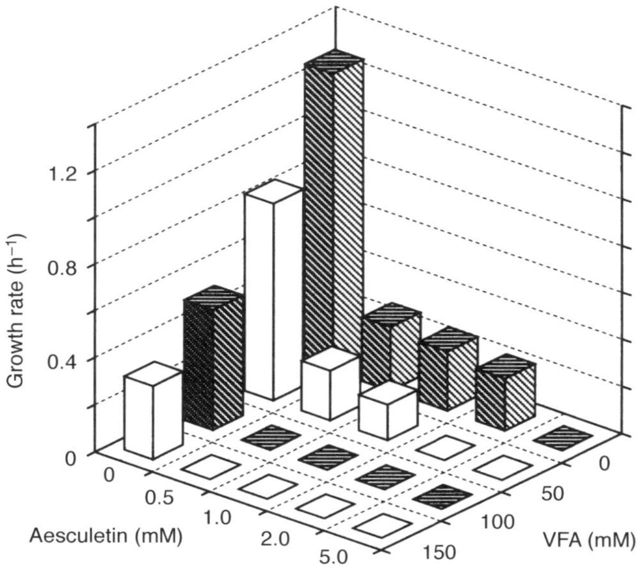

Fig. 6.4. Effects of aesculetin and aesculetin plus VFA on the rate of growth of *E. coli* O157 strain NCTC 12900 (data from Duncan *et al.*, 1998).

bacteria monitored in these studies were total coliforms, it is likely that the effects reflect the trend for EHEC counts. Brown *et al.* (1997) have shown that withholding feed from experimentally infected, weaned calves (6–8 weeks old) increased faecal shedding of *E. coli* O157, and Cray *et al.* (1998) showed that experimentally infected calves were more susceptible to infection if they were starved prior to infection.

Dargatz *et al.* (1997) examined faecal samples from cattle from 100 feedlots in 13 American states and showed that feeding barley increased the incidence of faecal contamination, while feeding soy meal decreased the incidence of detection of EHEC in faecal samples. In some studies, horizontal transmission of infection from experimentally infected animals to non-dosed animals was also found (Cray and Moon, 1995; Kudva *et al.*, 1995). Recent colonization and loss of EHEC did not appear to prevent recolonization.

Kudva *et al.* (1995) showed that, when sheep were changed from lucerne pellets to native sagebrush–bunch grass, all the animals tested positive for EHEC within 7 days of the dietary change. This may have resulted from horizontal transmission or from some animals previously being wrongly identified as non-carriers. Once fed the sagebrush–bunch grass, the animals continued to shed EHEC for 15 days, after which time all the animals tested negative. The animals remained negative despite several dietary changes, which included withholding feed for 24 h and reconfining animals in dry lots and refeeding with the lucerne pellets. Kudva *et al.* (1997) showed that, when animals experienced a dietary change, there was a significantly larger number of EHEC positive ewes at 4 days after the change-over. Thus it seems that dietary stress appears to contribute significantly to EHEC carriage. Nagy and Tengerdy (1968) reported that the essential oils extracted from sagebrush had antimicrobial activity, but whether this activity could selectively affect *E. coli* was not tested.

The effect of aesculin, as described above, suggests that some dietary-plant secondary compounds may have a selective inhibitory effect on *E. coli*. It is possible that reported effects of feeding cottonseed in reducing shedding of *E. coli* O157 are related to the presence in this plant of pigments and antimicrobial factors in cottonseed oil, although Rasmussen *et al.* (Chapter 3, this volume) reported that gossypol had little effect on the growth of *E. coli*. Feeding forage legumes has also been reported to decrease shedding of *E. coli*: these plants are especially rich in plant secondary compounds, including coumarins (Murray *et al.*, 1982).

FATE OF EHEC IN ANIMAL FAECES

Wallace (Chapter 12, this volume) has reviewed the fate of *E. coli* in animal faeces. It is clear, from our understanding of the interactions which occur between *E. coli* and other gut microorganisms, that the fate of *E. coli* in faeces may be influenced by the presence of other microorganisms or products that may be coexcreted. In the case of *P. aeruginosa*, for example, the phenazine pigment pyocyanin is much more active in the presence of oxygen than under anaerobic conditions (Hassan and Fridovitch, 1980). The coexcretion of *P. aeruginosa* with *E. coli* would be expected to reduce the survival of the latter bacterium upon exposure of faeces to air. Differences between animals in the presence of bacteria expressing inhibitory activity towards *E. coli* could contribute to animal-to-animal differences in the survival of this pathogen, either in the gut or following faecal shedding.

PROSPECTS FOR CONTROL

It is apparent that our knowledge of the microbial ecology of *E. coli* O157 in the ruminant gut is inadequate. To achieve any control over the proliferation of *E. coli* within the gut, it is important to know in much greater detail the sites of maximal colonization and the conditions under which *E. coli* can replicate and survive. Furthermore, it is still not clear to what extent *E. coli* O157 strains differ from other *E. coli* strains found in the ruminant gut in traits relevant for survival, and to what extent competition between different *E. coli* strains determines the population size of this serogroup. While Diez-Gonzalez *et al.* (1998) found larger acid-tolerant *E. coli* populations in the colon than in the rumen and some *E. coli* O157 strains are acid-tolerant, it is not clear whether this necessarily applies to the behaviour of a wide range of *E. coli* O157 strains.

In general, however, several practical avenues for dietary or other manipulations appear to be worth considering.

1. Removal of causative or contributory factors. The identification of dietary and other factors that may contribute to enhanced numbers or survival of *E. coli*, such as certain growth promoters or electron acceptors, as suggested by Rasmussen *et al.* (Chapter 3, this volume), is an essential part of a strategic approach to control the spread of this bacterium.
2. Creation of an unfavourable environment for survival of *E. coli* through elevation of VFA. In principle, there are two ways to approach this – through direct supplementation of the diet with VFA or by stimulating VFA production from commensal anaerobes through supply of appropriate substrates that are unavailable to *E. coli*. Since it is hard to envisage VFA supplementation at the levels needed being a practical approach economically or in terms of palatability, the second approach is more likely. However, maintaining high VFA concentrations during the period of feed withdrawal immediately before slaughter or during transport to slaughterhouses might be practicable – through the use of soluble additives to drinking-water, for example – as it is during this phase that numbers of *E. coli* are thought to increase (Rasmussen *et al.*, Chapter 3, this volume). To increase VFA concentrations by feeding bulk solids, the substrates required, such as plant cell-wall polysaccharides, are those that normally make up the bulk of the ruminant diet. Therefore, this approach simply equates to maintenance of feed supply and appears at odds with the need to reduce faecal contamination during the period prior to slaughter. It is also far from clear whether this approach would lead to suppression of *E. coli* in all regions of the gut, particularly in sites close to the gut wall or within the small intestine, where obligate anaerobes are less abundant.
3. Delivery of selective, non-clinical antimicrobial agents. The findings that some plant metabolites might have a selective effect on the survival of *E. coli* suggests that some production diets rich in such compounds may be useful, or that the compounds themselves might be used as supplements for short periods to further reduce the numbers of *E. coli* in the gut, ideally in combination with other measures. Here, efficacy, practicality and cost remain to be evaluated. Furthermore, bacteria exposed to such compounds may become resistant. It has recently been argued that exposure of bacteria to certain disinfectants may result in the appearance of antibiotic-resistant mutants, as bacteria employ the same systems for the efflux of these different compounds (Moken *et al.*, 1998).
4. Deprivation of essential nutrients for growth of *E. coli*. Probably the most attractive means of suppressing the growth of *E. coli* is to feed diets for

which this bacterium competes poorly for nutrients. Here, our lack of knowledge of what *E. coli* grows on in the gut is critical, although it is reasonable to suppose that this contributes to the low numbers of *E. coli* in animals fed fibre, compared with grain (Diez-Gonzalez *et al.*, 1998). The inhibitory effect of fluorescein on *E. coli* recorded above is of interest in this respect, as this pigment is known to sequester iron.

5. Competition for gut-wall attachment sites. The outcome of investigations on the localization of *E. coli* in the ruminant gut (Dean-Nystrom *et al.*, Chapter 4, this volume) is critical, as at present it is not clear whether this strategy would be valid.

6. The use of probiotics/bacteriocins. The successful use of probiotic mixtures (Zhao *et al.*, 1998; Harmon *et al.*, Chapter 5, this volume) is encouraging. The main questions are whether probiotics will prove reliable and robust enough to work in animals in different feeding and husbandry regimes and the need for more mechanistic studies to be carried out on their mode(s) of action. Although the present authors believe that some of the commensal strains of *E. coli* in this probiotic preparation may produce colicins active against *E. coli* O157 strains, this clearly needs further investigation.

7. Immunization. Ruminants carry circulating antibodies to enterobacteria and to some anaerobic rumen (and colonic) bacteria, and there is evidence to suggest that the caecum is one site of antibody production in ruminants (Sharpe *et al.*, 1975). Whether immunization of animals becomes a practical option for the reduction of shedding of *E. coli* O157 may depend on the location of these bacteria within the ruminant gut and, in particular, the extent to which they colonize the colonic mucosa (Dean-Nystrom *et al.*, Chapter 4, this volume).

ACKNOWLEDGEMENT

The Rowett Research Institute is funded by the Scottish Office Agriculture, Environment and Fisheries Department.

REFERENCES

Bradley, D.E. and Howard, S.P. (1991) Colicinogeny of O157:H7 enterohemorrhagic *Escherichia coli* and the shielding of colicin and phage receptors by their O-antigenic side chains. *Canadian Journal of Microbiology* 37, 97–104.

Brecher, A.S., Moehlam, T.A. and Hann, W.D. (1991) Utilisation of chymotrypsin as a sole carbon and (or) nitrogen source by *Escherichia coli*. *Canadian Journal of Microbiology* 38, 290–295.

Brown, C.A., Harmon, B.G., Zhao, T. and Doyle, M.P. (1997) Experimental *Escherichia coli* O157:H7 carriage in calves. *Applied and Environmental Microbiology* 63, 27–32.

Brownlie, L.E. and Grau, F.H. (1967) Effect of food intake on the growth and survival of salmonellas and *Escherichia coli* in the bovine rumen. *Journal of General Microbiology* 46, 125–134.

Caprioli, A., Donelli, G., Falbo, V., Passi, C., Pagano, A. and Mantovani, A. (1991) Antimicrobial resistance and production of toxins in *Escherichia coli* strains from wild ruminants and the alpine marmot. *Journal of Wildlife Diseases* 27, 324–327.

Cheng, K.J., Bailey, C.B.M., Hironaka, R. and Costerton, J.W. (1979) A technique for depletion of bacteria adherent to the epithelium of the bovine rumen. *Canadian Journal of Animal Science* 59, 207–209.

Cheng, K.J., Stewart, C.S., Dinsdale, D. and Costerton, J.W. (1984) Electron microscopy of bacteria involved in the digestion of plant cell walls. *Animal Feed Science and Technology* 10, 93–120.

Cheng, K.J., McAllister, T.A., Mathiesen, S.D., Blix, A.S., Orpin, C.G. and Costerton, J.W. (1993) Seasonal changes in the adherent microflora of the rumen in high-arctic Svalbard reindeer. *Canadian Journal of Microbiology* 39, 101–108.

Cray, W.C. and Moon, H.W. (1995) Experimental infection of calves and adult cattle with *Escherichia coli* O157:H7. *Applied and Environmental Microbiology* 61, 1586–1590.

Cray, W.C., Casey, T.A., Bosworth, B.T. and Rasmussen, M.A. (1998) Effect of dietary stress on faecal shedding of *Escherichia coli* O157:H7 in calves. *Applied and Environmental Microbiology* 64, 1975–1979.

Dargatz, D.A., Wells, S.J., Thomas, L.A., Hancock, D.D. and Garber, L.P. (1997) Factors associated with the presence of *Escherichia coli* O157 in faeces of feedlot cattle. *Journal of Food Protection* 5, 466–470.

Davies, D., Theodorou, M.K., Lawrence, M.I. and Trinci, A.P.J. (1993) Distribution of anaerobic fungi in the digestive tract of cattle and their survival in faeces. *Journal of General Microbiology* 139, 1395–1400.

Dean-Nystrom, E.A., Bosworth, B.A., Moon, H.W. and O'Brien, A.D. (1998) Bovine infection with shiga toxin-producing *Escherichia coli.* In: Kaper, J.B. and O'Brien, A.D. (eds) Escherichia coli *O157:H7 and Other Shiga Toxin-producing* E. coli *Strains.* ASM, Washington, DC, pp. 261–267.

Dehority, B.A. and Grubb, J.A. (1981) Bacterial population adherent to the epithelium on the roof of the dorsal rumen of sheep. *Applied and Environmental Microbiology* 41, 1424–1437.

Demeyer, D.I. (1981) Rumen microbes and digestion of plant cell walls. *Agriculture and Environment* 6, 295–337.

Diez-Gonzalez, F. and Russell, J.B. (1997) The ability of *Escherichia coli* O157:H7 to decrease its intracellular pH and resist the toxicity of acetic acid. *Microbiology* 143, 1175–1180.

Diez-Gonzalez, F., Callaway, T.R., Kizoulis, M.G. and Russell, J.B. (1998) Grain feeding and the dissemination of acid-resistant *Escherichia coli* from cattle. *Science* 281, 1666–1668.

Duncan, S.H., Scott, K.P., Stewart, C.S., Flint, H.J., Thomson-Carter, F. and Pennington, T.H. (1997a) The fate of *Escherichia coli* O157 isolates under simulated rumen conditions and the use of a *gfp*-labelled isolate for ecological studies. In: *Reproduction, Nutrition and Development, Supplement: Rumen Microbial Ecosystem Symposium Abstracts,* p. 31.

Duncan, S.H., Doherty, C.J., Govan, J.R.W. and Stewart, C.S. (1997b) Rumen isolates of *Pseudomonas aeruginosa* antagonistic to an *Escherichia coli* O157 strain. In: *Abstracts 97th Annual Meeting American Society for Microbiology, Miami,* p. 419.

Duncan, S.H., Flint, H.J. and Stewart, C.S. (1998) Inhibitory activity of gut bacteria against *Escherichia coli* O157 mediated by dietary plant metabolites. *FEMS Microbiology Letters* 164, 283–288.

Fliegerova, K. (1993) Multiresistant strains of *Escherichia coli* isolated from the rumen of young calves. *Folia Microbiologica* 38, 363–366.

Flint, H.J., Duncan, S.H. and Stewart, C.S. (1987) Transmissible antibiotic resistance in strains of *Escherichia coli* isolated from the ovine rumen. *Letters in Applied Microbiology* 5, 47–49.

Galfi, P., Neogrady, S., Semjen, G., Bardocz, S. and Pusztai, A. (1998) Attachment of different *Escherichia coli* O157 strains to cultured rumen epithelial cells. *Veterinary Microbiology* 61, 191–197.

Gibson, G.R. and Wang, X. (1994) Regulatory effects of bifidobacteria on the growth of other colonic bacteria. *Journal of Applied Bacteriology* 77, 412–420.

Gibson, S.A.W., McFarlane, C., Hay, S. and MacFarlane, G.T. (1989) Significance of microflora in proteolysis in the colon. *Applied and Environmental Microbiology* 55, 679–683.

Grau, F.H. and Brownlie, L.E. (1965) Occurrence of salmonellas in the bovine rumen. *Australian Veterinary Journal* 41, 321–323.

Gustafson, R.H. and Bowen, R.E. (1997) Antibiotic use in animal agriculture. *Journal of Applied Microbiology* 83, 531–541.

Hassan, H.M. and Fridovitch, I. (1980) Mechanism of the antibiotic action of pyocyanine. *Journal of Bacteriology* 141, 156–163.

Heim, R., Pracher, D.C. and Tsien, R.Y. (1994) Wavelength mutations and post-translational autooxidation of green fluorescent protein. *Proceedings of the National Academy of Sciences USA* 91, 12501–12504.

Hinton, A., Jr and Hume, M.E. (1995) Antibacterial activity of the metabolic by-products of a *Veillonella* species and *Bacterioides fragilis*. *Anaerobe* 1, 121–127.

Howe, K., Linton, A.H. and Osborne, A.D. (1976) A longitudinal study of *Escherichia coli* in cows and calves with special reference to the distribution of O-antigen types and antibiotic resistance. *Journal of Applied Bacteriology* 40, 331–340.

Hungate, R.E. (1966) *The Rumen and its Microbes.* Academic Press, New York.

Klieve, A.V. and Swain, R.A. (1993) Estimation of ruminal bacteriophage numbers by pulsed-field gel electrophoresis and laser densitometry. *Applied and Environmental Microbiology* 59, 2299–2303.

Kudva, I.T., Hatfield, P.G. and Hovde, C.J. (1995) Effect of diet on the shedding of *Escherichia coli* O157:H7 in a sheep model. *Applied and Environmental Microbiology* 61, 1363–1370.

Kudva, I.T., Hunt, C.W., Williams, C.J., Nance, U.M. and Hovde, C.J. (1997) Evaluation of dietary influences on *Escherichia coli* O157:H7 shedding by sheep. *Applied and Environmental Microbiology* 63, 3878–3886.

McCowan, R.P., Cheng, K.J., Bailey, C.B.M. and Costerton, J.W. (1978) Adhesion of bacteria to epithelial surfaces within the reticulorumen of cattle. *Applied and Environmental Microbiology* 35, 149–155.

Mann, S.O. and Orskov, E.R. (1973) The effect of rumen and post-rumen feeding of carbohydrates on the caecal microflora of sheep. *Journal of Applied Bacteriology* 36, 475–484.

Mann, S.O., Masson, F.M, and Oxford, A.E. (1954) Facultative anaerobic bacteria from the sheep's rumen. *Journal of General Microbiology* 10, 142–149.

Maxwell, F.J., Duncan, S.H. and Stewart, C.S. (1998) Characterisation of a porcine isolate of *Bifidobacterium boum* inhibitory to *Escherichia coli.* In: *Proceedings, 8th International Symposium on Microbial Ecology, Halifax, Nova Scotia*, p. 230.

Mead, L.J. and Jones, G.A. (1981) Isolation and presumptive identification of adherent epithelial bacteria ('epimural bacteria') from the ovine rumen wall. *Applied and Environmental Microbiology* 41, 1020–1028.

Moken, M.C., McMurry, L.M. and Levy, S.B. (1998). Selection of multiple antibiotic-resistant (Mar) mutants of *Escherichia coli* by using the disinfectant pine oil: roles of the *mar* and the *acr*AB loci. *Antimicrobial Agents and Chemotherapy* 41, 2770–2772.

Mueller, R.E., Ianotti, E.L. and Asplund, J.M. (1984) Isolation and identification of adherent epimural bacteria during succession in young lambs. *Applied and Environmental Microbiology* 47, 724–730.

Murinda, S.E., Roberts, R.F. and Wilson, R.A. (1996) Evaluation of colicins for inhibitory activity against diarrheagenic *Escherichia coli* strains, including serotype O157:H7. *Applied and Environmental Microbiology* 62, 3196–3202.

Murray, R.D.H., Mendez, J. and Brown, S.A. (1982) *The Natural Coumarins.* John Wiley & Sons, Chichester.

Murray, R.M., Bryant, A.M. and Leng, R.A. (1978) Methane production in the rumen and lower gut of sheep given lucerne chaff: effect of level of intake. *British Journal of Nutrition* 39, 337–345.

Nagy, J.G. and Tengerdy, R.P. (1968) Antibacterial action of essential oils of *Artemisia* as an ecological factor. *Applied Microbiology* 16, 441–444.

Pugsley, A.P. (1985) *Escherichia coli* K12 strains for use in the identification and characterisation of colicins. *Journal of General Microbiology* 131, 369–376.

Rasmussen, M.A., Cray, W.C., Casey, T.A. and Whipp, S.C. (1993) Rumen contents as a reservoir of enterohemorrhagic *Escherichia coli. FEMS Microbiology Letters* 114, 79–84.

Riley, M.A. and Gordon, D.M. (1996) The ecology and evolution of bacteriocins. *Journal of Industrial Microbiology* 17, 151–158.

Russell, J.B. and Wallace, R.J. (1997) Energy yielding and consuming reactions. In: Hobson, P.N. and Stewart, C.S. (eds) *The Rumen Microbial Ecosystem*, 2nd edn. Blackie, London, pp. 246–282.

Scott, K.P. and Flint, H.J. (1995) Transfer of plasmids between strains of *Escherichia coli* under rumen conditions. *Journal of Applied Bacteriology* 78, 189–193.

Scott, K.P., Mercer, D.K., Glover, L.A. and Flint, H.J. (1998) The green fluorescent protein as a visible marker for lactic acid bacteria in complex ecosystems. *FEMS Microbiology Ecology* 26, 219–230.

Sharpe, M.E., Latham, M.J. and Reiter, B. (1975) The immune response of the host animal to bacteria in the rumen and caecum. In: McDonald, I.W. and Warner, A.C.I. (eds) *Digestion and Metabolism in the Ruminant.* University of New England, Armidale, pp. 193–204.

Stewart, C.S. (1975) Some effects of phosphate and volatile fatty acid salts on the growth of rumen bacteria. *Journal of General Microbiology* 89, 319–326.

Stewart, C.S., Flint, H.J. and Bryant, M.P. (1997) The rumen bacteria. In: Hobson, P.N. and Stewart, C.S. (eds) *The Rumen Microbial Ecosystem.* Blackie, London, pp. 10–72.

Synge, B. (1997) *E. coli* O157 – consequences for the veterinary surgeon in practice. *Journal of the British Cattle Veterinary Association* 5, 209–212.

Tan, Y. and Riley, M.A. (1996) Rapid invasion by colicinogenic *Escherichia coli* with novel immunity functions. *Microbiology* 142, 2175–2180.

Tombolini, R., Unge, A., Davey, M.E., de Bruijin, F.J. and Jansson, J.K. (1997) Flow cytometric and microscopic analysis of GFP-tagged *Pseudomonas fluorescens* bacteria. *FEMS Microbiology Ecology* 22, 17–28.

Trinci, A.P.J., Davies, D.R., Gull, K., Lawrence, M., Nielsen, B.B., Rickers, A. and Theodorou, M.K. (1993) Anaerobic fungi in herbivorous mammals. *Mycological Research* 98, 129–152.

Ulyatt, M.J., Dellow, D.W., Reid, C.S.W. and Bauchop, T. (1975). Structure and function of the large intestine of ruminants. In: McDonald, I.W. and Warner, A.C.I. (eds) *Digestion and Metabolism in the Ruminant*. University of New England, Armidale, pp. 119–133.

Van Gylswyk, N.O., Wejdemar, K. and Kulander, K. (1992) Comparative growth rates of various rumen bacteria in clarified rumen fluid from cows and sheep fed different diets. *Applied and Environmental Microbiology* 58, 99–105.

Van Soest, P.J. (1994) *Nutritional Ecology of the Ruminant*, 2nd edn. Comstock, Ithaca, New York, 476 pp.

Veirheijden, J.H.M., Van Meirt, A.S.J.P.A.M., Schotman, A.J.H. and Van Duin, C.T.M. (1983) Pathophysiological aspects of *Escherichia coli* mastitis in ruminants. *Veterinary Research Communications* 7, 229–236.

Wallace, R.J. and Brammall, M.L. (1985) The role of different species of bacteria in the hydrolysis of protein in the rumen. *Journal of General Microbiology* 131, 821–832.

Wallace, R.J., Falconer, M.L. and Bhargava, P.K. (1989) Toxicity of volatile fatty acids at rumen pH prevents enrichment of *Escherichia coli* by sorbitol in rumen contents. *Current Microbiology* 19, 277–281.

Wolin, M.J. (1969) Volatile fatty acids and the inhibition of *Escherichia coli* growth by rumen fluid. *Applied Microbiology* 17, 83–87.

Wolin, M.J., Miller, T. and Stewart, C.S. (1997) Microbe–microbe interactions. In: Hobson, P.N. and Stewart, C.S. (eds) *The Rumen Microbial Ecosystem*. Blackie, London, pp. 467–491.

Wood, B.J.B. (ed.) (1992) *The Lactic Acid Bacteria in Health and Disease*. Elsevier, London, pp. 151–339.

Wood, J., Scott, K.P., Avgustin, G., Newbold, C.J. and Flint, H.J. (1998) Estimation of the relative abundance of different *Bacteroides/Prevotella* ribotypes in gut samples by restriction enzymes profiling of PCR amplified 16S rDNA sequences. *Applied and Environmental Microbiology* 64, 3683–3689.

Zhao, T., Doyle, M.P., Harmon, B.G., Brown, C.A., Mueller, P.O.E. and Parks, A.H. (1998) Reduction of carriage of enterohaemorrhagic *Escherichia coli* O157:H7 in cattle by inoculation with probiotic bacteria. *Journal of Clinical Microbiology* 36, 641–647.

7

Animal Studies in Scotland

B.A. Synge

SAC, Veterinary Science Division, Drummond Hill, Inverness, UK

INTRODUCTION

Work in Scotland studying verocytotoxigenic *Escherichia coli* (VTEC) O157 has been ongoing since the first UK isolation in calves (Synge and Hopkins, 1992). A bovine reservoir of infection had been suspected since the first described human outbreak was linked to the consumption of minced beef in the USA (Riley *et al.*, 1983). Research funding has recently been increased following the world's worst-ever outbreak, which occurred in central Scotland in 1996, when 496 people were known to be affected and 21 adults died. Previously, in a study carried out in Scotland in 1992/93, cited by Reilly (1996), of 139 cases investigated, 59% of patients were admitted to hospital; of these, 15% developed haemorrhagic uraemic syndrome (HUS) and four people (5%) died.

The isolation rates of VTEC O157 in Scotland are shown in Fig. 7.1. Over the last 10 years, there has been a steady increase in the number of human cases and the rate per 100,000 of population has been consistently four times higher in Scotland than in England and Wales or Northern Ireland (H. Smith, personal communication). There is a steady rise in isolation rates in these regions also. It is not known if there are real geographical reasons for the higher rates in Scotland or whether Scotland has just experienced the problem earlier. Other countries have reported high incidences. In Canada, for example, there were between three and six cases per 100,000 population each year from 1990 to 1995 (Spika *et al.*, 1998), slightly higher than in Scotland at this time.

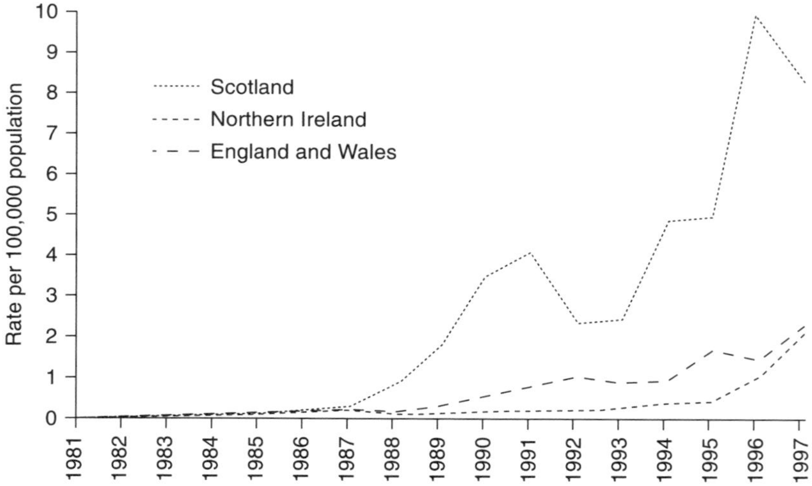

Fig. 7.1. Isolation rates of VTEC O157 in the UK 1981–1997. (Sources: Laboratory of Enteric Pathogens, CPHL Colindale, London. Scottish Centre for Infection and Environmental Health, Glasgow.)

CATTLE AS A SOURCE OF VTEC *E. COLI* O157

A bovine reservoir of VTEC is now widely recognized. Isolations from healthy cattle have been reported in North America (Martin *et al.*, 1986; Borczyk *et al.*, 1987; Wilson *et al.*, 1994) and from other countries – for example, Germany (Montenegro, 1990). Isolates of VTEC O157 have been reported in the UK in abattoir surveys (Chapman *et al.*, 1989, 1992) and in farm-animal surveys (Synge and Hopkins, 1992). Only rarely, however, has the animal source of a human case of VTEC O157 infection been demonstrated (Chapman *et al.*, 1993; Renwick *et al.*, 1993; Synge *et al.*, 1993).

Outbreaks of VTEC O157 infection associated with eating undercooked hamburgers have been reported in North America (Riley *et al.*, 1983) and in the UK (Anon., 1991), along with other food-borne outbreaks implicating dairy produce, such as unpasteurized milk (Chapman *et al.*, 1993) and yoghurt (Morgan *et al.*, 1993). Other routes of transmission have been associated with contaminated drinking-water supplies or handling or eating raw vegetables grown in ground on which farm manure had been spread (J. Curnow, personal communication).

An early study by the author involved investigation of cattle herds which might have been the source of human infection. Epidemiological surveillance of VTEC infection in Scotland is based on the routine weekly reporting of isolates of *E. coli* O157 by hospital laboratories to the Scottish Centre for Infection and Environmental Health, Glasgow (Sharp *et al.*, 1994). A detailed questionnaire form was completed for every human case in an attempt to identify possible sources of infection, and individual herds were identified. Faeces samples were collected from 40 herds where epidemiological information suggested involvement of cattle.

The numbers of samples collected were sufficient to give a 90% probability of isolating the organism, assuming 5% prevalence of detectable faecal carriage of *E. coli* O157. For this study, the more sensitive isolation technique of immunomagnetic separation (IMS) (Chapman *et al.*, 1994) was used. In addition to the phage typing and identification of genes encoding verocytotoxin production, isolates were compared at the reference laboratory in Aberdeen by pulsed-field gel electrophoresis (PFGE). The Salmonella Reference Laboratory in Glasgow carried out plasmid profiling and fingerprinting of the plasmid nucleic acid.

The study was more revealing than expected. In ten out of 19 human incidents investigated, the *E. coli* O157 isolated from cattle was indistinguishable from an isolate in an associated human case. Features of the isolates, such as the verocytotoxins produced, the phage type and the PFGE and plasmid profiles, corresponded in all these cases. In four herds, VTEC O157 of a different type was isolated and in a further 26 herds no VTEC O157 was isolated.

Phage type 2 was encountered in seven incidents, while phage types 49, 54 and 28 were each seen once only. The first link established between cattle and humans was in Orkney (Synge *et al.*, 1993). VTEC O157 had been isolated from a child with diarrhoea and medical investigation noted that there was a farm adjacent to the child's house. The child had visited the farm and the family pet dogs roamed freely through the cattle sheds and dung-heap. On visiting the farm, 84 samples were collected and all were screened for VTEC O157. One sample from a dung pat yielded the organism. Typing of the organism showed it to be indistinguishable from the human isolate. Both isolates were VT1-negative and VT2-positive, both were phage type 49, both had the unusual plasmid profile described as 90b:4 and the genomes of the isolates were indistinguishable by PFGE.

A sample of the other incidents investigated are now described. Incident no. 3 was a dairy herd in Ayrshire, at which the 53-year-old farmer's wife regularly fed calves and drank raw milk. She developed severe bloody diarrhoea, requiring admission to hospital. Incident no. 6 involved a suckler herd in Borders region, where an 8-month-old child was regularly exposed to a cattle environment when he was taken daily in a pushchair to the cowshed where his parents worked. Following the onset of bloody diarrhoea, the child developed HUS.

Incident no. 9 was a major epidemiological investigation following a major community outbreak in Lothian, associated with a milk-processing plant (Upton and Coia, 1994). Cattle on 18 dairy farms (herd nos 9–26) supplying the plant were investigated. In only one of the these (herd no. 26) was VTEC O157 isolated. The organism was recovered from 16 of the 35 faecal samples examined and was indistinguishable from the human isolates.

The complexity of the situations that can be encountered was demonstrated by incident no. 10. Following bloody diarrhoea in a 15-month-old child in Dumfriesshire who had been admitted to hospital, three herds adjacent to the child's home (27–29, two dairy and one suckler) were investigated. In two herds (27 and 28), VTEC O157 of matching phage and verotoxin type to the human case was isolated. In one of these herds (28) and a third herd (29), VTEC O157 of a different type was also isolated. There was considerable regular contact with cattle faeces in the environment surrounding the house.

In addition to isolations from cattle faeces, VTEC O157 was isolated from a hard cheese on two occasions that were epidemiologically linked to a human outbreak. The organism was not isolated from the milk used to make the cheese or from the cows that produced the milk.

The possible methods of spread of infection were investigated in each case and, where cattle were implicated, the possible methods of spread are summarized in Table 7.1.

OTHER ANIMALS AS A SOURCE OF INFECTION

Sheep have been shown to shed VTEC O157 (Chapman *et al.*, 1996) and, in two human incidents in Scotland, newly lambed ewes were implicated as a source of infection (Allison *et al.*, 1997). Goats, horses and domestic geese have also been associated with zoonoses in Scotland. Horses have also been implicated in Wales (Chalmers *et al.*, 1997). Experimentally, day-old chickens were infected and the hens shed the organisms for 11 months (Schoeni and Doyle, 1994). The organism has been isolated from wild birds (mainly gulls) by sampling droppings at landfill sites and on intertidal sediments (Wallace *et al.*, 1997). Deer could be another reservoir (Rice *et al.*, 1995). Recently, media attention has turned in Scotland to the applications of sewage sludge and slaughterhouse waste to pasture as a possible health hazard or source of infection for livestock.

PREVALENCE STUDIES

Surveys to estimate the prevalence of VTEC O157 in animals are listed in a review (Armstrong *et al.*, 1996), showing a wide range in values, from 0.28

Table 7.1. Incidents related to possible sources of infection.

No. of incidents	Source
1	Improperly pasteurized milk
2	Raw milk on direct contact
7	Direct contact or contamination of food by persons handling the cattle

to 9.5%. The variation is partly due to the sensitivity of the method of isolation and partly to the differing groups of animals studied.

An initial survey in 1992/93, using sorbitol MacConkey agar to screen faeces and rectal swabs submitted to all the veterinary investigation centres in Scotland, detected VTEC O157 in 0.25% of 5237 cattle samples (Synge and Hopkins, 1996). At this stage, the organism was not found in other animals. A similar study by the Veterinary Laboratories Agency in 1994/95 in England and Wales found VTEC O157 in 0.83% of 6495 bovine faeces samples (Richards *et al.*, 1998). This study used the more sensitive method of IMS, as described by Chapman *et al.* (1994). As a result of a recommendation by the Pennington Group (1997), the Scottish Office commissioned the specification for a statistically based prevalence study in beef cattle. The study is designed to assess the prevalence of herds shedding VTEC O157. Approximately 900 herds producing finished cattle will be sampled over 2 years. Farms included may be dairy, beef suckler or specialist finishing units. A subobjective is to determine the within-herd prevalence on positive farms.

There appears to be a higher prevalence in young animals. In the initial study in Scotland, which found 0.25% prevalence, 0.4% calves under 2 months excreted, while 0.12% young stock (2 months to 2 years) and zero adults were excreting. In the USA, a study showed 0.2% adults and 0.65% weaned calves to be shedding (Hancock *et al.*, 1994).

FACTORS AFFECTING THE SHEDDING OF VTEC O157 BY CATTLE

When visiting farms in the above study, the opportunity will be taken to collect epidemiological information relating to the geographical location and management of the cattle, and it is intended to establish if any associations can be found with increased shedding of the organism.

In a separate study, funded by the Ministry of Agriculture, Fisheries and Food, 32 herds are each being studied over a period of 1 year. Cohorts of beef suckler cows are being sampled before and after specific events, such as calving, turnout, housing, changes in feed, etc., to try to establish if any management factor has an effect on shedding. In a single beef suckler herd in Orkney studied over a year, there was a small peak of shedding in May, with a larger peak in the autumn. This is in agreement with the findings in an English dairy herd (Mechie *et al.*, 1997).

CONCLUSIONS

Cattle have been clearly established as an important, but possibly not the main, source of VTEC O157 for humans. Sheep have been shown to be a risk at lambing time, while goats and horses have also been incriminated.

Pigs and poultry have not yet been shown to be infected with VTEC O157 in Scotland. Work is in progress to establish the prevalence in Scottish beef cattle and factors that affect shedding. The role of wildlife and environmental factors that influence the infection of cattle needs further investigation.

ACKNOWLEDGEMENT

SAC receives financial support from the Scottish Office Agriculture, Environment and Fisheries Department.

REFERENCES

Allison, L., Thomson-Carter, F., Gray, D., Rusbridge, S. and MacLennan, M. (1997) Human cases of *E. coli* O157:H7 infection associated with exposure to lambing ewes. In: *Association of Veterinary Teachers and Research Workers 51st Scientific Meeting*, p. 28.

Anon. (1991) Haemorrhagic colitis: *Escherichia coli* O157. *PHLS Communicable Disease Report* 1, 1.

Armstrong, G.L., Hollingsworth, J. and Morris, J.G., Jr (1996) Emerging foodborne pathogens: *Escherichia coli* O157:H7 as a model of entry of a new pathogen into the food supply of the developed world. *Epidemiological Reviews* 18, 29–51.

Borczyk, A., Karmali, M.A., Lior, H. and Duncan, L.M.C. (1987) Bovine reservoir for verotoxin-producing *Escherichia coli* O157:H7. *Lancet* i, 98.

Chalmers, R.M., Salmon, R.L., Willshaw, G.A., Cheasty, T., Looker, N., Davies, I. and Wray, C. (1997) Vero-cytotoxin producing *Escherichia coli* O157 in a farmer handling horses. *Lancet* 349, 1816.

Chapman, P.A., Wright, D.J. and Norman, P. (1989) Verotoxin-producing *Escherichia coli* infections in Sheffield: cattle as a possible source. *Epidemiology and Infection* 102, 439–445.

Chapman, P.A., Siddons, C.A., Wright, D.J., Norman, P., Fox, J. and Crick, E. (1992) Cattle as a source of verotoxigenic *Escherichia coli* O157. *Veterinary Record* 131, 323–324.

Chapman, P.A., Wright, D.J. and Higgins, R. (1993) Untreated milk as a source of verotoxigenic *Escherichia coli* O157. *Veterinary Record* 133, 171–172.

Chapman, P.A., Wright, D.J. and Siddons, C.A. (1994) A comparison of immunomagnetic separation and direct culture for the isolation of verocytotoxin producing *Escherichia coli* O157 from bovine faeces. *Journal of Medical Microbiology* 40, 424–427.

Chapman, P.A., Siddons, C.A. and Harkin, M.A. (1996) Sheep as a potential source of verocytotoxin-producing *Escherichia coli* O157. *Veterinary Record* 138, 23–24.

Hancock, D.D., Besser, T.E., Kinsel, M.L., Tarr, P.I., Rice, D.H. and Paros, M.G. (1994) The prevalence of *Escherichia coli* O157:H7 in dairy and beef cattle in Washington state. *Epidemiology and Infection* 113, 199–207.

Martin, M.L., Shipman, L.D. and Wells, J.G. (1986) Isolation of *Escherichia coli* O157:H7 from dairy cattle associated with two cases of haemolytic uraemic syndrome. *Lancet* ii, 1043.
Mechie, S.C., Chapman, P.A. and Siddons, C.A. (1997) A fifteen month study of *Escherichia coli* O157:H7 in a dairy herd. *Epidemiology and Infection* 118, 17–25.
Montenegro, M.A., Buelte, M. and Trumpf, T. (1990) Detection and characterisation of fecal verotoxin-producing *Escherichia coli* from healthy cattle. *Journal of Clinical Microbiology* 28, 1417–1421.
Morgan, D., Newman, C.P., Hutchinson, D.N., Walker, A.M., Rowe, B. and Majid, F. (1993) Verotoxin producing *Escherichia coli* O157 infections associated with the consumption of yoghurt. *Epidemiology and Infection* 111, 181–187.
Pennington Group (1997) *Report on the Circumstances Leading to the 1996 Outbreak of Infection with* E. coli *O157 in Central Scotland, the Implications for Food Safety and the Lessons to be Learned.* HMSO, Edinburgh, 58 pp.
Reilly, W.J. (1996) Verotoxigenic *Escherichia coli* O157 in Scotland. In: *Society for Veterinary Epidemiology and Preventive Medicine, Proceedings, Glasgow,* pp. 60–71.
Renwick, S.A., Wilson, J.B., Clarke, R.C., Lior, H., Borczyck, A.A., Spika, J., Rahn, K., McFadden, K., Brouwer, A., Copps, A., Anderson, N., Alves, D. and Karmali, M.A. (1993) Evidence of direct transmission of *Escherichia coli* O157:H7 infection between calves and a human. *Journal of Infectious Diseases* 168, 792–793.
Rice, D.H., Hancock, D.D. and Besser, T.E. (1995) Verotoxigenic *Escherichia coli* O157 colonisation of wild deer and range cattle. *Veterinary Record* 137, 524.
Richards, M.S., Corkish, A.D., Sayers, A.R., McLaren, I.M., Evans, S.J., Gibbens, J.C. and Wray, C. (1998) Studies on the presence of verocytotoxic *Escherichia coli* O157 in bovine faeces in England and Wales and on beef carcass in abattoirs in the United Kingdom. *Epidemiology and Infection* 120, 187–192.
Riley, L.W., Remis, R.S., Helgerson, S.D., McGee, H.B., Wells, J.G., Davis, B.R., Herbert, R.J., Olcott, E.S., Johnson, L.M., Hargrett, N.T., Blake, P.A. and Cohen, M.L. (1983) Haemorrhagic colitis associated with a rare *Escherichia coli* serotype. *New England Journal of Medicine* 308, 681–685.
Schoeni, J.L. and Doyle, M.P. (1994) Variable colonisation of chickens perorally inoculated with *Escherichia coli* O157:H7 and subsequent contamination of eggs. *Applied and Environmental Microbiology* 60, 2958–2962.
Sharp, J.C.M., Coia, J.E., Curnow, J. and Reilly, W.J. (1994) *Escherichia coli* O157 infections in Scotland. *Journal of Medical Microbiology* 40, 3–9.
Spika, J.S., Khakhria, R., Michel, P., Milley, D., Wilson, J. and Waters, J. (1998) Shiga toxin-producing *Escherichia coli* infections in Canada. In: Kaper, J.B. and O'Brien, A.D. (eds) Escherichia coli *O157:H7 and Other Shiga Toxin-producing* E. coli *Strains.* American Society for Microbiology, Washington DC.
Synge, B.A. and Hopkins, G.F. (1992) Verotoxigenic *Escherichia coli* O157 in Scottish calves. *Veterinary Record* 130, 583.
Synge, B.A. and Hopkins, G.F. (1996) Verocytotoxin producing *E. coli* O157 – zoonotic implications. In: *XIX World Buiatrics Congress Proceedings, Edinburgh.* BCVA, pp. 633–637.
Synge, B.A., Hopkins, G.F., Reilly, W.J. and Sharp, J.C.M. (1993) Possible link between cattle and *E. coli* O157 infection in a human. *Veterinary Record* 133, 507.

Upton, P. and Coia, J.E. (1994) Outbreak of *Escherichia coli* O157 associated with pasteurised milk supply. *Lancet* 344, 1015.

Wallace, J.S., Cheasty, T. and Jones, K. (1997). Isolation of verocytotoxin-producing *Escherichia coli* O157 from wild birds. *Journal of Applied Microbiology* 82, 399–404.

Wilson, J.B., Clarke, R.C., Renwick, S., Rahn, K., Johnson, R.P., Alves, D., Karmali, M.A., Lior, H., McEwan, S.A. and Spika, J. (1994). Verocytotoxigenic *Escherichia coli* infection on dairy farms in southern Ontario. In: Karmali, M.A. and Goglio, A.G. (eds) *Proceedings 2nd International Symposium and Workshop on Verocytotoxin-producing Escherichia coli Infections (VTEC 94).* Elsevier, Bergamo, Italy, pp. 61–64.

8

Escherichia coli O157: 14 Years' Experience in Sheffield, UK

P.A. Chapman

Public Health Laboratory, Sheffield, UK

INTRODUCTION

Verocytotoxigenic *Escherichia coli* (VTEC) are now well documented as a cause of symptoms ranging from mild non-bloody diarrhoea to haemorrhagic colitis (HC) and haemolytic uraemic syndrome (HUS). *E. coli* O157 is by far the most common VTEC serogroup that causes infections in humans. In the first documented outbreak of HC caused by *E. coli* O157 (Riley *et al.*, 1983), which occurred in Michigan and Oregon, USA, in 1982, there was a strong epidemiological association between infection and prior consumption of ground beef from one chain of fast-food restaurants. *E. coli* O157 was also isolated from beef patties from one of the suspect food outlets. The first association of HUS with prior VTEC infection was made in Toronto, Canada, by Karmali *et al.* (1983, 1985), who found evidence of VTEC infection in 30 out of 40 cases of HUS, but in none of 40 age- and sex-matched healthy control patients. Since these initial reports, outbreaks and sporadic cases of HUS and HC associated with VTEC infection, particularly caused by serogroup O157, have been reported worldwide. Reported outbreaks of *E. coli* O157 infection have often been very severe, with high mortality rates in the elderly. In one outbreak, due to undercooked beef, which occurred in a residential home in Ontario, Canada, in September 1985, 55 residents and 18 staff were affected; of the 55 residents affected, six died in the early stages of HC and a further 12 developed HUS, of whom 11 died (Carter *et al.*, 1987). A high incidence in HUS of subsequent renal and neurological sequelae has also been a feature of outbreaks of *E. coli* O157 infection: of 35 children affected in an outbreak in the West Midlands in 1982/83, 23 needed renal dialysis, three died, six developed chronic renal failure (CRF) alone and three developed CRF together with other complications (Taylor *et al.*, 1986). In January 1993, a large outbreak of HC caused by *E. coli* O157 and associated with the ingestion of undercooked fast-food hamburgers occurred in the Seattle–Tacoma area of Washington in the USA (Centers for Disease Control, 1993).

Reported cases of HUS in both North America and the UK are increasing steadily and HUS is now the single commonest cause of acute renal failure in children in these countries (British Paediatric Surveillance Unit, 1989; Karmali, 1989). At present, *E. coli* O157 infections appear to be more common in the USA, Canada and the UK than elsewhere in the world. It is unclear whether this simply reflects that these countries have better developed epidemiological and microbiological investigation infrastructures, necessary to identify outbreaks and sporadic cases of infection, which might go unnoticed elsewhere. In North America, *E. coli* O157 infection is markedly seasonal, occurring most commonly from midsummer to mid-autumn (Karmali, 1989). The seasonality in the UK is still marked but appears to be slightly earlier, which is difficult to explain.

Strains of *E. coli* first isolated from diarrhoeal cattle in Argentina in 1977 were later shown to be *E. coli* O157 (Ørskov *et al.*, 1987); these are probably the first documented isolates of the organism from cattle. Argentina has a higher incidence of childhood HUS than many other countries and the possibility of this being linked to *E. coli* O157 infections from a bovine reservoir cannot be ignored (Lopez *et al.*, 1989). *E. coli* O157 have also been isolated from healthy cattle, while attempting to find a source of human infections, in Canada (Borczyk *et al.*, 1987a), the USA (Martin *et al.*, 1986) and England (Chapman *et al.*, 1989, 1993a, b, 1994).

ESCHERICHIA COLI O157 INFECTIONS IN SHEFFIELD

Introduction

We first identified cases of human infection by *E. coli* O157 in the Sheffield area in June 1984. At that time, specific methods for the selective isolation of *E. coli* O157 did not exist and cases were identified by the very laborious procedure of culture on MacConkey agar and screening of many individual colonies for verocytotoxin production by a Vero cell assay. Since the summer of 1986, we have investigated 12 outbreaks of *E. coli* O157 infection in the Sheffield area. The outbreaks are summarized in Table 8.1. The frustrations experienced during the early investigations motivated us to develop better and more sensitive methods for detection and typing of the organism. *E. coli* O157 was isolated from a suspect food source for the first time in the UK in Sheffield in 1993. In addition to investigating outbreaks, the improved methods have also been used for large surveillance studies in our area. This review of our experiences over the last 14 years is divided

Table 8.1. Outbreaks of *E. coli* O157 infection in Sheffield, 1986–1997.

Time	Culture-confirmed cases	Population	Source	Reference
1986–1987	35	Community	Not identified	Chapman *et al.* (1989)
1989	45	Community	Not identified	Chapman *et al.* (1990)
February 1992	5	Institutional	Person-to-person	Unpublished data
May/June 1992	5	Community	Beef from local abattoir	Chapman *et al.* (1993a)
May 1993	7	Community	Unpasteurized milk	Chapman *et al.* (1993b)
November 1994	9	Family	Potatoes/person-to-person	Chapman *et al.* (1997a)
September 1995	7	Community	Contact with infected calves	Unpublished results
April/May 1997	23	Community	Not definitely identified – possibly milk	Unpublished results
June/July 1997	5	Family	Contact with infected calves	Unpublished results
July/August 1997	3	Community	Contact with infected cow, pony, goats, sheep and pigs	Unpublished results

into three parts: outbreak investigations, method development and surveillance studies. This division is purely arbitrary, as the three areas of work have been inextricably linked.

Outbreak investigations

Outbreaks during 1986–1987

During the 2-year period 1986–1987, *E. coli* O157 was isolated from 30 patients presenting with bloody diarrhoea and from five cases of HUS (Chapman *et al.*, 1989). All isolations were made by inoculating faecal samples on to sorbitol MacConkey agar (SMAC) and all isolates were stored at −70°C for future reference. Retrospective typing of the strains by a combination of plasmid profile analysis, toxin genotyping and phage typing showed that small point-source outbreaks almost certainly occurred in both years. A source of the infections was not definitely identified. However, *E. coli* O157 was isolated from faecal samples taken from two of 207 cattle immediately after slaughter at a South Yorkshire abattoir (Chapman *et al.*, 1989); these were the first isolates from cattle in the UK. Typing by the above procedures showed them to be indistinguishable from the strains isolated from some of the human cases; a bovine source of the infections, therefore, could not be ruled out.

Outbreaks during 1989

During the summer of 1989, we investigated 43 cases of *E. coli* O157 infection. Typing of strains as above indicated that point-source outbreaks of 15 cases in late May/early June and 19 cases in late July had probably occurred (Chapman *et al.*, 1990). The remaining nine cases were apparently sporadic cases caused by unrelated types. A questionnaire about food history, eating habits and lifestyle was completed for each patient and for a number of control patients who had not been ill. Three separate case–control studies were performed: (i) all cases compared with unmatched controls; (ii) the cases occurring in May/June compared with age- and sex-matched controls; and (iii) the cases occurring in July compared with age- and sex-matched controls. Risk factors for infection were not determined by any of the studies (Chapman *et al.*, 1990).

Outbreaks during 1992

In February 1992, five cases of *E. coli* O157 infection occurred in a residential home for the elderly. The cases occurred over a 3-week period and two of the patients died. The source of infection for the initial case was not identified, but the time intervals between this and subsequent cases suggested that person-to-person transmission might have occurred.

In late May/early June, a further five cases occurred over a 10-day period. When cases were questioned, it appeared that they had all consumed meat products from the same mobile butcher. Although samples were not available directly from the butcher, the abattoir in South Yorkshire from which he habitually obtained his meat was identified. During investigation of the abattoir, *E. coli* O157 was isolated from 84 (4%) of 2103 bovine rectal swabs; of these 84, 78 (93%) were verocytotoxigenic (VT^+), the most common phage types being 2 and 8, the types implicated in the cluster of human cases. Positive cattle, which were roughly equal numbers of prime beef and culled dairy animals, originated from diverse geographical areas within England. *E. coli* O157 was isolated from seven (30%) of 23 carcasses of rectal swab-positive cattle and from two (8%) of 25 carcasses of rectal swab-negative cattle (Chapman *et al.*, 1993a). During August, a strain of *E. coli* O157 belonging to phage type 1, producing both VT1 and VT2 and harbouring 92- and 6.6-kb plasmids, was isolated from rectal faeces of a cow at slaughter and from the carcass of the same animal 1 day later. We had never isolated this strain previously in the Sheffield area, but, within the following 10 days, three cases of human infection occurred in the community caused by *E. coli* O157 strains with the same characteristics.

Outbreaks during 1993

In May 1993, a cluster of seven cases of HC and HUS caused by *E. coli* O157 infection occurred in a small, well-defined geographical area of north-west Sheffield. Initial epidemiological evidence suggested that these cases may have been linked to consumption of untreated milk from one farm. Using enrichment culture and a newly developed immunomagnetic separation (IMS) technique, we isolated *E. coli* O157 from ten of 105 milking cows, from one sample of farmyard slurry and from one of ten milk samples taken from the individual milking jars used for the rectal swab-positive cattle. All the isolates of *E. coli* O157 harboured a single 92-kb plasmid, produced VT2 but not VT1, and were of phage type 2 (Chapman *et al.*, 1993b). This was the first incident of *E. coli* O157 infection in the UK in which a suspect food source was microbiologically confirmed.

Carriage of *E. coli* O157 by the cattle in the herd was monitored over the 15-month period immediately following the outbreak to examine seasonal, age and management factors affecting faecal excretion of the organism (Mechie *et al.*, 1997). Between May 1993 and July 1994, 26 visits were made to the farm to collect a total of 3593 rectal swabs from cows, heifers and calves and 329 milk samples. *E. coli* O157 was isolated from 153 (4.3%) of 3593 bovine rectal swabs. The maximum prevalence at any one visit was 14% in lactating cows, 40% in non-lactating cows, 56% in calves and 68% in heifers. The prevalence in lactating cows, which was significantly lower than in the other groups, peaked during May–July 1993, again briefly after the cattle were housed during November 1993 and then again during May 1994. Excretion rates of *E. coli* O157 in lactating cows were highest during the first month after calving, falling during lactation and rising to another peak at 7 months post-partum. This was possibly due to changes in diet introduced at these times; such changes in diet have been shown to markedly affect the excretion of *E. coli* O157 in a sheep model (Kudva *et al.*, 1995, 1997). Between November 1993 and May 1994, there was no evidence of excretion of *E. coli* O157 in any group. Of the animals which excreted *E. coli* O157, 87 (74%) did so on only one occasion, but 23 (32%) of 73 cows and heifers and seven (16%) of 44 calves which excreted the organism did so on more than one occasion. *E. coli* O157 was not isolated from milk taken from the bulk tank, but it was isolated from individual milk samples (one milk jar and one forestream milk) from two animals previously shown to be faecal excreters of the organism. All isolates of *E. coli* O157 obtained were of the same phage type, plasmid profile and toxin genotype. More recent examination of the strains by pulsed-field gel electrophoresis (PFGE) (Thomson-Carter *et al.*, 1993) and a restriction fragment length polymorphism technique (Samadpour *et al.*, 1993) indicated that the colonizing strain remained the same throughout the study. This is in contrast to other studies that have shown that the strain present in a herd changed frequently (Faith *et al.*, 1996).

Outbreaks during 1994

In November 1994, an outbreak of *E. coli* O157 infection occurred which affected four families (Chapman *et al.*, 1997a). Several weeks elapsed before epidemiological investigations suggested a putative link between the four families, and this delay almost certainly had an adverse effect on the outcome of standard laboratory investigations. Three members of family A, who had diarrhoea on 20 October, lived on a small arable farm that had ten cattle. Manure from the animals was used to fertilize the ground for growing potatoes, which were then offered for retail sale, unwashed, directly from the farm. The mother from family B bought potatoes, which were covered with manure, from family A in early November and over the subsequent 10 days she became ill with diarrhoea and her daughter and son both became ill with bloody diarrhoea. The mother from family C visited family B while the daughter from the latter family was symptomatic; the mother developed diarrhoea several days later. The mother and two sons from family D visited family B while the son from the latter family was symptomatic; the first son developed bloody diarrhoea 6 days later, which progressed to development of HUS. Direct culture of faecal samples on cefixime rhamnose (CR)-SMAC failed to isolate *E. coli* O157 from any of the symptomatic patients, and direct culture on cefixime tellurite (CT)-SMAC isolated the organism from only one patient. In contrast, a combination of isolation of *E. coli* O157 by IMS (Chapman and Siddons, 1996a) and detection of *E. coli* O157-specific secretory immunoglobulin A (IgA) by an enzyme immunoassay (Siddons and Chapman, 1993) suggested *E. coli* O157 infection in all eight symptomatic patients, but not in any of the family members who were not ill. The outbreak clearly illustrated the need to use the most sensitive methods available during both the investigation and the follow-up of cases of *E. coli* O157 infection. Two children who excreted the organism for 60 and 89 days, respectively, were the only two patients who did not develop a secretory IgA response. Further work is ongoing to test the hypothesis that this prolonged excretion may be due to failure to produce specific secretory antibody.

Reports on the length of the period of excretion of *E. coli* O157 following infection differ widely and probably reflect differences both in methodology and in populations studied. According to Tarr *et al.* (1990), patients rapidly stop excreting the organism after illness, as determined by direct culture on plain SMAC, whereas Karch *et al.* (1995) used DNA hybridization to detect shedding of the organism for up to 62 days in HC patients and for up to 124 days in HUS patients. Excretion of the organism may also be prolonged in young children (Belongia *et al.*, 1993; Shah *et al.*, 1996). IMS was used in the present study and we have previously shown this to be more sensitive than direct culture for the isolation of *E. coli* O157 from human faecal samples from several different categories of patient (Chapman and Siddons, 1996a); this has subsequently been confirmed by others (Cubbon *et al.*, 1996; Karch *et al.*, 1996).

Outbreaks during 1995–1997

In September 1995, seven cases of *E. coli* O157 infection were identified in seven children in a small area, again in north-west Sheffield. Three of the seven had visited young calves on a local farm. Indistinguishable strains of *E. coli* O157 were isolated from faecal samples from two of the calves. Secondary person-to-person spread probably accounted for the other cases (Sheffield Public Health Laboratory (PHL), unpublished results).

In 1997 there were 67 culture-confirmed cases of *E. coli* O157 infection in the Sheffield area, more than in any previous year. Despite intensive epidemiological investigations, we were unable to identify any definite food sources of the organism. However, 23 cases that occurred in a small area, again in north-west Sheffield, were caused by a strain which had been previously uncommon in Sheffield. Indistinguishable strains of *E. coli* O157 were isolated from milking cows on a farm within the geographical area of the infections; although the farm sold unpasteurized milk locally, a definite link with the cases was not established (Sheffield PHL, unpublished results).

Two incidents of three cases in early June and a further two cases in July occurred in children who had visited open farms in the area, and again indistinguishable strains of *E. coli* O157 were isolated from faecal samples from calves at the farms. A further three cases of infection occurred in August in children who had visited a city farm within central Sheffield. Indistinguishable strains of *E. coli* O157 were isolated from faecal samples taken from a cow, a pony, two different breeds of goat, two different breeds of sheep and three different breeds of pigs (Sheffield PHL, unpublished results). Although *E. coli* O157 has been isolated previously from the faeces of healthy pigs and piglets with diarrhoea (Linggood and Thompson, 1987;

Gannon *et al.*, 1988), the majority of these strains have been VT^-, have produced heat-labile or heat-stable enterotoxin and have belonged to H antigen types other than H7; they have not, therefore, been characteristic of those *E. coli* O157 strains most commonly isolated from humans. We are not aware of any previous reports of the isolation of VT^+ *E. coli* O157 from pigs. We also isolated *E. coli* O157 from samples of finished compost (composted animal manure and vegetable waste), which was both sold at the farm shop and included in potting compost for plants for sale. Studies of the survival of *E. coli* O157 in compost are planned.

DIAGNOSTIC METHODS FOR *ESCHERICHIA COLI* O157

Culture on solid media

Strains of *E. coli* O157 do not normally ferment sorbitol, whereas many other serogroups of *E. coli* do (Wells *et al.*, 1983; Pai *et al.*, 1984) and SMAC has become widely used for their isolation (March and Ratnam, 1986; Smith *et al.*, 1987; Walker *et al.*, 1988). However, reports of its selectivity have varied widely. Using SMAC, Smith *et al.* (1987) isolated *E. coli* O157 from 22% of faecal samples examined, whereas Walker *et al.* (1988) isolated the organism from only 0.5%; this disparity is more likely to reflect differences between highly selected samples sent to a reference laboratory and unselected samples examined in a clinical diagnostic laboratory than between methods used for isolation. In common with Walker *et al.* (1988), we have found sorbitol-non-fermenting (SNF) organisms other than *E. coli* O157 to be more common and more troublesome than early reports from the USA had suggested (Chapman *et al.*, 1989). The major problem organisms encountered in human faecal samples are SNF *E. coli* of serogroups other than O157 and *Proteus* spp.; in animal faecal samples and food samples, additional problem organisms may be *Escherichia hermanii* and *Aeromonas* spp. (Borczyk *et al.*, 1987b; Lior and Borczyk, 1987). Our efforts to develop better culture media therefore initially focused on controlling the growth of these other organisms.

Our first modification of SMAC (Chapman *et al.*, 1991) used fermentation of both sorbitol and rhamnose to provide better discrimination between *E. coli* O157 and other *E. coli*, and cefixime, a third-generation cephalosporin antibiotic, because it is more inhibitory to *Proteus* spp. than to *E. coli* (Stone *et al.*, 1989; Wise *et al.*, 1990). SMAC was compared with CR-SMAC for the primary isolation of *E. coli* O157 from 1763 human faecal samples. During this comparison, 411 (23.3%) organisms isolated on SMAC required further investigation, whereas only 178 did so from CR-SMAC. This offered a significant saving of time and cost for a busy diagnostic laboratory. Seven isolates of *E. coli* O157 grew on both media. However, in one instance, when six non-fermenting colonies were examined from each medium, only one colony from SMAC was *E. coli* O157, whereas all colonies from CR-SMAC were *E. coli* O157; in this case, the organism could easily have been missed using SMAC medium. *E. hermanii* is an SNF organism which may be present in foodstuffs, and which may cross-react antigenically with *E. coli* O157 (Borczyk *et al.*, 1987b; Lior and Borczyk, 1987). Strains of *E. hermanii* used during the development and those isolated from food since have all fermented rhamnose and would therefore have been excluded from further investigation using CR-SMAC. The only drawback with the medium is that rhamnose is an expensive sugar, which adds significantly to the cost of laboratory investigations.

In a further improvement to SMAC, we used potassium tellurite as an additional selective agent and omitted the rhamnose, to develop CT-SMAC (Zadik *et al.*, 1993). Tellurite has been used traditionally as a selective agent for other toxigenic bacteria, such as *Corynebacterium diphtheriae* and *Vibrio cholerae*. In our initial studies of CT-SMAC, a concentration of potassium tellurite of 2.5 mg l^{-1} allowed the growth of all strains of VT^{+} *E. coli* O157 tested, but completely inhibited the growth of 67% of other strains of *E. coli* (including VT^{-} *E. coli* O157) and 97% of strains of *Proteus* spp., *Morganella* spp., *Aeromonas* spp. and *Providencia* spp. A comparison was made of CR-SMAC and CT-SMAC for the isolation of *E. coli* O157 from swabs of rectal faeces taken from cattle immediately after slaughter (Zadik *et al.*, 1993). Of 391 samples screened on CT-SMAC medium, 26 yielded isolates of *E. coli* O157, whereas CR-SMAC yielded only nine isolates. However, some more recently reported strains of sorbitol-fermenting VT^{+} *E. coli* O157 (Aleksic *et al.*, 1992) isolated from cases of HUS in Germany (kindly supplied by Professor S. Aleksic, Hamburg) are sensitive to tellurite and so do not grow on CT-SMAC.

Another feature of *E. coli* O157 is that, unlike most other *E. coli*, they do not produce β-glucuronidase. The fluorogenic substrate 4-methylumbelliferyl β-D-glucuronide (MUG) and the chromogenic substrate 5-bromo-4-chloro-3-indoxyl-β-D-glucuronide (BCIG) have therefore been advocated for incorporation into culture media for the detection of *E. coli* O157 (Szabo *et al.*, 1986; Okrend *et al.*, 1990; Thompson *et al.*, 1990). However, the extremely high cost of these substrates would probably preclude their use in the majority of diagnostic laboratories.

Enrichment culture

While direct culture may be a suitable technique for the isolation of *E. coli* O157 from the faeces of patients with acute illness, where the organism is likely to be the predominant organism in the sample, more sensitive methods are needed for its isolation from food and environmental samples, in which numbers of the organism may be low. Standard methods for the selective isolation of *E. coli* from food have used growth at 44°C as a selective factor. However, *E. coli* O157 have an upper temperature for growth of 41°C in selective *E. coli* broth (Raghubeer and Matches, 1990) and grow only poorly at temperatures higher than this in non-selective media (Doyle and Schoeni, 1984). Standard methods are therefore ineffective for the isolation of *E. coli* O157 from food, and specific methods are needed.

Doyle and colleagues (Doyle and Schoeni, 1987; Padhye and Doyle, 1991a) have described a modified tryptone broth (mTSB), supplemented with a phosphate buffer, bile salts and either novobiocin or acriflavine. After enrichment culture of samples in mTSB, with shaking at 37°C for 24 h, the cultures were serially diluted in phosphate-buffered saline (PBS) from 10^{-5} to 10^{-7} before inoculation on to SMAC medium. Using this technique, *E. coli* O157 was isolated from a wide range of uncooked meats, although the rationale for a prolonged incubation and the subsequent dilution of the culture was not explained. A modification of the *E. coli* medium used in standard methods for food and water microbiology in the USA has also been described (Raghubeer and Matches, 1990). However, such media containing lactose are possibly best avoided for the enrichment culture of *E. coli* O157, as many other organisms that are common in the alimentary tract of humans and animals can metabolize lactose to compounds that are inhibitory to the growth and survival of the organism (Hinton *et al.*, 1991, 1992). In particular, *Enterococcus* spp. can metabolize lactose to form lactic acid, which in turn can be metabolized by *Veillonella* spp. to propionic acid and acetic acid. These three acids are inhibitory to the growth of *E. coli* O157 (Hinton *et al.*, 1991, 1992) and, indeed, both lactic acid and acetic acid have been reported as effective agents for the destruction of the organism on contaminated carcasses (Dickson, 1991; Abdul-Raouf *et al.*, 1993).

In an attempt to improve enrichment culture for isolation of *E. coli* O157 from food, we studied the minimum inhibitory concentrations (MICs) of various antimicrobial agents for over 300 *E. coli* O157 strains and a wide range of other organisms which we had commonly isolated from food samples. We found a combination of vancomycin, cefsulodin and cefixime, to inhibit Gram-positive organisms, *Aeromonas* spp. and *Proteus* spp., respectively, to be an effective supplement to buffered peptone water for the enrichment culture of *E. coli* O157. Using this medium (BPW-VCC) and incubation at 37°C for 6 h, a time that we had found to be optimum for recovery of the organism from inoculated beef samples, we isolated the organism from naturally contaminated beef carcasses for the first time in 1992 (Chapman *et al.*, 1993a). Despite our previous successful use of potassium tellurite as a selective agent in the solid CT-SMAC medium (Zadik *et al.*, 1993), we found it to be ineffective as a selective agent in liquid media. This is probably due to antagonism of tellurite metabolism both by the widely used phosphate buffer system and by the rapid development of anaerobic conditions in the enrichment culture (Tomas and Kay, 1986). Our attempts to solve this problem have so far been unsuccessful (Chapman, 1994).

Immunomagnetic separation

In 1992, we began, jointly with colleagues from Dynal, Oslo, Norway, to develop and improve an IMS technique for the selective concentration of *E. coli* O157 from enrichment cultures. Enrichment culture in BPW-VCC, followed by IMS with paramagnetic beads coated with an antibody against *E. coli* O157 (Dynabeads anti-*E. coli* O157, Dynal) and culture of beads on CT-SMAC, was approximately 100-fold more sensitive than direct culture on CR-SMAC or CT-SMAC for detection of *E. coli* O157 in inoculated bovine faecal samples (Chapman *et al.*, 1994). This increase in sensitivity was confirmed during subsequent monitoring of a dairy herd, when *E. coli* O157 was isolated from 84 (8.2%) of 1024 rectal swabs taken from cattle over a 4-month period; 23 (27.4%) of the 84 strains were isolated by both direct culture and IMS, whereas 61 (72.6%) of the 84 strains were isolated by IMS only (Chapman *et al.*, 1994). Using the IMS technique, *E. coli* O157 was isolated from two of 279 forestream milk samples from individual cattle in this dairy herd (Chapman *et al.*, 1993b; Mechie *et al.*, 1997); neither strain was isolated by direct subculture of the enrichment medium on to CT-SMAC. Inclusion of an IMS step after enrichment culture of minced beef in BPW-VCC again enhanced the sensitivity about 100-fold, when compared with direct subculture on to CT-SMAC, to a detection limit of about two *E. coli* O157 per gram of beef (Wright *et al.*, 1994).

Enrichment culture in BPW-VCC, followed by IMS, was compared with direct inoculation of CR-SMAC and CT-SMAC for isolation of *E. coli* O157 from human faecal samples. The organism was isolated from 25 (3.6%) of 690 samples by IMS but from only 15 (2.1%) by CT-SMAC and 12 (1.7%) by CR-SMAC (Chapman and Siddons, 1996a). The difference in sensitivity of detection was at its most marked on screening repeat samples from known cases and samples from asymptomatic contacts, when, of 12 strains isolated by IMS, only five were isolated by direct culture. However, when applied to the detection of *E. coli* O157 from human faeces, the IMS technique has not been free of problems. For reasons that we are unable to explain, far more SNF organisms appear to adhere non-specifically to the beads than happens with other sample types, and we are currently investigating this problem further.

Immunoassays as alternatives to culture techniques

There are several alternatives to traditional culture techniques for the identification of VTEC in samples. Detection of free faecal verocytotoxin (VT) by Vero-cell assay has been used with success as a diagnostic method (Karmali *et al.*, 1985; Chapman *et al.*, 1989; Ritchie *et al.*, 1992). However, routine use of cells suffers from the drawbacks of microbial contamination of cell monolayers and interference in the assay by a number of other microbial toxins which are active against cultured Vero cells (Chapman, 1994). Detection of free faecal VT may also be performed by enzyme immunoassays of different formats (Ashkenazi and Cleary, 1989; Acheson *et al.*, 1990), but, although these are more rapid to perform and less subjective than cell culture assays, they lack sensitivity.

Enzyme immunoassays and immunoblot techniques for the detection of *E. coli* O157 antigen have been described as methods for the detection of the organism in enrichment cultures of food and environmental samples (Doyle and Schoeni, 1987; Szabo *et al.*, 1990; Padhye and Doyle, 1991b; Sernowski and Ingham, 1992). Although sensitive, these methods may be time-consuming, technically demanding, expensive and prone to give false-positive results that cannot be confirmed by culture (Sernowski and Ingham, 1992). We have evaluated two commercially available enzyme immunoassays for the detection of *E. coli* O157 in bovine faecal samples and in artificially and naturally contaminated samples of raw beef products (Chapman and Siddons, 1996b; Chapman *et al.*, 1997b). Both assays gave a sensitivity of detection equal to that of enrichment culture in BPW-VCC, followed by IMS and CT-SMAC. However, both were prone to give false-positive results that could not be confirmed by our normal culture method; in some cases, these positive results were shown to be due to sorbitol-fermenting VT^- *E. coli* O157, which were present in the sample, and, in others, the enrichment cultures appeared to react equally well in other enzyme immunoassays for different antigens.

Typing of strains of *E. coli* O157

Further subdivision of *E. coli* O157 strains is necessary during outbreak investigations. A phage-typing scheme has been developed in Canada (Ahmed *et al.*, 1987; Khakhria *et al.*, 1990) and has been used by the national reference laboratories of England and Wales, and Scotland for the typing of *E. coli* O157 isolates submitted to them (Frost *et al.*, 1989; Krause *et al.*, 1996); the latter group concluded, however, that phage typing alone did not provide sufficient discrimination between strains. Several groups, including ourselves, have described plasmid analysis of strains of *E. coli* O157. Ratnam *et al.* (1988) examined 174 isolates from geographically diverse locations in Canada and the USA and found that most strains belonged to one of only three plasmid types; in contrast, strains from diverse locations in the UK showed considerable variation in plasmid profile (Frost *et al.*, 1989). In our studies of human and bovine isolates from the Sheffield area between 1987 and 1993, there was considerable variation in plasmid profile and toxin genotype within strains from several different single phage types. Phage type 4, for example, contained strains of two different toxin genotypes and five different plasmid profiles (Chapman *et al.*, 1993a). A combination of phage type, toxin genotype and plasmid profile provides more useful information than any one scheme used alone. Using such a combination, we were able to show that 94% of human isolates of *E. coli* O157 matched strains isolated from cattle during 1987 to 1993 (Chapman and Siddons, 1994). Other techniques, such as PFGE (Thomson-Carter *et al.*, 1993) and detection of restriction fragment length polymorphisms by hybridization with lambda-phage DNA (Samadpour *et al.*, 1993), may provide better discrimination than other typing schemes and we have occasionally found these useful in our studies (Chapman *et al.*, 1997a). Development of PFGE and various polymerase chain reaction (PCR)-based typing schemes is in progress at Sheffield PHL.

ESCHERICHIA COLI O157 SURVEILLANCE IN SHEFFIELD

In April 1995, we began a programme of surveillance of *E. coli* O157 (funded by the Department of Health) which proposed to monitor the prevalence of the organism in: (i) faecal samples collected from cattle, pigs, sheep and poultry at slaughter; (ii) a wide variety of raw meat products collected from various retail outlets; and (iii) faecal samples from human patients with acute uncomplicated diarrhoea. This surveillance programme was undertaken to determine: (i) if carriage by cattle of *E. coli* O157 was seasonal and, if so, whether this season corresponded to that observed in human infections in the Sheffield area; (ii) if the rates of carriage of *E. coli* O157 were different in prime beef cattle and dairy cattle; (iii) if other food animals were potential sources of *E. coli* O157; and (iv) if there was a relationship between acute non-bloody diarrhoea and *E. coli* O157 in the Sheffield area. Isolation of *E. coli* O157 during all the surveillance work was by enrichment culture in BPW-VCC, IMS and culture of beads on CT-SMAC. The aims of the surveillance were to elucidate further the descriptive epidemiology of *E. coli* O157 infections in the Sheffield area and thus to indicate areas for possible intervention and control.

Samples of rectal faeces were collected immediately after slaughter from 400 cattle each month for a 1-year period and from 1000 each of sheep, pigs and poultry over the same period. *E. coli* O157 was isolated from 752 (15.7%) of 4800 cattle, 22 (2.2%) of 1000 sheep and four (0.4%) of 1000 pigs, but not from any of 1000 chickens. Of the cattle sampled, 1840 (38.4%) were prime beef animals, 1661 (34.6%) were dairy animals being culled and the status could not be determined for the other 1299 (27%) animals. *E. coli* O157 was found in 246 (13.4%) of the 1840 beef cattle and 268 (16.1%) of the 1661 dairy cattle. The monthly prevalence of *E. coli* O157 in cattle varied from 4.8% to 36.8% and was at its highest in spring and late summer. Seventeen of the 22 isolates from sheep were also made over the summer period. All *E. coli* O157 isolates from sheep and 749 (99.6%) of the 752 *E. coli* O157 isolates from cattle were VT$^+$, as determined by Vero-cell assay and DNA hybridization, *eae*A gene$^+$, contained a 92-kb plasmid and were thus typical of strains causing infections in humans. In contrast, isolates from pigs were VT^-, *eae*A $gene^-$ and did not contain a 92-kb plasmid and would, therefore, be unlikely to be a source of infection for humans (Chapman *et al.*, 1997c).

The overall prevalence of *E. coli* O157, in this study 15.7%, is far higher than that reported in previous studies from the UK and USA (Chapman *et al.*, 1989, 1993a; Synge and Hopkins, 1993; Hancock *et al.*, 1994). There may be several reasons for this. There may have been a genuine increase in prevalence of *E. coli* O157 in the cattle population, a hypothesis possibly supported by the rising incidence of *E. coli* O157 infections in humans in the UK and USA over the same period. The season during which studies were conducted may also have had an effect on prevalence figures. However, it is also likely that the higher isolation rates achieved could have been a result of the more sensitive IMS method used in our study. In our previous dairy-herd study (Chapman *et al.*, 1994; Mechie *et al.*, 1997), *E. coli* O157 was isolated from about four times as many bovine rectal swabs by IMS than by direct culture; this fourfold increase in sensitivity could largely explain the increase from the 4% prevalence, as detected by direct culture, in cattle at slaughter in 1992 (Chapman *et al.*, 1993a) to the 15.7% prevalence reported from the same abattoir in this later surveillance. *E. coli* O157 was found in a slightly higher percentage of dairy cattle (16.1%) than of beef cattle (13.4%), in contrast to findings in Washington State, USA (Hancock *et al.*, 1994). There was marked month-to-month variation in the prevalence of *E. coli* O157 in cattle, with rates being highest in spring and late summer. During the period of this study, clusters of human cases of *E. coli* O157 infections were observed in May–June and also in September, a seasonal distribution remarkably similar to that for the isolation of the organism from cattle.

We also isolated *E. coli* O157 from 2.2% of 1000 sheep. Although insufficient numbers were isolated to determine any variation in seasonal prevalence, 17 were isolated in the period June–September. Since the commencement of this study, the isolation of *E. coli* O157 from sheep in Idaho has also been reported and in this study all were isolated in the summer months (Kudva *et al.*, 1996). Isolates from sheep in our study and in Idaho appear typical of those causing infections in humans, and further studies of the prevalence of *E. coli* O157 in sheep are needed. *E. coli* O157 was not isolated from 1000 chickens, indicating a prevalence of < 0.25%. Two case–control studies (Salmon *et al.*, 1989; Salmon and Smith, 1994) have statistically indicated poultry meat as a possible risk factor for infection by *E. coli* O157, although neither was confirmed microbiologically. In feeding studies performed on young chickens, three groups in the USA (Beery *et al.*, 1985; Stavric *et al.*, 1993; Schoeni and Doyle, 1994) have shown that even very low inocula of *E. coli* O157 lead to rapid colonization of the caecum and excretion of large numbers of the organism in the faeces for up to 3 months. A possible criticism of these experimental colonization studies is that all three groups used the same highly atypical strain of *E. coli* O157 which was resistant to nalidixic acid 200 mg l^{-1}. While the use of such a strain may facilitate subsequent laboratory detection of the organism, the results obtained should be interpreted with caution and further studies with more typical strains of *E. coli* O157 are probably needed. However, despite the limited experimental evidence suggesting that chickens may act as a reservoir of the organism, there have not been, to date, any microbiologically confirmed cases of *E. coli* O157 infection from a poultry source.

Our surveillance of food samples is ongoing to determine the prevalence of *E. coli* O157 in retail beef and lamb products. We examined 2062 samples collected from retail outlets in South Yorkshire during April to September 1996. Samples of 25 g were examined by enrichment culture and IMS, as described above. *E. coli* O157 was isolated from 26 (5.9%) of 431 samples of lamb products and from 25 (1.5%) of 1631 samples of beef products (Chapman *et al.*, 1996). *E. coli* O157 was isolated most frequently from lamb burgers (15 (7.2%) of 208 samples) and, on 15 separate occasions when samples of minced beef, beefburger, minced lamb and lamb burger from an individual retailer were examined, the organism was isolated only from the lamb burger. Strains of *E. coli* O157 isolated from lamb were biochemically typical of *E. coli* O157, were either serotype O157:H7 or nonmotile, hybridized with DNA probes specific for VT genes, contained the large 92-kb plasmid characteristic of VTEC and belonged to a range of plasmid types (Chapman *et al.*, 1996).

Work is continuing in an attempt to explain why the organism is apparently more prevalent in lamb products than in beef products in our area, despite a much higher prevalence in healthy cattle than in healthy sheep. Lamb and other foods of ovine origin have not been reported as sources of *E. coli* O157 infection in humans, but our findings indicate that lamb products, particularly lamb burgers, are a potential vehicle of transmission of the organism to humans.

REFERENCES

Abdul-Raouf, U.M., Beuchat, L.R. and Ammar, M.S. (1993) Survival and growth of *Escherichia coli* O157:H7 in ground, roasted beef as by pH, acidulants, and temperature. *Applied and Environmental Microbiology* 59, 2364–2368.

Acheson, D.W.K., Keusch, G.T., Lightowlers, M. and Donohue-Rolfe A. (1990) Enzyme-linked immunosorbent assay for shigatoxin and shiga-like toxin II using P1 glycoprotein from hydatid cysts. *Journal of Infectious Diseases* 161, 134–137.

Ahmed, R., Bopp, C., Borczyk, A. and Kasatiya, S. (1987) Phage typing scheme for *Escherichia coli* O157:H7. *Journal of Infectious Diseases* 155, 805–809.

Aleksic, S., Karch, H. and Bockemuhl, J. (1992) A bio-typing scheme for shiga-like (vero) toxin-producing *Escherichia coli* O157 and a list of cross reactions between O157 and other Gram-negative bacteria. *Zentrablatt Bakteriology* 276, 221–230.

Ashkenazi, S. and Cleary, T.G. (1989) Rapid method to detect shiga toxin and shiga-like toxin I based on binding to globotriosyl ceramide (Gb_3) their natural receptor. *Journal of Clinical Microbiology* 27, 1145–1150.

Beery, J.T., Doyle, M.P. and Schoeni, J.L. (1985) Colonization of chicken cecae by *Escherichia coli* associated with hemorrhagic colitis. *Applied and Environmental Microbiology* 49, 310–315.

Belongia, E.A., Osterholm, M.T., Soler, J.T., Ammend, D.A., Braun, J.E. and MacDonald K.L. (1993) Transmission of *Escherichia coli* O157:H7 infection in Minnesota child care facilities. *Journal of the American Medical Association* 269, 883–888.

Borczyk, A.A., Karmali, M.A., Lior, H. and Duncan, L.M.C. (1987a) Bovine reservoir for verotoxin-producing *Escherichia coli* O157:H7. *Lancet* i, 98.

Borczyk, A.A., Lior, H. and Ciebin, B. (1987b) False positive identifications of *Escherichia coli* O157 in foods. *International Journal of Food Microbiology* 4, 347–349.

British Paediatric Surveillance Unit (BPSU) (1989) *Third Annual Report 1988–1989.* BPSU, London.

Carter, A.O., Borczyk, A.A., Carlson, J.A.K., Harvey, B., Hockin, J.C., Karmali, M.A., Kriskna, C., Korn, D.A. and Lior, H. (1987) A severe outbreak of *Escherichia coli* O157:H7-associated haemorrhagic colitis in a nursing home. *New England Journal of Medicine* 317, 1496–1500.

Centers for Disease Control (1993) Update: multistate outbreak of *Escherichia coli* O157:H7 infections from hamburgers – western United States, 1992–1993. *Morbidity and Mortality Weekly Report* 42, 258–263.

Chapman, P.A. (1994) Isolation, identification and typing of Vero cytotoxin-producing *Escherichia coli. PHLS Microbiology Digest* 111, 13–17.

Chapman, P.A. and Siddons, C.A. (1994) A comparison of strains of *Escherichia coli* O157 from humans and cattle in Sheffield, United Kingdom. *Journal of Infectious Diseases* 170, 251–252.

Chapman, P.A. and Siddons, C.A. (1996a) A comparison of immunomagnetic separation and direct culture for the isolation of verocytotoxin-producing *Escherichia coli* O157 from cases of bloody diarrhoea, non-bloody diarrhoea and asymptomatic contacts. *Journal of Medical Microbiology* 44, 267–271.

Chapman, P.A. and Siddons, C.A. (1996b) Evaluation of a commercial enzyme immunoassay (EHEC-Tek) for detecting *Escherichia coli* O157 in beef and beef products. *Food Microbiology* 13, 175–182.

Chapman, P.A., Wright, D.J. and Norman, P. (1989) Verotoxin-producing *Escherichia coli* infections in Sheffield: cattle as a possible source. *Epidemiology and Infection* 102, 439–445.

Chapman, P.A., Jewes, L., Siddons, C.A., Norman, P. and George, S.L. (1990) Verocytotoxin-producing *Escherichia coli* infections in Sheffield: 1985–1989. *Public Health Laboratory Service Microbiology Digest* 7, 163–166.

Chapman, P.A., Siddons, C.A., Zadik, P.M. and Jewes, L. (1991) An improved selective medium for the isolation of *Escherichia coli* O157. *Journal of Medical Microbiology* 35, 107–110.

Chapman, P.A., Siddons, C.A., Wright, D.J., Norman, P., Fox, J. and Crick, E. (1993a) Cattle as a possible source of verocytotoxin-producing *Escherichia coli* O157 infections in man. *Epidemiology and Infection* 111, 439–447.

Chapman, P.A., Wright, D.J. and Higgins, R. (1993b) Untreated milk as a source of verotoxigenic *E. coli* O157. *Veterinary Record* 133, 171–172.

Chapman, P.A., Wright, D.J. and Siddons, C.A. (1994) A comparison of immunomagnetic separation and direct culture for the isolation of verocytotoxin-producing *Escherichia coli* O157 from bovine faeces. *Journal of Medical Microbiology* 40, 424–427.

Chapman, P.A., Siddons, C.A., Cerdan Malo, A.T. and Harkin, M.A. (1996) Lamb products as a potential source of verocytotoxin-producing *Escherichia coli* O157. *Veterinary Record* 139, 427–428.

Chapman, P.A., Siddons, C.A., Manning, J. and Cheetam, C. (1997a) An outbreak of infection due to verocytotoxin-producing *Escherichia coli* O157: the influence of laboratory methods on the outcome of the investigation. *Epidemiology and Infection* 119, 113–119.

Chapman, P.A., Cerdan Malo, A.T., Siddons, C.A. and Harkin, M. (1997b) Use of commercial enzyme immunoassays and immunomagnetic separation systems for detecting *Escherichia coli* O157 in bovine fecal samples. *Applied and Environmental Microbiology* 63, 2549–2553.

Chapman, P.A., Siddons, C.A., Cerdan Malo, A.T. and Harkin, M.A. (1997c) A one year study of *Escherichia coli* O157 in cattle, pigs, sheep and poultry. *Epidemiology and Infection* 119, 245–250.

Cubbon, M.D., Coia, J.E., Hanson, M.F. and Thomson-Carter, F. (1996) A comparison of immunomagnetic separation, direct culture and polymerase chain reaction for the detection of verocytotoxin-producing *Escherichia coli* in human faeces. *Journal of Medical Microbiology* 44, 219–222.

Dickson, J.S. (1991) Control of *Salmonella typhimurium, Listeria monocytogenes* and *Escherichia coli* O157:H7 on beef and a model spray chilling system. *Journal of Food Science* 56, 191–193.

Doyle, M.P. and Schoeni, J.L. (1984) Survival and growth characteristics of *Escherichia coli* associated with hemorrhagic colitis. *Applied and Environmental Microbiology* 48, 855–856.

Doyle, M.P. and Schoeni, J.L. (1987) Isolation of *Escherichia coli* O157:H7 from retail fresh meats and poultry. *Applied and Environmental Microbiology* 53, 2394–2396.

Faith, N.G., Shere, J.A., Brosch, R., Arnold, K.W., Ansay, S.E., Lee, M.S., Luchansky, J.B. and Kaspar, C.W. (1996) Prevalence and clonal nature of *Escherichia coli* O157:H7 on dairy farms in Wisconsin. *Applied and Environmental Microbiology* 62, 1519–1525.

Frost, J.A., Smith, H.R., Willshaw, G.A., Scotland, S.M., Gross, R.J. and Rowe, B. (1989) Phage typing of vero-cytotoxin (VT) producing *Escherichia coli* O157 isolated in the United Kingdom. *Epidemiology and Infection* 103, 73–81.

Gannon, V.P.J., Gyles, C.L. and Friendship, R.W. (1988) Characteristics of verotoxigenic *Escherichia coli* from pigs. *Canadian Journal of Veterinary Research* 52, 331–337.

Hancock, D.D., Besser, T.E., Kinsell, M.L., Tarr, P.I., Rice, D.H. and Paros, M.G. (1994) The prevalence of *Escherichia coli* O157.H7 in dairy and beef cattle in Washington State. *Epidemiology and Infection* 113, 199–207.

Hinton, A., Spates, G.E., Corrier, D.E., Hume, M.E., Deloach, J.R. and Scanlan, C.M. (1991) *In vitro* inhibition of *Salmonella typhimurium* and *Escherichia coli* O157:H7 by bacteria isolated from the cecal contents of adult chickens. *Journal of Food Protection* 54, 496–501.

Hinton, A., Corrier, D.E. and Deloach, J.R. (1992) *In vitro* inhibition of *Salmonella typhimurium*, and *Escherichia coli* O157:H7 by an anaerobic Gram-positive coccus from the cecal contents of adult chickens. *Journal of Food Protection* 55, 162–166.

Karch, H., Russmann, H., Schmidt, H., Schwarzkopf, A. and Heesemann, J. (1995) Long-term shedding and clonal turnover of enterohemorrhagic *Escherichia coli* O157 in diarrheal diseases. *Journal of Clinical Microbiology* 33, 1602–1605.

Karch, H., Janetzki-Mittmann, C., Aleksic, S. and Datz, M. (1996) Isolation of enterohemorrhagic *Escherichia coli* O157 strains from patients with hemolytic–uremic syndrome by using immunomagnetic separation, DNA-based methods and direct culture. *Journal of Clinical Microbiology* 34, 516–519.

Karmali, M.A. (1989) Infection by verocytotoxin-producing *Escherichia coli. Clinical Microbiology Reviews* 2, 15–38.

Karmali, M.A., Steele, B.T., Petric, M. and Lim, C. (1983) Sporadic cases of haemolytic–uraemic syndrome associated with faecal cytotoxin and cytotoxin-producing *Escherichia coli* in stools. *Lancet* i, 619–620.

Karmali, M.A., Petric, M., Lim, C., Fleming, P.C., Arbus, G.S. and Lior, H. (1985) The association between idiopathic hemolytic uraemic syndrome and infection by verotoxin-producing *Escherichia coli. Journal of Infectious Diseases* 151, 775–782.

Khakhria, R., Duck, D. and Lior, H. (1990) Extended phage typing scheme for *Escherichia coli* O157:H7. *Epidemiology and Infection* 105, 511–520.

Krause, U., Thomson-Carter, F.M. and Pennington, T.H. (1996) Molecular epidemiology of *Escherichia coli* O157:H7 by pulsed field gel electrophoresis and comparison with that of phage typing. *Journal of Clinical Microbiology* 34, 959–961.

Kudva, I.T., Hatfield, P.G. and Hovde C.J. (1995) Effect of diet on the shedding of *Escherichia coli* O157:H7 in a sheep model. *Applied and Environmental Microbiology* 61, 1363–1370.

Kudva, I.T., Hatfield, P.G. and Hovde, C.J. (1996) *Escherichia coli* O157:H7 in microbial flora of sheep. *Journal of Clinical Microbiology* 34, 431–433.

Kudva, I.T., Hunt, C.W., Williams, C.J., Nance, U.M. and Hovde, C.J. (1997) Evaluation of dietary influences on *Escherichia coli* O157:H7 shedding by sheep. *Applied and Environmental Microbiology* 63, 3878–3886.

Linggood, M.A. and Thompson, J.M. (1987) Verotoxin production among porcine strains of *Escherichia coli* and its association with oedema disease. *Journal of Medical Microbiology* 25, 359–362.

Lior, H. and Borczyk, A.A. (1987) False positive identifications of *Escherichia coli* O157. *Lancet* i, 333.

Lopez, E.L., Diaz, M., Grinstein, S., Devoto, S., Mendilaharzu, F., Murray, B.E., Ashkenazi, S., Rubeglio, E., Woloj, M., Vasquez, M., Turco, M., Pickering, L.K. and Cleary, T.G. (1989) Hemolytic uremic syndrome and diarrhea in Argentine children: the role of shiga-like toxins. *Journal of Infectious Diseases* 160, 469–475.

March, S.B. and Ratnam, S. (1986) Sorbitol MacConkey medium for the detection of *Escherichia coli* O157:H7 associated with hemorrhagic colitis. *Journal of Clinical Microbiology* 23, 869–872.

Martin, M.L., Shipman, L.D., Wells, J.G., Potter, M.E., Hedberg, K., Wachsmuth, I.K., Tauxe, R.V., Davis, J.P., Arnold, J. and Tilleli, J. (1986) Isolation of *Escherichia coli* O157:H7 from dairy cattle associated with two cases of haemolytic uraemic syndrome. *Lancet* ii, 1043.

Mechie, S.C., Chapman, P.A. and Siddons, C.A. (1997) A fifteen month field study of *Escherichia coli* O157 in a dairy herd. *Epidemiology and Infection* 118, 17–25.

Okrend, A.J.G., Rose, B.E. and Lattuada, C.P. (1990) Use of 5-bromo-4-chloro-3-indoxyl-β-D-glucuronide in MacConkey sorbitol agar to aid the isolation of *Escherichia coli* O157:H7 from ground beef. *Journal of Food Protection* 53, 941–943.

Ørskov, F., Ørskov, I. and Villar, J.A. (1987) Cattle as a reservoir of verotoxin-producing *Escherichia coli* O157:H7. *Lancet* ii, 276.

Padhye, N.V. and Doyle, M.P. (1991a) Rapid procedure for detecting entero-hemorrhagic *Escherichia coli* O157:H7 in food. *Applied and Environmental Microbiology* 57, 2693–2698.

Padhye, N.V. and Doyle, M.P. (1991b) Production and characterization of a monoclonal antibody specific for enterohemorrhagic *Escherichia coli* of serotypes O157:H7 and 026:H11. *Journal of Clinical Microbiology* 29, 99–103.

Pai, C.H., Gordon, R., Simms, H.V. and Bryan, L.E. (1984) Sporadic cases of hemorrhagic colitis associated with *Escherichia coli* O157:H7. *Annals of Internal Medicine* 101, 738–742.

Raghubeer, E.V. and Matches, J.R. (1990) Temperature range for growth of *Escherichia coli* O157:H7 and selected coliforms in *E. coli* medium. *Journal of Clinical Microbiology* 28, 803–805.

Ratnam, S., March, S.B., Ahmed, R., Bezanson, G.S. and Kasatiya, S. (1988) Characterisation of *Escherichia coli* serotype O157:H7. *Journal of Clinical Microbiology* 26, 2006–2012.

Riley, L.W., Remis, R.S., Helgerson, S.D., McGee, H.B., Wells, J.G., Davis, B.R., Herbert, R.J., Olcott, E.S., Johnson, L.M., Hargrett, N.T., Blake, P.A. and Cohen, M.L. (1983) Haemorrhagic colitis associated with a rare *Escherichia coli* serotype. *New England Journal of Medicine* 308, 681–685.

Ritchie, M., Partington, S., Jessop, J. and Kelly, M.T. (1992) Comparison of direct shiga-like toxin assay and sorbitol MacConkey agar culture for laboratory diagnosis of enterohemorrhagic *Escherichia coli* infection. *Journal of Clinical Microbiology* 30, 461–464.

Salmon, R.L. and Smith, R.M.M. (1994) How common is *Escherichia coli* O157 and where is it coming from? Total population surveillance in Wales 1990–1993. In: Karmali, M.A. and Goglio, A.G. (eds) *Recent Advances in Verocytotoxin-producing* Escherichia coli *Infections*. Elsevier Science BV, Amsterdam, The Netherlands, pp. 73–75.

Salmon, R.L., Farrell, I.D., Hutchison, J.G.P., Coleman, D.J., Gross, R.J., Fry, N.K., Rowe, B. and Palmer, S.R.A. (1989) A christening party outbreak of haemorrhagic colitis and haemolytic–uraemic syndrome associated with *Escherichia coli* O157:H7. *Epidemiology and Infection* 103, 249–254.

Samadpour, M., Grimm, L.M., Desai, B., Alfi, D., Ongerth, J.E. and Tarr, P.I. (1993) Molecular epidemiology of *Escherichia coli* O157:H7 strains by bacteriophage l restriction fragment length polymorphism analysis: application to a multistate foodborne outbreak and a day-care center cluster. *Journal of Clinical Microbiology* 31, 3179–3183.

Schoeni, J.L. and Doyle, M.P. (1994) Variable colonization of chickens perorally inoculated with *Escherichia coli* O157:H7 and subsequent contamination of eggs. *Applied and Environmental Microbiology* 60, 2958–2962.

Sernowski, L.P. and Ingham, S.C. (1992) Frequency of false presumptive positive results obtained using a commercial ELISA kit to screen retail ground beef for *Escherichia coli* O157:H7. *Journal of Food Protection* 55, 846.

Shah, S., Hoffman, R., Shillam, P. and Wilson, B. (1996) Prolonged fecal shedding of *Escherichia coli* O157:H7 during an outbreak at a day care center. *Clinical Infectious Diseases* 23, 835–836.

Siddons, C.A. and Chapman, P.A. (1993) Detection of serum and faecal antibodies in haemorrhagic colitis caused by *Escherichia coli* O157. *Journal of Medical Microbiology* 39, 408–415.

Smith, H.R., Rowe, B., Gross, R.J., Fry, N.K. and Scotland, S.M. (1987) Haemorrhagic colitis and Vero-cytotoxin-producing *Escherichia coli* in England and Wales. *Lancet* i, 1062–1065.

Stavric, S., Buchanan, B. and Gleeson, T.M. (1993) Intestinal colonization of young chicks with *Escherichia coli* O157:H7 and other verotoxin-producing serotypes. *Journal of Applied Bacteriology* 74, 557–563.

Stone, J.W., Linong, G., Andrews, J.M. and Wise, R. (1989) Cefixime, in-vitro activity, pharmacokinetics and tissue penetration. *Journal of Antimicrobial Chemotherapy* 23, 221–228.

Synge, B.A. and Hopkins, G.F. (1993) Verotoxigenic *Escherichia coli* O157 in Scottish calves. *Veterinary Record* 130, 583.

Szabo, R.A., Todd, E.C. and Jean, A. (1986) A method to isolate *Escherichia coli* O157:H7 from food. *Journal of Food Protection* 49, 768–772.

Szabo, R.A.E., Todd, E., MacKenzie, J., Parrington, L. and Armstrong, A. (1990) Increased sensitivity of the rapid hydrophobic grid membrane filter enzyme labelled antibody procedure for *Escherichia coli* O157 detection in foods and bovine feces. *Applied and Environmental Microbiology* 56, 3546–3549

Tarr, P.I., Neill, M.A., Clausen, C.R., Watkins, S.L., Christie, D.L. and Hickman, R.O. (1990) *Escherichia coli* O157:H7 and the haemolytic uremic syndrome: importance of early cultures in establishing etiology. *Journal of Infectious Diseases* 162, 553–556.

Taylor, C.M., White, R.H.R., Winterborn, M.H. and Rowe, B. (1986) Haemolytic-uraemic syndrome: clinical experience of an outbreak in the West Midlands. *British Medical Journal* 292, 1513–1516.

Thompson, J.S., Hodge, D.S. and Borczyk, A.A. (1990) Rapid biochemical test to identify vero-cytotoxin-positive strains of *Escherichia coli* serotype O157. *Journal of Clinical Microbiology* 28, 2165–2168.

Thomson-Carter, F.M., Carter, P.E. and Pennington, T.H. (1993) Pulsed field gel electrophoresis in the analysis of bacterial populations. In: Kroll, R.G., Gilmour, A. and Sussman, M. (eds) *New Techniques in Food and Beverage Microbiology*. Blackwell Scientific Publications, Oxford, pp. 251–264.

Tomas, J.M. and Kay, W.W. (1986) Tellurite susceptibility and non-plasmid mediated resistance in *Escherichia coli*. *Antimicrobial Agents and Chemotherapy* 30, 127–131.

Walker, C.W., Upson, R. and Warren, R.E. (1988) Haemorrhagic colitis: detection of verotoxin-producing *Escherichia coli* in a clinical microbiology laboratory. *Journal of Clinical Pathology* 41, 80–84.

Wells, J.G., Davis, B.R., Wachsmuth, I.K., Riley, L.W., Remis, R.S., Sokolov, R. and Morris, G.K. (1983) Laboratory investigation of hemorrhagic colitis associated with a rare *Escherichia coli* serotype. *Journal of Clinical Microbiology* 18, 518–520.

Wise, R., Andrews, J.M., Ashby, J.P. and Thorner, D. (1990) *In vitro* activity of Bay v 322, a new cephalosporin, compared with activities of other agents. *Antimicrobial Agents and Chemotherapy* 34, 813–818.

Wright, D.J., Chapman, P.A. and Siddons, C.A. (1994) Immunomagnetic separation as a sensitive method for isolating *Escherichia coli* O157 from food samples. *Epidemiology and Infection* 113, 31–39.

Zadik, P.M., Chapman, P.A. and Siddons, C.A. (1993) Use of tellurite for the selection of verocytotoxigenic *Escherichia coli* O157. *Journal of Medical Microbiology* 39, 155–158.

Escherichia coli O157 and Other Types of Verocytotoxigenic *E. coli* (VTEC) Isolated from Humans, Animals and Food in Germany

9

L. Beutin

Robert Koch Institute, Division of Emerging Bacterial Pathogens, Berlin, Germany

INTRODUCTION

The first known human isolates of verocytotoxigenic *Escherichia coli* (VTEC) belonging to serogroup O157 in Germany were from patients with bloody diarrhoea and haemolytic uraemic syndrome (HUS) and date back to 1987 (Wuthe, 1987; Aleksic *et al.*, 1992). In the same year, VTEC O157:H7 were isolated for the first time from cattle (Montenegro *et al.*, 1990). Since that time, VTEC have been more intensively examined for in human patients, animal populations and food in Germany. From the beginning, most studies did not focus on detection of VTEC O157 alone, but employed methods suitable for detection of all VTEC types, such as verocytotoxin (VT)-specific DNA probes, polymerase chain reaction (PCR) techniques, enzyme-linked immunosorbent assays (ELISAs) and the Vero cell toxicity test. As a result of these studies, VTEC belonging to different serotypes were detected in faeces of healthy domestic animals, such as cattle, sheep, goats and pigs, and a number of different VTEC types were isolated from stools of human patients with diarrhoea or HUS in Germany.

Retrospective investigations of old *E. coli* strain collections revealed that VTEC were already present in animals and humans in Germany more than 30 years ago. Thus, the oldest VTEC isolate from cattle (O113:H21, VT2) dates back to 1965 (Beutin and Müller, 1998) and the oldest human VTEC isolate (O114:H4, VT1) was from a diarrhoeic patient in 1967 (Beutin *et al.*, 1990). The finding that VTEC were already present in the 1960s was also reported for other European countries, such as Belgium, Denmark, the UK and Italy (Pohl, 1991; summarized in Beutin and Müller, 1998).

VTEC IN HUMANS

VTEC surveillance and estimated VTEC incidence in Germany

There are currently no established nationwide surveillance systems for HUS or for human infections with *E. coli* O157 and other VTEC types in Germany. Since 1996, three of the 16 German federal states (Bundesländer) made it mandatory to notify specifically human infections with all types of VTEC within their regions. Work is in progress to establish an HUS and VTEC surveillance network for the whole country by legislation and by concerted action between federal health institutes (Anon., 1997a). VTEC infections in humans and HUS became mandatory notifiable diseases in Germany in November 1998.

Epidemiological investigations on VTEC incidence in humans and animals in Germany are mainly performed in national reference laboratories and in some specialized public health and university institutes. The results of these studies give an estimate of the significance of VTEC O157 and other VTEC types in human patients, animals and food in Germany.

During the last few years, VTEC O157 and other VTEC types have been isolated from infected humans living in rural and urban areas in different parts of Germany (Beutin *et al.*, 1994a, b, 1996a; Bockemühl and Karch, 1996; Bockemühl *et al.*, 1997). It was a general observation that the VTEC detection rates from human patients had increased over this time. It is not known, however, to what degree this finding reflects a real increase in VTEC infections of humans. In part, this observation might be attributed to the increased surveillance and improved diagnosis of these pathogens, which was facilitated by the introduction of commercially available diagnostic tests (VT ELISA, VTEC reversed passive latex agglutination (RPLA) test) for detection of verotoxins VT1 and VT2 in routine laboratories (Anon., 1997a; Beutin *et al.*, 1998a).

Several studies were performed to determine the VTEC incidence in different groups of human patients. For the paediatric population in the area of Würzburg (Bavaria), the incidence of VTEC infections was calculated as 33 hospitalized patients per 100,000 for children less than 6 years of age (Huppertz *et al.*, 1996). The estimated incidence of VTEC infections in humans varied from 0.3 to 1.2 per 100,000 population between different federal states, with voluntary notification up to 2.5 per 100,000 in Bavaria (mandatory notification) in 1997. A significantly higher incidence of 13 VTEC-infected humans per 100,000 population was calculated on the basis of a laboratory-based sentinel study performed on 3670 diarrhoeic patients (Anon., 1998).

Outbreaks of VTEC infections have been less frequently observed in Germany compared with the USA or the UK. However, significantly higher incidence rates of VTEC O157 infections and HUS cases in children were observed in some regions of Germany (Münsterland 1994, Bavaria 1995/96 and Lower Saxony 1997) and these were related to local outbreaks. Contaminated raw milk and meat products were suspected as possible vehicles of transmission of infections (Anon., 1996a, b, 1997b; Störmann *et al.*, 1996).

A well-documented outbreak of VTEC O157:H7 occurred in August 1992 in a day-care centre in northern Germany and was related to person-to-person spread. The outbreak affected 39 children, two adults and four asymptomatic carriers (Reida *et al.*, 1994). Person-to-person transmission and asymptomatic carriership of VTEC was found to be common in small outbreaks in families involving adults and children (Ludwig *et al.*, 1996, 1997; Pulz, 1997; Beutin *et al.*, 1998a). Although most VTEC infections in Germany are reported as sporadic, outbreak investigations are not always performed. It is therefore likely that a certain number of infections which are registered as sporadic could be part of small unidentified outbreaks (Karch *et al.*, 1990; Pulz, 1997; Beutin *et al.*, 1998a, b).

Outbreaks with non-O157 VTEC have been rarely reported. Unpasteurized milk contaminated with VTEC O22:H8 was identified as the source of a family outbreak in 1989 causing HUS in a 4-year-old girl, whereas all other family members were asymptomatic excreters of the pathogen (Bockemühl *et al.*, 1990). Two unrelated outbreaks in families with diarrhoeal episodes were caused by VTEC O145:H− strains carrying the genes for VT2 and intimin (*eae*$^+$) in Berlin and VTEC Orough (VT1$^+$, *eae*$^+$) in Augsburg (Bavaria) in 1996 (Beutin *et al.*, 1998a).

VTEC in diarrhoeic humans

A number of studies have been performed in order to determine the frequency of VTEC infections in groups of hospitalized and ambulant patients with diarrhoea. Table 9.1 summarizes the data obtained from investigations on a total of 13,564 human diarrhoeic patients, which were performed between 1988 and 1996. The studies differed from each other in sample size, patient groups and their geographical origin, but also in the detection methods used for identification of VTEC in stool specimens. VTEC-infected patients were observed in all studies; however, the VTEC incidence varied from 0.7% to 9.3% between different surveys and patient groups. The average incidence of VTEC-infected patients was 2.6%. VTEC O157 strains were isolated from patients in all except one of the studies, but less frequently than non-O157 VTEC strains. The incidence of VTEC O157 infections in diarrhoeic humans varied from 0.1% to 2.7%.

Infections with sorbitol-fermenting (SF)-VTEC O157:H− strains were frequently reported in patients living in Bavaria (Gunzer *et al.*, 1992; Karch *et al.*, 1997; Pulz, 1997). Six of 12 VTEC O157 strains isolated from humans

Table 9.1. VTEC from diarrhoeic humans.

Patients (age group)	No. examined	Patients with VTEC (%)	Patients with VTEC O157 (%)	Geographical region and time period	Method of investigation (reference)
Diarrhoeic, hospitalized	668	62 (9.3)	18[a] (2.7)	Germany, 1988–1991	VT-gene probes (Gunzer *et al.*, 1992)
Diarrhoeic	2,165	50 (2.3)	28[a] (1.3)	Germany, 1988–1991	Vero cell test, VT-gene probes (Beutin *et al.*, 1994a)
Diarrhoeic	802	42 (5.2)	1 (0.1)	Bavaria, 1989–1992	VT-gene probes (Rüssmann, 1992)
Diarrhoeic, hospitalized (0–1 year)	282	2 (0.7)	0	Berlin, 1991/92	Vero cell test (Hübner *et al.*, 1997)
Diarrhoeic, hospitalized (2 months–16 years)	468	13[b] (2.8)	2[c] (0.6)	Würzburg, Bavaria, 1994	VT-PCR (Huppertz *et al.*, 1996)
Diarrhoeic children	2,320	22 (1.0)	7 (0.3)	Würzburg, Bavaria, 1991–1993 and 1995	VT-PCR (Karch *et al.*, 1997)
Diarrhoeic and contact persons	2,712	53[d] (2.0)	12[c] (0.4)	Bavaria, 1995/96	VT-ELISA; VT-PCR (Pulz, 1997)
Diarrhoeic	477	5 (1.0)	1 (0.2)	Berlin, 1995/96	VT-PCR, Vero cell test, VT-ELISA, enterohaemolysin agar (Beutin *et al.*, 1997)
Diarrhoea	3,670	108 (2.9)	12 (0.3)	Germany, 1997	VT-PCR (Anon., 1998)
Total	13,564	357 (2.6)	81 (0.6)		

[a] Five were from HUS patients.
[b] Three were from nosocomial infections.
[c] One was from HUS.
[d] Three were from HUS patients.

in northern Bavaria were SF (Pulz, 1997) and the majority of the VTEC O157 isolates from patients in the area of Würzburg were of the SF type (Karch *et al.*, 1997).

Although *E. coli* O157 is the most important VTEC type found in patients with bloody diarrhoea or HUS in Germany, an increasing number of non-O157 VTEC serotypes have been found to be associated with human illness (Bockemühl and Karch, 1996; Karch *et al.*, 1997; Pulz, 1997, Beutin *et al.*, 1998a). However, severe diarrhoea and HUS were closely associated with VTEC types carrying additional virulence markers, such as the genes for intimin (*eae*) and for enterohaemolysin production (enterohaemorrhagic *E. coli* (EHEC)-*hly*), properties which are also characteristic for human virulent VTEC O157:H7 strains. Among this group of virulent non-O157 VTEC strains, the serotypes O26:[H11]; O103:H2; O111:H−; O118:H16 and O145:[H28]) were most common in human patients (Bockemühl and Karch, 1996; Bockemühl *et al.*, 1997; Karch *et al.*, 1997; Pulz, 1997; Beutin *et al.*, 1998a).

In contrast, other serotypes of non-O157 VTEC which are negative for the *eae* gene and, in some cases, also for enterohaemolysin have been rarely implicated in severe human illness but have been more frequently found in asymptomatic carriers or in uncomplicated cases of diarrhoea and in adult patients (Pulz, 1997; Beutin *et al.*, 1998a). Further work is necessary to investigate the epidemiological importance of the different non-O157 VTEC-types and to determine their possible role in human infections and disease.

VTEC in humans with HUS

VTEC infections can result in the development of HUS, particularly in young infants and elderly patients. Enteropathic HUS (D^+ HUS) caused by VTEC is generally preceded by gastrointestinal illness such as diarrhoea, abdominal pain and vomiting (Griffin and Tauxe, 1991; Anon., 1995). The prevalence of VTEC in HUS patients and the VTEC types associated with HUS in Germany have been the subject of different studies. In contrast to VTEC-associated diarrhoea, *E. coli* O157 were found to dominate in D^+ HUS patients with VTEC infection. Thus, VTEC of serogroup O157 were detected in 70–80% of the VTEC-excreting HUS patients examined in Germany between 1993 and 1996 (Beutin *et al.*, 1994a, 1996a; Bockemühl and Karch, 1996; Bockemühl *et al.*, 1997). The majority of D^+ HUS patients were young children with a peak incidence in the age between 0 and 4 years and only a few cases were associated with adults (Beutin *et al.*, 1996a; Anon., 1997a; Bockemühl *et al.*, 1997). Table 9.2 summarizes the results obtained from four different investigations made on HUS patients in Germany. VTEC could be isolated from the stools of 145 (28.0%) of 518 HUS patients and 112 (77.2%) of the 145 VTEC-positive stool samples from HUS patients yielded VTEC of serotype O157:H7 or O157:H−. Among the VTEC O157 isolates

Table 9.2. VTEC from HUS patients.

No. of HUS patients in study	HUS patients, geographical origin	Patients with VTEC isolate (%)	Patients with VTEC O157 isolate (%)	Numbers of VTEC O157/ total VTEC isolates (%)	Method of investigation (reference)
104	Germany, 1988–1991	33 (31.8)	26[a] (25.0)	26/33 (78.8)	VT-gene probes (Gunzer *et al.*, 1992)
44	Würzburg, Bavaria, 1992	12 (27.3)	8 (18.2)	8/12 (66.7)	VT-gene probes (Rüssmann, 1992)
347[b]	Germany, 1994/95	88 (25.4)	70 (20.1)[c]	70/88 (78.4)	VT-PCR, SMAC agar (Karch *et al.*, 1997)
23	Berlin, 1995/96	12 (52.2)	8 (34.7)	8/12 (66.7)	VT-PCR, Vero cell test, VT-ELISA, enterohaemolysin test (Beutin *et al.*, 1997)
518		145 (28.0)	112 (21.4)	112/145 (77.2)	

[a] Fourteen of 26 VTEC O157 isolates from patients were sorbitol-fermenting.
[b] Only 201 stool samples were microbiologically investigated; by analysis of patients' serum samples, an additional 20 patients (14%) were found to be positive for antibodies to *E. coli* O157.
[c] Eleven patients were infected with sorbitol-fermenting VTEC O157.
SMAC, sorbitol MacConkey agar.

from HUS patients from Bavaria, SF O157:H− strains accounted for 15.7% of all VTEC O157 isolates in one study (Karch *et al.*, 1997) and 53.8% in another study (Gunzer *et al.*, 1992).

Besides VTEC O157, an increasing number of different non-O157 VTEC strains have been isolated from HUS cases (Table 9.3). With a few exceptions, the non-O157 VTEC strains from HUS patients were positive for the *eae* gene and for enterohaemolysin. The most frequent non-O157 VTEC groups from HUS patients were O26, O111, O103, O145 and O-rough (Bockemühl *et al.*, 1997; Karch *et al.*, 1997; Beutin *et al.*, 1998a). VTEC belonging to other serotypes were isolated only from single cases.

VTEC in humans not suffering from diarrhoea or HUS

A few non-diarrhoeic human control groups have been investigated for faecal VTEC. VTEC were not detected in 205 healthy infants aged between 0 and 2 years (Beutin *et al.*, 1989) or in 171 healthy humans of different ages (Rüssmann, 1992). Similarly, VTEC were not found in a survey of 323 hospitalized, non-diarrhoeic paediatric patients, which served as a control group for a study on diarrhoeic patients (Huppertz *et al.*, 1996). In another study, one (0.5%) of 184 hospitalized patients who were negative for diarrhoea and HUS excreted VTEC (Gunzer *et al.*, 1992).

In contrast to these findings, asymptomatic carriers of VTEC were more frequently found in outbreak investigations, among persons who were in close contact with infected patients, generally in adults, in children consuming raw milk and in patients recovering from VTEC infections. In

Table 9.3. Non-O157 VTEC isolated from HUS patients in Germany.

Serotype	Number of cases reported	Reference
O26:H11; NM	12	Rüssmann, 1992; Bockemühl *et al.*, 1997; Karch *et al.*, 1997; L. Beutin *et al.* (unpublished)
O111:NM; NT	6	Karch *et al.*, 1997; Beutin *et al.*, 1998a; Bitzan *et al.*, 1988
O103:H2	3	Bockemühl *et al.*, 1997; Beutin *et al.*, 1998a
O145:H28; NM	2	Beutin *et al.*, 1996a, 1998a
O-rough:H11; NM	2	Beutin *et al.*, 1997; Karch *et al.*, 1997
Others*	7	*

* VTEC O2:H6; O8:H21; O69:H−; O119:H5 (Karch *et al.*, 1997), O22:H8 (Bockemühl *et al.*, 1990); O15:H2 and O118:H16 (Beutin *et al.*, 1997, 1998a) were isolated from single cases of HUS in Germany.
NM, non-motile; NT, non-typable.

these investigations, epidemiologically related strains of VTEC O157:H7 or O157:H− could be isolated from both the stools of asymptomatic carriers and from diseased humans (Reida *et al.*, 1994; Karch *et al.*, 1995; Pulz, 1997; Beutin *et al.*, 1998b; Pulz *et al.*, 1998).

Surveillance of VTEC infections in Bavaria revealed high proportions of non-diarrhoeic human excreters. In 1997, 30% of 300 reported cases of human VTEC infections could be attributed to non-diarrhoeic excreters (Anon., 1998). A survey in northern Bavaria on 2712 children and adults with and without diarrhoeal disease, including investigations of single cases and outbreaks, showed that 60% (32 of 53) of VTEC-infected humans were asymptomatic excreters (Pulz, 1997). Asymptomatic carriers were more frequently found among adults and the VTEC strains associated with these cases were more often found to be negative for the *eae* gene and for enterohaemolysin (Pulz, 1997). Another survey was performed in Lower Saxony on 1697 asymptomatic children and 175 adults from different day-care centres. Consumption of certified raw milk was known for 1019 children, and 15 (0.8%) human excreters shedding VTEC O157, O111, O145 and other types were detected in this study (Pulz *et al.*, 1998).

An association between VTEC serotypes, virulence markers, age of patients and severity of disease was also found by investigation of 89 non-O157 VTEC-infected humans from different parts of Germany in 1996. The association for *eae*$^{+}$ VTEC was with severe diarrhoeal disease, HUS and young age, while *eae*$^{-}$ VTEC were more associated with clinically uncomplicated cases and adult patients (Beutin *et al.*, 1998a).

VTEC IN ANIMALS

VTEC in cattle

Cattle are one of the most important reservoirs for VTEC and most of the studies performed on VTEC in animal populations in Germany have been done with bovines. Between 1987 and 1996, six separate investigations on VTEC in cattle were conducted with animals in different parts of Germany. A total of 1596 cattle were examined and the results of the studies are summarized in Table 9.4.

Most of the investigations were performed with healthy animals (calves, bulls and dairy cows). Healthy and diarrhoeic calves were compared in only one study (Wieler *et al.*, 1992). In most cases, VTEC were detected by DNA–DNA hybridization of faecal coliforms with VT1- and VT2-specific DNA probes, using the colony blot technique (Bülte *et al.*, 1990; Wieler *et al.*, 1992; Gallien *et al.*, 1994). Other detection methods used were a VT-colony immunoblot (Richter *et al.*, 1997) and the Vero cell toxicity test (Beutin *et al.*, 1993). Up to 35 colonies per animal were investigated, depending on the particular study (Table 9.4).

Table 9.4. VTEC from cattle.

Cattle investigated	No. animals examined	Animals with VTEC (%)	Animals with VTEC O157 (%)	Reference	Method of VTEC detection
Cattle (bulls and dairy cows)	259	28 (10.8)	2 (0.8)	Montenegro *et al.*, 1990	VT-gene probes
Dairy cows	82	10 (12.2)	0	Bülte *et al.*, 1990	VT-gene probes
Slaughtered bulls	212	20 (9.4)	0	Bülte *et al.*, 1990	VT-gene probes
Diarrhoeic calves	232	7 (3.0)	0	Wieler *et al.*, 1992	VT-gene probes, retrospective investigation for 1989
Diarrhoeic calves	150	0	0	Wieler *et al.*, 1992	VT-gene probes, retrospective investigation for 1985–1988
Diarrhoeic calves	73	16 (21.9)	0	Wieler *et al.*, 1992	VT-gene probes
Calves	101	13 (12.9)	0	Wieler *et al.*, 1992	VT-gene probes
Cattle	142	30 (21.1)	0	Beutin *et al.*, 1993	Vero cell test
Healthy and diseased cattle	141	6 (5.0)	0	Gallien *et al.*, 1994	VT-gene probes
Cattle (bulls and dairy cows)	204	97 (47.0)	0	Richter *et al.*, 1997	VT-colony immunoblot
Total	1596	227 (14.2)	2 (0.12)		

A specific selection for VTEC O157 was performed in one investigation only by use of a modified hemorrhagic colitis (HC) agar, but no VTEC O157 were isolated (Bülte *et al.*, 1990). VTEC O157 were only detected in one of the studies, where two (0.8%) of 259 cattle were found to excrete VTEC O157:H7 (Montenegro *et al.*, 1990). Since all other studies were negative for VTEC O157, the total frequency for this serotype was calculated as 0.12% of the 1596 cattle which were investigated. The low prevalence of VTEC O157 in cattle is in contrast to the high proportion of cattle excreting non-O157 VTEC types (Table 9.4). For these organisms, 227 (14.2%) of 1596 cattle were found positive. Non-O157 VTEC were as common in healthy as in diseased cattle. Absence or a low prevalence of VTEC was only found in a retrospective analysis of older bovine *E. coli* collections, where only one *E. coli* isolate per animal was tested (Wieler *et al.*, 1992). In all other studies, more *E. coli* isolates per animal were tested and 5.0–47.0% of cattle were found to excrete VTEC (Table 9.4). Even higher frequencies of cattle carrying VTEC (63.2%) were observed when the animals were repeatedly examined over a 6-month period (Beutin *et al.*, 1997). Occasionally, multiple VTEC serotypes occurred in single cattle and sheep (Montenegro *et al.*, 1990; Beutin *et al.*, 1993, 1997; Richter *et al.*, 1997). The high prevalence of VTEC in cattle and the finding that bovine colostra and sera usually contained antibodies against shiga toxins (Pirro *et al.*, 1995) indicate that cattle are frequently exposed to VTEC in their normal environment.

An analysis of the serotypes found among bovine VTEC isolates indicates a great serological diversity. The bovine VTEC isolates obtained from four separate studies could be assigned to 45 different O antigens and to O-untypable and O-rough strains (Table 9.5). However, only a few *E. coli* O groups (O22, O39, O82, O113, O116, O146, O153 and O156) were more frequent and commonly found in cattle populations of different origin. Some of these VTEC O groups (O22, O113, O116, O153 and O156) were also associated with cattle or beef products originating from others countries and time periods and might thus represent the VTEC types which are well adapted to their bovine host (Read *et al.*, 1990; Suthienkul *et al.*, 1990; Pohl, 1991; Tokhi *et al.*, 1993; Samadpour *et al.*, 1994; Zhao *et al.*, 1995; Blanco *et al.*, 1996; Sandhu *et al.*, 1995; Beutin and Müller, 1998). Longitudinal studies on separate bovine populations in Germany and in Sri Lanka revealed that typical bovine VTEC strains (O116 and O153) were predominating in the animals and were isolated over long time periods (Tokhi *et al.*, 1993; Beutin *et al.*, 1997). In contrast, many other 'transient' VTEC serotypes occurred only sporadically in a few animals and for a short time.

Among the 23 different flagellar (H) types found in the 45 bovine VTEC O groups, H types 2, 8 and 21 were the most frequent (Table 9.5). These three H types were associated each with 7–12 different *E. coli* O groups, indicating an H-type specificity for many bovine VTEC strains.

Most of the VTEC that were isolated from healthy cattle in Germany do not belong to those serotypes which are the known human-pathogenic EHEC

Table 9.5. Serotypes of VTEC from cattle.

Serogroup	H type	Number of animals	Reference
O2	25, 49	3	Beutin *et al.*, 1993; Richter *et al.*, 1997
O3	NM	1	Montenegro *et al.*, 1990
O4	4	1	Richter *et al.*, 1997
O8	2, 19, 25	3	Beutin *et al.*, 1993
O10	21	1	Montenegro *et al.*, 1990
O15	4	1	Richter *et al.*, 1997
O20	19	4	Beutin *et al.*, 1993; Richter *et al.*, 1997
O22	8, 16, 21	20	Montenegro *et al.*, 1990; Beutin *et al.*, 1993; Richter *et al.*, 1997
O35	21	2	Richter *et al.*, 1997
O38	16	1	Richter *et al.*, 1997
O39	7, 21, 40, 48	5	Montenegro *et al.*, 1990; Richter *et al.*, 1997
O43	2	1	Richter *et al.*, 1997
O46	2	2	Richter *et al.*, 1997
O68	NM	1	Richter *et al.*, 1997
O73	NT	1	Richter *et al.*, 1997
O74	NT, 29	2	Beutin *et al.*, 1997; Richter *et al.*, 1997
O75	8	1	Montenegro *et al.*, 1990
O76	21	2	Beutin *et al.*, 1993
O82	2, 8, 40	7	Montenegro *et al.*, 1990; Richter *et al.*, 1997
O84	28	1	Richter *et al.*, 1997
O87	16	4	Beutin *et al.*, 1993, 1997
O88	25	1	Richter *et al.*, 1997
O90	24	2	Beutin *et al.*, 1997
O91	10, 21, 49	4	Beutin *et al.*, 1997; Richter *et al.*, 1997
O104	21	1	Montenegro *et al.*, 1990
O105	18	1	Montenegro *et al.*, 1990
O110	2	2	Richter *et al.*, 1997
O113	4, 21	25	Montenegro *et al.*, 1990; Beutin *et al.*, 1993; Richter *et al.*, 1997
O116	21	24	Montenegro *et al.*, 1990; Beutin *et al.*, 1997; Richter *et al.*, 1997
O119	8	1	Richter *et al.*, 1997
O120	NM, 2, 18, 42	4	Beutin *et al.*, 1993; Richter *et al.*, 1997
O126	20, 21	2	Montenegro *et al.*, 1990
O130	38	2	Richter *et al.*, 1997
O131	2	1	Richter *et al.*, 1997
O136	12	2	Montenegro *et al.*, 1990
O139	8	1	Montenegro *et al.*, 1990
O146	21	6	Beutin *et al.*, 1993; Richter *et al.*, 1997
O147	11, 29	2	Richter *et al.*, 1997
O153	NM, 9, 19, 25	7	Beutin *et al.*, 1993; Richter *et al.*, 1997
O156	NM, 21, 46	6	Montenegro *et al.*, 1990; Beutin *et al.*, 1993; Richter *et al.*, 1997
O157	7	2	Montenegro *et al.*, 1990
O168	8	2	Richter *et al.*, 1997
O169	NT	1	Richter *et al.*, 1997
O170	8	2	Richter *et al.*, 1997
O171	2	9	Richter *et al.*, 1997

NM, non-motile; NT, non-typable.

groups. Interestingly, some of human-virulent *E. coli* types, such as VTEC O26, O111 and O118, occurred more frequently in calves with diarrhoea than in healthy adult cattle (Montenegro *et al.*, 1990; Wieler *et al.*, 1992, 1996; Beutin *et al.*, 1995, 1997; Richter *et al.*, 1997). Similar findings were reported from investigations made on healthy and diseased cattle in other countries (Pohl, 1991; Blanco *et al.*, 1996; Sandhu *et al.*, 1996). Corresponding to these findings, *eae*A$^+$ VTEC types were only detected at low frequencies (1–3%) in healthy adult cattle in Germany (Beutin *et al.*, 1995, 1997; Richter *et al.*, 1997), but were more prevalent in diarrhoeic and healthy calves (Blanco *et al.*, 1996; Sandhu *et al.*, 1996; Wieler *et al.*, 1996). Similar findings were reported for VTEC O157, which were more frequently found in calves and heifers than in adult cattle (Wells *et al.*, 1991; Sandhu *et al.*, 1995; Mechie *et al.*, 1997).

VTEC in sheeps and goats

A few studies have been performed on the prevalence of VTEC in sheep and goats (Beutin *et al.*, 1993, 1997; Gallien *et al.*, 1994). The results indicate that VTEC also occur very frequently in ruminant species other than cattle. The single examination of 135 sheep showed animals excreting VTEC at frequencies between 20.0% and 66.6%. Repeated examination of a flock of 25 sheep over a 6-month period resulted in detection of 88.0% VTEC-carrying animals (Beutin *et al.*, 1997). In goats, 56.1% of 66 animals, which were from four separate populations, were found to be positive for VTEC (Beutin *et al.*, 1993). However, *eae*$^+$ VTEC were rarely found and none of the VTEC isolates from sheep and goats belonged to serogroup O157, although VTEC O157 were occasionally isolated from sheep meat in Germany (Beutin *et al.*, 1996b).

Examination of VTEC serotypes from cattle, sheep and goats revealed remarkable differences, which could point to an animal-host serotype specifity for some VTEC types. VTEC from sheep could be attributed to 17 different O groups, to O-untypable and to O-rough strains (Beutin *et al.*, 1993, 1997). A few O groups (O5, O77, O91, O125, O128 and O146) were found to be present in many animals and in separate populations and some of these VTEC types (O125, O128 and O146) were found to predominate in a flock of sheep investigated in a longitudinal study (Beutin *et al.*, 1997). Interestingly, VTEC O5, O91 and O128 were also found among ovine VTEC that were isolated in the USA (Kudva *et al.*, 1997). It appears likely that VTEC from sheep and goats show a great serological diversity, similar to that found with VTEC from cattle, but the serotypes may differ between the different animal-host species. Despite the fact that most of the VTEC O groups were associated with a distinct animal host, some VTEC serogroups were found to occur in different animal species (Table 9.6). It has to be investigated whether these particular strains are heterogeneous for their clonal types and host specificity, despite possessing the same O antigen.

Table 9.6. Serogroups of VTEC isolated from different animal hosts.

O group	H types	Animal host	Reference
O74	NM, NT, 29	Cattle, goats	Beutin *et al.*, 1993, 1997; Richter *et al.*, 1997
O82	2, 8, 40	Cattle, goats	Montenegro *et al.*, 1990; Beutin *et al.*, 1993, 1997; Richter *et al.*, 1997
O87	16, 21	Cattle, sheep, goats	Beutin *et al.*, 1993, 1997
O90	NM, 21, 24	Cattle, sheep	Beutin *et al.*, 1993, 1997
O91	NM, 10, 21, 49	Cattle, sheep, pigs	Montenegro *et al.*, 1990; Beutin *et al.*, 1993, 1997; Richter *et al.*, 1997
O119	8, 25	Cattle, sheep	Beutin *et al.*, 1993; Richter *et al.*, 1997
O136	12, 20	Cattle, sheep	Montenegro *et al.*, 1990; Beutin *et al.*, 1993
O146	8, 21	Cattle, sheep	Beutin *et al.*, 1993, 1997; Richter *et al.*, 1997
O153	NM, 19, 25	Cattle, sheep	Beutin *et al.*, 1993; Richter *et al.*, 1997

NM, non-motile; NT, non-typable.

VTEC in pigs

A total of 567 healthy and diseased pigs was investigated in four different studies and VTEC were isolated from 124 (21.9%) of the animals (Table 9.7). VTEC O157 were not isolated from pigs but non-verotoxigenic *E. coli* O157 were found in one of the studies (Gallien *et al.*, 1994). The porcine *E. coli* O157 isolates were different from VTEC O157 in the absence of VT production and the carriage of fimbrial adhesins K88 and F107 (Wittig *et al.*, 1995) and such O157 strains are not clonally related to VTEC O157 (Whittam *et al.*, 1993). Most VTEC that were isolated from diseased pigs in Germany belonged to serogroups O138, O139, O147 and O149 (Appel *et al.*, 1989; Wittig *et al.*, 1995) and these O groups are known to be closely associated with the *E. coli* causing diarrhoea and oedema disease in pigs (Alexander, 1994; Hampson, 1994). VTEC were more prevalent in diseased than in healthy pigs (Appel *et al.*, 1989).

Interestingly, some of the VTEC types isolated from healthy pigs in Germany (O6, O9, O91, O100 and O-antigen non-typable (ONT)) were also found as contaminants in pork sausages in Britain (Smith *et al.*, 1991). VTEC from healthy pigs and pork sausages were serologically different from the porcine-pathogenic VTEC types (Beutin *et al.*, 1993; Hampson, 1994; Wittig *et al.*, 1995). Although porcine-pathogenic VTEC strains producing the verotoxin variant VT2e have only been rarely associated with diarrhoea and

Table 9.7. VTEC from pigs.

Pigs investigated	No. animals examined	Animals with VTEC (%)	Animals with VTEC O157 (%)	Reference	Method of investigation
Healthy pigs, all ages	26	1 (3.8)	0	Appel *et al.*, 1989	VT-gene probes
Diarrhoeic pigs, all ages	40	11 (27.5)	0	Appel *et al.*, 1989	VT-gene probes
Slaughtered pigs	75	5 (6.7)	0	Bülte *et al.*, 1990	VT-gene probes
Healthy pigs	120	9 (7.5)	0	Beutin *et al.*, 1993	Vero cell test, VT-gene probes
Healthy and diseased pigs	306	98 (32.0)	0	Gallien *et al.*, 1994	VT-gene probes
Total	567	124 (21.9)	0 (< 0.2)		

HUS in humans (Pierard *et al.*, 1991; Thomas *et al.*, 1994), the possible transmission of other porcine VTEC to animals and humans has to be investigated. This is of importance, since 3.8–7.5% of healthy pigs were found to carry VTEC belonging to different serotypes and VT types.

VTEC in chickens

Little is known on the occurrence of VTEC in chicken and poultry in Germany. The examination of rectal swabs taken from 144 chicken yielded no VTEC isolates (Beutin *et al.*, 1993). Absence of VTEC in retail chicken was found in a British study (Smith *et al.*, 1991), whereas 1–12% of poultry meat investigated in the USA and Thailand were positive for VTEC or tested positive with VT-specific gene probes (Doyle and Schoeni, 1987; Suthienkul *et al.*, 1990; Samadpour *et al.*, 1994). However, it is not clear whether the meat samples were contaminated with VTEC originating from chicken or from other sources. Further studies are necessary to explore poultry as a possible reservoir of VTEC in nature.

VTEC in cats and dogs

Very little is known yet on the role of VTEC in household pets, such as dogs and cats. Two studies on a total of 88 dogs were performed in Germany (Beutin *et al.*, 1993; Gallien *et al.*, 1994). In both studies, VTEC were isolated from healthy dogs at frequencies of 4.0% (Gallien *et al.*, 1994) and 4.8% (Beutin *et al.*, 1993). Only three isolates from dogs were serotyped and two O116:H− and one O17:H− strain were identified. VTEC were not found among *E. coli* isolated from dogs with gastroenteritis (Prada *et al.*, 1991) nor were they described as diarrhoeagenic agents in dogs (Peters, 1994). However, dogs could play a role as asymptomatic carriers of VTEC, since VTEC O157 were isolated from an asymptomatic dog that was in contact with a pony and a human excreting the same VTEC O157 strain (Trevena *et al.*, 1996).

VTEC expressing verotoxins VT1 or VT2 were not isolated from 94 cats that were investigated in Germany (Beutin *et al.*, 1993, 1995; Gallien *et al.*, 1994). An activity that was cytotoxic for Vero cells was found in some feline *E. coli* isolates, but these were negative for VT1 and VT2 genes when tested by DNA–DNA hybridization (Beutin *et al.*, 1993, 1995). VTEC have not been described so far as diarrhoeagenic agents in cats (Peters, 1994).

VTEC IN FOOD

Large outbreaks of VTEC O157 infections have been associated with consumption of contaminated foodstuffs, such as raw or undercooked meat and milk products, vegetables and water (World Health Organization, 1997). Studies on VTEC as contaminants of food in Germany were performed on raw milk, raw meat and raw-meat products. Raw milk samples originating from different parts of Germany were investigated for VTEC and contamination rates between < 0.4% and 12.9% were reported. No VTEC were isolated in an examination of 245 raw milk samples and 15 samples of raw-milk cheese (Kuntze *et al.*, 1996). One of 110 samples of certified raw milk (unpasteurized raw milk prepared for direct consumption) from northern Germany was found to contain VTEC (Bockemühl and Karch, 1996). In another study, five of 127 raw milk (3.9%) and three of 146 (2.1%) certified raw milk samples were found to contain VTEC (Klie *et al.*, 1997). Higher VTEC contamination rates of 8.0% were found in 50 samples (Bockemühl and Karch, 1996) and 12.2% in 180 samples of raw milk (Gallien *et al.*, 1998), which were from different parts of Germany. Different serotypes of VTEC were found in raw milk and among these were the human-pathogenic VTEC types O26:H11 and O157:H7 (Bockemühl *et al.*, 1990; Beutin *et al.*, 1996a; Bockemühl and Karch, 1996; Klie *et al.*, 1997; Gallien *et al.*, 1998). VTEC were also detected in raw-milk cheese and were isolated from 1.8% of 55 samples (Bülte *et al.*, 1996) and from 2.8% of 72 samples (Teufel *et al.*, 1998) examined.

Similar results were obtained by examination of raw meat and raw-meat products. VTEC were found in one of 120 samples of retail ground meat from grocery stores in Berlin (Geier, 1992). More recently, VTEC were detected in 12.3% of 105 samples of minced meat (Teufel *et al.*, 1998) and in 8.3% of 168 samples of raw sausage (Gallien *et al.*, 1998).

A large study for VTEC was performed in raw meat and meat products (1033 samples) (Bülte *et al.*, 1996). A total of 4484 *E. coli* colonies were isolated and tested by DNA–DNA hybridization, with gene probes specific for VT1 and VT2. Although many samples were highly contaminated with *E. coli*, only four (0.7%) of 567 beef samples and two of 78 lamb samples contained VTEC. In this study, *E. coli* O157 were not detected but were occasionally isolated from slaughtered cattle (Beutin *et al.*, 1996a). In contrast to the low prevalence of VTEC in meat samples, 72.4% of 87 lamb carcasses were found to be contaminated with VTEC (Bülte *et al.*, 1996). Some of the VTEC serotypes isolated from food carried the *eae* gene and were thus regarded as potential human pathogens (Bülte *et al.*, 1996).

CHARACTERISTICS OF VTEC O157 ISOLATED IN GERMANY

Two major different types of VTEC O157 strains have been described in Germany. The most common type is represented by sorbitol-non-fermenting, β-glucuronidase-negative VTEC O157:H7 and O157:H− strains. Such VTEC strains were isolated from faeces of diseased and healthy humans, from cattle, from bovine meat and milk samples and from sheep meat. The sorbitol-non-fermenting VTEC O157:H7 strains of different geographical origin, including isolates from Germany, are of clonal origin (Whittam *et al.*, 1993). The sorbitol-non-fermenting VTEC O157:H7 and O157:H− strains from Germany and from other countries were also similar for their VT types, presence of the *eae* gene and production of enterohaemolysin (O'Brien *et al.*, 1993; Beutin *et al.*, 1994b; Anon., 1995; Heuvelink *et al.*, 1995; Krause *et al.*, 1996; Thomas *et al.*, 1996).

Table 9.8 summarizes the properties of 106 VTEC O157 strains from human patients in different parts of Germany. The strains were isolates from 1996 and 1997 and were typed at the Robert Koch Institute in Berlin. Interestingly, 104 (98.1%) of the 106 VTEC O157 isolates were positive for VT2 or for VT1 and VT2. In contrast, only two (1.9%) of the 106 isolates were found to be positive for VT1 only. A similar pattern of the VT types was found in VTEC O157 strain collections from different geographical areas (Heuvelink *et al.*, 1995; Krause *et al.*, 1996; Thomas *et al.*, 1996).

Three (2.8%) of the 106 VTEC O157 analysed in our laboratory were found to ferment sorbitol promptly and were positive for β-glucuronidase (Table 9.8). SF-VTEC O157 were first isolated in 1988 from children in Bavaria with HUS (Karch *et al.*, 1990; Aleksic *et al.*, 1992). In the following years, SF-VTEC O157 were frequently detected in human patients with diarrhoea and HUS in Bavaria (Gunzer *et al.*, 1992; Bockemühl and Karch, 1996; Karch *et al.*, 1997; Pulz, 1997). In contrast, most VTEC O157 strains which were from patients from other parts of Germany were of the sorbitol-non-fermenting type (Beutin *et al.*, 1993, 1994a; Bockemühl and Karch, 1996; this work).

SF-VTEC O157 are *eae*$^+$ but they differ from sorbitol-non-fermenting VTEC O157 in some other important properties. SF-VTEC O157 are non-motile and negative for expression of haemolysin, although they carry the genes for the plasmid-encoded EHEC haemolysin, which confers the enterohaemolytic phenotype in many VTEC strains (Karch *et al.*, 1993; Bockemühl *et al.*, 1997). In contrast, 102 (99.0%) of 103 sorbitol-non-fermenting VTEC O157 analysed in our laboratory were positive for enterohaemolysin on washed sheep-blood, enterohaemolysin agar plates (Table 9.8). Moreover, in contrast to sorbitol-non-fermenting VTEC O157, SF-VTEC O157 strains are positive for β-glucuronidase and do not grow on cefixime tellurite sorbitol MacConkey agar (CT-SMAC), a medium which is widely used as a selective medium for detection of VTEC O157 strains (Gunzer *et al.*, 1992; Karch *et al.*, 1996, 1997; this work). These properties make it difficult to detect SF-VTEC O157 by diagnostic procedures that were developed for specific detection of VTEC O157 strains.

CONCLUSIONS

Numerous studies on the occurrence of VTEC in humans and animals have shown that these organisms are widespread in many regions of the world.

Table 9.8. Properties of VTEC O157 isolated in 1996 and 1997 from human patients in Germany.

Relevant properties	O157	H7	H−	VT1	VT2	VT1 + VT2	Sorbitol-non-fermenting	Enterohaemolysin-positive
Numbers of strains	106	63	43	2	69	35	103	102[a]
Percentage of total	(100)	59.4	40.6	1.9	65.1	33.0	97.2	96.2

[a] All sorbitol-fermenting strains and one sorbitol-non-fermenting O157 strain were negative for haemolysis.

In Germany, as in many other countries, *E. coli* O157 and non-O157 VTEC have been isolated from humans, animals and food and the strains belonging to the VTEC group are characterized by their serotype diversity and by a broad spectrum of mammalian host species.

Certain VTEC strains have been shown to cause disease in animals and humans. *Eae*A^{+} VTEC were found to be more prevalent in healthy and diarrhoeic calves than in adult cattle and were also associated with diarrhoeal disease and HUS, particularly in children. In contrast, *eae*$^{-}$ VTEC were found to predominate in healthy adult cattle, sheep and goats and were less frequently or not associated with human virulence.

The findings that many cattle, sheep and goats are colonized with VTEC and that certain VTEC types appear to be closely associated with their bovine host species indicate that VTEC are a natural part of the intestinal flora of cattle and other ruminants. The significance of this finding is not clear, but it appears possible that VTEC may play a role in the intestinal ecology of ruminants which is still not understood. It appears unlikely that VTEC were only recently introduced into domestic farm animals, since they were already present in cattle more than 30 years ago. Moreover, the finding that VTEC have been isolated from wild deer (Rice *et al.*, 1995), from ruminants living in a zoological garden (Beutin *et al.*, 1993) and from bovines in regions of the world that differ widely in their climate, environment and agriculture makes it unlikely that VTEC were only recently introduced into ruminant species.

Although more than 150 different VTEC serotypes have been described in cattle, only relatively few of these are associated with severe illness in humans. VTEC O157 were found to be most frequent in patients with bloody diarrhoea and HUS in Germany, which is in contrast to the low prevalence of these organisms in animals or food. This could indicate that person-to-person transmission is the most important mode of infection with VTEC O157 in the human population in Germany. This might be equally true for SF-VTEC O157 strains, which have not been detected in animals so far.

In addition to VTEC O157, some other non-O157 VTEC types have been incriminated as human pathogens. Some of these, such as VTEC O26 and O111 strains, are known to be pathogens of calves and humans and have been isolated worldwide for many decades. However, other types of non-O157 VTEC have only more recently been described to cause illness in humans. In Germany, new virulent VTEC types, such as O103:H2 and O118:H16, have been described as emerging pathogens in humans and calves. The emergence of new VTEC types could be an indicator of a continuous evolution in the VTEC reservoir, which results in the spread of former rare or unknown VTEC types in animals and humans. In view of the possible changes in the type spectrum of human-pathogenic VTEC and in regard to the different VTEC types which are implicated in human disease, serotype-independent diagnostic tests for VTEC infections are necessary, particularly in paediatric patients, as a risk group.

ACKNOWLEDGEMENTS

I am grateful to F. Fehrenbach, Robert Koch Institute (Berlin), R.D. Hess, University of Freiburg, Germany, and H.R. Smith, Central Public Health Laboratory, London, for critical reading of the manuscript.

REFERENCES

Aleksic, S., Karch, H. and Bockemühl, J. (1992) A biotyping scheme for shiga-like (Vero) toxin-producing *Escherichia coli* O157 and a list of serological cross-reactions between O157 and other gram-negative bacteria. *Zentralblatt für Bakteriologie* 276, 221–230.

Alexander, T.J.L. (1994) Neonatal diarrhoea in pigs. In: Gyles, C.L. (ed.) Escherichia coli *in Domestic Animals and Humans.* CAB International, Wallingford, pp. 151–170.

Anon. (1995) *Report on Veroxytotoxin-producing* Escherichia coli. Advisory Committee on the Microbiological Safety of Food, HMSO, London.

Anon. (1996a) Häufung von EHEC Erkrankungen in Bayern. *Robert Koch-Institut, Epidemiologisches Bulletin* 20, 137–138.

Anon. (1996b) Outbreak of EHEC infections in Bavaria. *WHO Surveillance Programme for Control of Foodborne Infections and Intoxications in Europe Newsletter* 49/50, 1–2.

Anon. (1997a) Zum Aufbau einer Surveillance für enterohämorrhagische *E. coli* (EHEC) in Deutschland. *Robert Koch-Institut, Epidemiologisches Bulletin* 39, 269–273.

Anon. (1997b) Zum Auftreten von EHEC-Infektionen in Niedersachsen. *Robert Koch-Institut, Epidemiologisches Bulletin* 46, 319–322.

Anon. (1998) Zur Situation bei ausgewählten meldepflichtigen Infektionskrankheiten im Jahr 1997. Teil 1: Gastroenteritiden (II). *Robert Koch-Institut, Epidemiologisches Bulletin* 9, 55–59.

Appel, G., Ewald, C., Heer, A., von Mickwitz, G., Aleksic, S., Rüssmann, H., Meyer, T. and Karch, H. (1989) Vorkommen und Bedeutung von Verotoxin-(Shiga-like toxin)-produzierenden *Escherichia coli* Stämmen beim Schwein. *Tierärztliche Umschau* 44, 410–420.

Beutin, L. and Müller, W. (1998) Cattle and verotoxigenic *Escherichia coli* (VTEC), an old relationship? *Veterinary Record* 142, 283–284.

Beutin, L., Montenegro, M.A., Orskov, I., Orskov, F., Prada, J., Zimmermann, S. and Stephan, R. (1989) Close association of verotoxin (shiga-like toxin) production with enterohemolysin production in strains of *Escherichia coli. Journal of Clinical Microbiology* 27, 2559–2564.

Beutin, L., Orskov, I., Orskov, F., Zimmermann, S., Prada, J., Gelderblom, H., Stephan, R. and Whittam, T. (1990) Clonal diversity and virulence factors in strains of *Escherichia coli* of the classic enteropathogenic serogroup O114. *Journal of Infectious Diseases* 162, 1329–1334.

Beutin, L., Geier, D., Steinrück, H., Zimmermann, S. and Scheutz, F. (1993) Prevalence and some properties of verotoxin (shiga-like toxin)-producing *Escherichia coli* in seven different species of healthy domestic animals. *Journal of Clinical Microbiology* 31, 2483–2488.

Beutin, L., Aleksic, S., Bockemühl, J., Schwarzkopf, A. and Karch, H. (1994a) Zur Epidemiologie von Infektionen durch enterohämorrhagische *E. coli* (EHEC) in der Bundesrepublik Deutschland im Jahr 1993. *Bundesgesundheitsblatt* 37, 410–414.

Beutin, L., Aleksic, S., Zimmermann, S. and Gleier, K. (1994b) Virulence factors and phenotypical traits of verotoxigenic strains of *Escherichia coli* isolated from human patients in Germany. *Medical Microbiology and Immunology* 183, 13–21.

Beutin, L., Geier, D., Zimmermann, S. and Karch, H. (1995) Virulence markers of shiga-like toxin-producing *Escherichia coli* strains originating from healthy domestic animals of different species. *Journal of Clinical Microbiology* 33, 631–635.

Beutin, L., Zimmermann, S. and Gleier, K. (1996a) Zur Epidemiologie und Diagnostik von Infektionen durch enterohämorrhagische *E. coli* (EHEC) in der Bundesrepublik Deutschland. *Bundesgesundheitsblatt* 39, 326–331.

Beutin, L., Knollmann-Schanbacher, G., Rietschel, W. and Seeger, H. (1996b) Animal reservoirs of *Escherichia coli* O157:[H7]. *Veterinary Record* 139, 70–71.

Beutin, L., Horbach, I., Zimmermann, S. and Gleier, K. (1997) Vergleich verschiedener diagnostischer Methoden zum Nachweis von Verotoxin (Shiga-Toxin) bildenden *Escherichia coli* Stämmen (VTEC) aus klinischen Stuhlproben. *Journal of Laboratory Medicine* 21, 537–546.

Beutin, L., Zimmermann, S. and Gleier, K. (1998a) Human infections with shiga toxin-producing *Escherichia coli* other than serogroup O157 in Germany. *Emerging Infectious Diseases* 4, 635–639.

Beutin, L., Kontny, I. and Kuttner-May, S. (1998b) Aufdeckung von Ausbrüchen bei Infektionen mit enterohämorrhagischen *Escherichia coli* (EHEC) O157. *Bundesgesundheitsblatt* 41, 253–256.

Bitzan, M., Karch, H., Altrogge, H., Strehlau, J. and Bläker, F. (1988) Hemolytic–uremic syndrome associated with a variant Shiga-like cytotoxin of *Escherichia coli* O111. *Pediatric Infectious Disease Journal* 7, 128–132.

Blanco, M., Blanco, J.E., Blanco, J., Gonzalez, E.A., Mora, A., Prado, C., Fernandez, L., Rio, M., Ramos, J. and Alonso, M.P. (1996) Prevalence and characteristics of *Escherichia coli* serotype O157:H7 and other verotoxin-producing *E. coli* in healthy cattle. *Epidemiology and Infection* 117, 251–257.

Bockemühl, J. and Karch, H. (1996) Zur aktuellen Bedeutung der enterohämorrhagischen *Escherichia coli* (EHEC) in Deutschland (1994–1995). *Bundesgesundheitsblatt* 39, 290–296.

Bockemühl, J., Karch, H., Rüssmann, H., Aleksic, S., Wiß, R. and Emmrich, P. (1990) Shiga-like toxin (Verotoxin)-produzierende *Escherichia coli* O22:H8. *Bundesgesundheitsblatt* 33, 3–6.

Bockemühl, J., Karch, H. and Tschäpe, H. (1997) Infektionen des Menschen durch enterohämorrhagische *Escherichia coli* (EHEC) in Deutschland, 1996. *Bundesgesundheitsblatt* 40, 194–197.

Bülte, M., Montenegro, M.A., Helmuth, R., Trumpf, T. and Reuter, G. (1990) Nachweis von Verotoxin-bildenden *E. coli* (VTEC) bei gesunden Rindern und Schweinen mit dem DNS–DNS-Koloniehybridisierungsverfahren. *Berliner und Münchener Tierärztliche Wochenschrift* 103, 380–384.

Bülte, M., Heckötter, S. and Schwenk, P. (1996) Enterohämorrhagische *E. coli* (EHEC)-aktuelle Lebensmittelinfektionserreger auch in der Bundesrepublik Deutschland? *Fleischwirtschaft* 76, 88–91.

Doyle, M.P. and Schoeni, J.L. (1987) Isolation of *Escherichia coli* O157:H7 from retail fresh meats and poultry. *Applied and Environmental Microbiology* 53, 2394–2396.

Gallien, P., Klie, H., Lehmann, S., Protz, D., Helmuth, R., Schäfer, R. and Ehrler, M. (1994) Nachweis verotoxinbildender *E. coli* in Feldisolaten von Haus- und landwirtschaftlichen Nutztieren in Sachsen-Anhalt. *Berliner und Münchener Tierärztliche Wochenschrift* 107, 331–334.

Gallien, P., Klie, H., Richter, H., Timm, M., Karch, H., Perlberg, K.-W., Teufel, P. and Protz, D. (1998) Detection of STEC (VTEC) in foods and characterization of isolates. In: *Book of Abstracts: 4th World Congress on Foodborne Infections and Intoxications.* Federal Health Institute for Protection of Consumers and Veterinary Medicine, Berlin, p. 83.

Geier, D. (1992) Untersuchungen zur Möglichkeit des Nachweises verotoxischer *E. coli* (VTEC-Stämme) über Enterohämolysin als epidemiologisches Merkmal bei unterschiedlichen Nutz- und Heimtieren sowie Hackfleisch in Berlin. MD thesis, Faculty of Veterinary Medicine, Free University of Berlin.

Griffin, P.M. and Tauxe, R.V. (1991) The epidemiology of infections caused by *Escherichia coli* O157:H7, other enterohemorrhagic *E. coli*, and the associated hemolytic uremic syndrome. *Epidemiologic Reviews* 13, 60–98.

Gunzer, F., Böhm, H., Rüssmann, H., Bitzan, M., Aleksic, S. and Karch, H. (1992) Molecular detection of sorbitol-fermenting *Escherichia coli* O157 in patients with hemolytic–uremic syndrome. *Journal of Clinical Microbiology* 30, 1807–1810.

Hampson, D.J. (1994) Postweaning *Escherichia coli* diarrhoea in pigs. In: Gyles, C.L. (ed.) Escherichia coli *in Domestic Animals and Humans.* CAB International, Wallingford, pp. 171–191.

Heuvelink, A.E., von de Kar, N.C.A.J., Meis, J.F.G.M., Monnens, L.A.H. and Melchers, W.J.G. (1995) Characterization of verocytotoxin-producing *Escherichia coli* O157 isolates from patients with haemolytic uraemic syndrome in Western Europe. *Epidemiology and Infection* 115, 1–14.

Hübner, H., Stück, B. and Beutin, L. (1997) Zur aktuellen Bedeutung von darmpathogenen *Escherichia coli* als Erreger von gastrointestinalen Erkrankungen bei Neugeborenen und Säuglingen in einer Berliner Kinderklinik. In: *Abstracts 4: Deutscher Kongreß für Infektions- und Tropenmedizin, Berlin, Chemotherapie Journal* 6 (Suppl. 15), 54.

Huppertz, H.-I., Busch, D., Schmidt, H., Aleksic, S. and Karch, H. (1996) Diarrhea in young children associated with *Escherichia coli* non-O157 organisms that produce Shiga-like toxin. *Journal of Pediatrics* 128, 341–346.

Karch, H., Wiß, R., Gloning, H., Emmrich, P., Aleksic, S. and Bockemühl, J. (1990) Hämolytisch-urämisches Syndrom bei Kleinkindern durch Verotoxin-produzierende *Escherichia coli. Deutsche Medizinische Wochenschrift* 115, 489–495.

Karch, H., Böhm, H., Schmidt, H., Gunzer, F., Aleksic, S. and Heesemann, J. (1993) Clonal structure and pathogenicity of shiga-like toxin-producing, sorbitol-fermenting *Escherichia coli* O157:H. *Journal of Clinical Microbiology* 31, 1200–1205.

Karch, H., Rüssmann, H., Schmidt, H., Schwarzkopf, A. and Heesemann, J. (1995) Long-term shedding and clonal turnover of enterohemorrhagic *Escherichia coli* O157 in diarrheal diseases. *Journal of Clinical Microbiology* 33, 1602–1605.

Karch, H., Janetzki-Mittmann, C., Aleksic, S. and Datz, M. (1996) Isolation of enterohemorrhagic *Escherichia coli* O157 strains from patients with hemolytic–uremic syndrome by using immunomagnetic separation, DNA-based methods, and direct culture. *Journal of Clinical Microbiology* 34, 516–519.

Karch, H., Huppertz, H.-I., Bockemühl, J., Schmidt, H., Schwarzkopf, A. and Lissner, R. (1997) Shiga toxin-producing *Escherichia coli* infections in Germany. *Journal of Food Protection* 60, 1454–1457.

Klie, H., Timm M., Richter, H., Gallien, P., Perlberg, K.-W. and Steinrück, H. (1997) Nachweis und Vorkommen von Verotoxin- bzw. Shigatoxin-bildenden *Escherichia coli* (VTEC bzw. STEC) in Milch. *Berliner und Münchener Tierärztliche Wochenschrift* 110, 337–341.

Krause, U., Thomson-Carter, F.M. and Pennington, T.H. (1996) Molecular epidemiology of *Escherichia coli* O157:H7 by pulsed-field gel electrophoresis and comparison with that by bacteriophage typing. *Journal of Clinical Microbiology* 34, 959–961.

Kudva, I.T., Hatfield, P.G. and Hovde, C.J. (1997) Characterization of *Escherichia coli* O157:H7 and other shiga-toxin-producing *Escherichia coli* serotypes isolated from sheep. *Journal of Clinical Microbiology* 35, 892–899.

Kuntze, U., Becker, H., Märtelbauer, E., Baumann, C. and Burow, H. (1996) Nachweis von verotoxin-bildenolen *E. coli*-stämmen in rohmilch und rohmilch käse. *Archiv für Lebens-Mittelhygiene* 47, 129–152.

Ludwig, K., Ruder, H., Rott, H.D. and Karch, H. (1996) Outcome of an enterohaemorrhagic *Escherichia coli* O157 infection in monozygotic twins. *Lancet* 347, 196–197.

Ludwig, K., Ruder, H., Bitzan, M., Zimmermann, S. and Karch, H. (1997) Outbreak of *Escherichia coli* O157:H7 infection in a large family. *European Journal of Clinical Microbiology and Infectious Diseases* 16, 238–241.

Mechie, S.C., Chapman, P. and Siddons, C.A. (1997) A fifteen month study of *Escherichia coli* O157:H7 in a dairy herd. *Epidemiology and Infection* 118, 17–25.

Montenegro, M.A., Bülte, M., Trumpf, T., Aleksic, S., Reuter, G., Bulling, E. and Helmuth R. (1990) Detection and characterization of fecal verotoxin-producing *Escherichia coli* from healthy cattle. *Journal of Clinical Microbiology* 28, 1417–1421.

O'Brien, A.D., Melton, A.R., Schmitt, C.K., McKee, M.L., Batts, M.L. and Griffin, D.E. (1993) Profile of *Escherichia coli* O157:H7 pathogen responsible for hamburger-borne outbreak of hemorrhagic colitis and hemolytic uremic syndrome in Washington. *Journal of Clinical Microbiology* 31, 2799–2801.

Peeters, J.E. (1994) *Escherichia coli* infections in rabbits, cats, dogs, goats and horses. In: Gyles, C.L. (ed.) Escherichia coli *in Domestic Animals and Humans.* CAB International, Wallingford, pp. 151–170.

Pierard, D., Huyghens, L., Lauwers, S. and Lior, H. (1991) Diarrhoea associated with *Escherichia coli* producing porcine oedema disease verotoxin. *Lancet* 338, 762.

Pirro, F., Wieler, L.H., Failing, K., Bauerfeind, R. and Baljer, G. (1995) Neutralizing antibodies against Shiga-like toxins from *Escherichia coli* in colostra and sera of cattle. *Veterinary Microbiology* 43, 131–141.

Pohl, P. (1991) Les *Escherichia coli* verotoxinogènes isolées des bovins. *Annales de Médecine Vétérinaire* 135, 569–576.

Prada, J., Baljer, G., De Rycke, J., Steinrück, H., Zimmermann, S., Stephan, R. and Beutin, L. (1991) Characteristics of α-hemolytic strains of *Escherichia coli* isolated from dogs with gastroenteritis. *Veterinary Microbiology* 29, 59–73.

Pulz, M. (1997) Zur Epidemiologie und aktuellen Bedeutung enterohämorrhagischer *Escherichia coli* (EHEC) in Nordbayern (1996). *Gesundheitswesen* 59, 656–660.

Pulz, M., Vogelsang, E., Fuchs, T., Hinz, S., von Hase, U., Fritsch, W., Windorfer, A. and Karch, H. (1998) Shiga toxin-producing *Escherichia coli* (STEC) in Weser-Ems kindergartens receiving certified raw milk. In: *Book of Abstracts. 4th World Congress on Foodborne Infections and Intoxications.* Federal Health Institute for Protection of Consumers and Veterinary Medicine, Berlin, p. 82.

Read, S.C., Gyles, C.L., Clarke, R.C., Lior, H. and McEwen, S. (1990) Prevalence of verocytotoxigenic *Escherichia coli* in ground beef, pork and chicken in southwestern Ontario. *Epidemiology and Infection* 105, 11–20.

Reida, P., Wolff, M., Pöhls, H.-W., Kuhlmann, W., Lehmacher, A., Aleksic, S., Karch, H. and Bockemühl, J. (1994) An outbreak due to enterohaemorrhagic *Escherichia coli* O1578:H7 in a children day care center characterized by person-to-person transmission and environmental contamination. *Zentralblatt Bakteriologie* 281, 534–543.

Rice, D.H., Hancock, D.D. and Besser, T.E. (1995) Verotoxigenic *E. coli* O157 colonisation of wild deer and range cattle. *Veterinary Record* 137, 524.

Richter, H., Klie, H., Timm, M., Gallien, P., Steinrück, H., Perlberg, K.-W. and Protz, D. (1997) Verotoxin-bildende *E. coli* (VTEC) im Kot von Schlachtrindern in Deutschland. *Berliner und Münchener Tierärztliche Wochenschrift* 110, 121–128.

Rüssmann, H. (1992) Nachweis von Shiga-like Toxin-produzierenden *Escherichia coli* in Stuhl- und Milchproben mit Gensonden. MD thesis, University of Würzburg.

Samadpour, M., Ongerth, J.E., Liston, J., Tran, N., Nguyen, D., Whittam, T.S., Wilson, R.A. and Tarr, P.I. (1994) Occurrence of shiga-like toxin-producing *Escherichia coli* in retail fresh seafood, beef, lamb, pork, and poultry from grocery stores in Seattle, Washington. *Applied and Environmental Microbiology* 60, 1038–1040.

Sandhu, K.S., Clarke, R.C., McFadden, K., Brouwer, A., Louie, M., Wilson, J., Lior, H. and Gyles, C.L. (1996) Prevalence of the *eae*A gene in verotoxigenic *Escherichia coli* strains from dairy cattle in southwest Ontario. *Epidemiology and Infection* 116, 1–7.

Smith, H.R., Cheasty, T., Roberts, D., Thomas, A. and Rowe, B. (1991) Examination of retail chickens and sausages in Britain for Vero cytotoxin-producing *Escherichia coli. Applied and Environmental Microbiology* 57, 2091–2093.

Störmann, J., Bulla, M., Kuwertz-Bröking, E. and Karch, H. (1996) Zunahme von Erkrankungen an hämolytisch-urämischen Syndrom (HUS) durch enterohämorrhagische *E. coli* (EHEC) im Münsterland/Emsland 1994. *Monatsschrift Kinderheilkunde* 144, 1242–1247.

Suthienkul, O., Brown, J.E., Seriwatana, J., Tienthongdee, S., Sastravaha, S. and Echeverria, P. (1990) Shiga-like-toxin-producing *Escherichia coli* in retail meats and cattle in Thailand. *Applied Environmental Microbiology* 56, 1135–1139.

Teufel, P., Bräunig, J., Ellerbroek, L., Gallien, P., Perlberg, K.-W., Richter, H., Klie, H., Timm, M., Wichmann-Schauer, H. and Bartelt, E. (1998) Detection of Verotoxin-producing *E. coli* (VTEC) in minced meat and soft cheese. In: *Book of Abstracts. 4th World Congress on Foodborne Infections and Intoxications.* Federal Health Institute for Protection of Consumers and Veterinary Medicine, Berlin, p. 208.

Thomas, A., Cheasty, T., Chart, H. and Rowe, B. (1994) Isolation of vero-cytotoxin-producing *Escherichia coli* serotype O9ab:H− carrying VT2 variant gene sequences from a patient with haemolytic–uraemic syndrome. *European Journal of Clinical Microbiology and Infectious Diseases* 13, 1074–1076.

Thomas, A., Cheasty, T., Frost, J.A., Chart, H., Smith, H.R. and Rowe, B. (1996) Vero cytotoxin-producing *Escherichia coli*, particularly serogroup O157, associated with human infections in England and Wales: 1992–4. *Epidemiology and Infection* 117, 1–10.

Tokhi, M., Peiris, J.S.M., Scotland, S.M., Willshaw, G.A., Smith, H.R. and Cheasty, T. (1993) A longitudinal study of vero cytotoxin producing *Escherichia coli* in cattle calves in Sri Lanka. *Epidemiology and Infection* 110, 197–208.

Trevena, W.B., Hooper, R.S., Wray, C., Willshaw, G.A., Cheasty, T. and Domingue, G. (1996) Vero cytotoxin-producing *Escherichia coli* O157 associated with companion animals. *Veterinary Record* 138, 400.

Wells, J.G., Shipman, L.D., Greene, K.D., Sowers, E.G., Green, J.H., Cameron, D.N., Downes, F.P., Martin, M.L., Griffin, P.M., Ostroff, S.M., Potter, M.E., Tauxe, R.V. and Wachsmuth, I.K. (1991) Isolation of *Escherichia coli* O157:H7 and other shiga-like-toxin-producing *E. coli* from dairy cattle. *Journal of Clinical Microbiology* 29, 985–989.

Whittam, T.S., Wolfe, M.L., Wachsmuth, K., Orskov, F., Orskov, I. and Wilson, R.A. (1993) Clonal relationships among *Escherichia coli* strains that cause hemorrhagic colitis and infantile diarrhea. *Infection and Immunity* 61, 1619–1629.

Wieler, L.H., Bauerfeind, R. and Baljer, G. (1992) Characterization of shiga-like toxin producing *Escherichia coli* (SLTEC) isolated from calves with and without diarrhea. *Zentralblatt Bakteriologie* 276, 243–253.

Wieler, L.H., Vieler, E., Erpenstein, C., Schlapp, T., Steinrück, H., Bauerfeind, R., Byomi, A. and Baljer, G. (1996) Shiga-toxin-producing *Escherichia coli* strains from bovines: association of adhesion with carriage of *eae* and other genes. *Journal of Clinical Microbiology* 34, 2980–2984.

Wittig, W., Klie, H., Gallien, P., Lehmann, S., Timm, M. and Tschäpe, H. (1995) Prevalence of fimbrial antigens F18 and K88 and of enterotoxins and verotoxins among *Escherichia coli* isolated from weaned pigs. *Zentralblatt Bakteriologie* 283, 95–104.

World Health Organization, Food Safety Unit, Consultations and Workshops (1997) *Prevention and Control of Enterohaemorrhagic* Escherichia coli *(EHEC) Infections: Report of a WHO Consultation.* Report No: WHO/FSF/FOS/97.6, WHO, Geneva, Switzerland.

Wuthe, H.-H. (1987) *Escherichia coli* O157:H7 bei hämorrhagischer Colitis. *Deutsche Medizinische Wochenschrift* 112, 1761–1762.

Zhao, T., Doyle, M.P., Shere, J. and Garber, L. (1995) Prevalence of enterohemorrhagic *Escherichia coli* O157:H7 in a survey of dairy herds. *Applied and Environmental Microbiology* 61, 1290–1293.

10

Human Infection with Verocytotoxigenic *Escherichia coli* Associated with Exposure to Farms and Rural Environments

R.P. Johnson,[1,4] J.B. Wilson,[2,5] P. Michel,[1] K. Rahn,[1] S.A. Renwick,[3] C.L. Gyles[4] and J.S. Spika[2]

[1]*Health Canada, Guelph Laboratory, Guelph, Ontario, Canada;* [2]*Health Canada, Laboratory Centre for Disease Control, Guelph, Ontario, Canada;* [3]*Canadian Food Inspection Agency, Nepean, Ontario, Canada;* [4]*Department of Pathobiology and* [5]*Population Medicine, University of Guelph, Guelph, Ontario, Canada*

INTRODUCTION

Verocytotoxigenic *Escherichia coli* (VTEC) are an important cause of uncomplicated diarrhoea, bloody diarrhoea (BD) and the haemolytic uraemic syndrome (HUS) in developed countries (Karmali, 1989; Griffin and Tauxe, 1991). Most reported outbreaks and sporadic cases of VTEC-associated illness in Canada, the USA and the UK are caused by *E. coli* O157:H7 (Griffin, 1998; Smith *et al.*, 1998; Spika *et al.*, 1998), reflecting both the probable predominance of this serotype in serious disease and the reliance on the relatively simple methods for detection of this serotype compared with non-O157 VTEC (Wilson *et al.*, 1997a). The incidence and importance of non-O157 VTEC infections in most countries are not known; however, many non-O157 VTEC have been isolated from sporadic cases of diarrhoea, BD and HUS, and several have been associated with disease outbreaks (Johnson *et al.*, 1996a; Robins-Browne *et al.*, 1998; Strockbine *et al.*, 1998).

The earliest reported outbreaks of *E. coli* O157:H7 infection were associated with consumption of ground beef (Riley *et al.*, 1983) or person-to-person spread (Johnson *et al.*, 1983). Since then, most information on transmission of VTEC has been derived from outbreak investigations (Slutzker *et al.*, 1998) and has emphasized the importance of foods, particularly ground beef, as sources of human VTEC infection (Wells *et al.*, 1983; Griffin and Tauxe, 1991; Griffin, 1998). Despite the serious public-health implications of outbreaks, most VTEC infections are sporadic (Wilson *et al.*, 1997b; Slutzker *et al.*, 1998). Risk factors for sporadic infection are less well defined, although consumption of inadequately cooked ground beef is again prominent (Parry *et al.*, 1998; Slutzker *et al.*, 1998; Spika *et al.*, 1998). However, in one Canadian study (Le Saux *et al.*, 1993), only 17% of cases were attributable to inadequately cooked ground beef, suggesting other sources of infection are also important.

Several case reports and epidemiological studies suggest that rural environments are important in the epidemiology of VTEC infections. Domestic and wild animals, particularly ruminants, are frequent hosts of VTEC and shed these organisms in their faeces. The environments of farming and wildlife areas also include soil, water and other sites where enteric organisms shed in faeces can be distributed and survive. Here, we present evidence from several Canadian and other studies relating to animals and rural environments as sources of human VTEC infection.

VTEC IN ANIMALS AND RURAL ENVIRONMENTS

The early associations between *E. coli* O157:H7 and cattle products quickly led to identification of cattle as natural hosts of VTEC O157 (Martin *et al.*, 1986; Borczyk *et al.*, 1987; Chapman *et al.*, 1989). Subsequent investigations have confirmed that a variety of animals, especially ruminants, may carry numerous serotypes of VTEC in their intestinal tracts. Most information on the prevalence and epidemiology of VTEC in animals and farm environments has been generated by microbiological testing of animal faeces and environmental sites to investigate risk factors for animal infections and entry of VTEC into the food-chain. Consequently, most of these studies do not directly assess prevalence at sites of contact between humans and animals involved in possible animal-to-human transmission. For example, farm residents and visitors, and others, such as abattoir workers, frequently contact the faeces and hides of animals, but there is little information on VTEC at these sites.

Prevalence of VTEC in animals

E. coli *O157:H7 in cattle*

E. coli O157:H7 appears to be widespread in cattle, but at low prevalence. Animal and herd prevalence estimates vary with study design, numbers of herds and cattle sampled, type and age of cattle, methodology and season.

In three surveys, involving up to nine selected dairy herds in Wisconsin, *E. coli* O157:H7 was isolated from faeces of 1.2–2.2% of cattle on 27.3–100% of farms (Wells *et al.*, 1991). Where higher numbers of farms were investigated on a single sampling, the prevalence rates were lower both in individual animals (0–0.7%) and farms (0–16%) (Synge and Hopkins, 1992; Hancock *et al.*, 1994; Wilson *et al.*, 1994; Garber *et al.*, 1995). Prevalence rates were higher in growing cattle, especially among newly weaned dairy calves, and during the summer (Hancock *et al.*, 1994; Wilson *et al.*, 1994; Garber *et al.*, 1995; Zhao *et al.*, 1995). In a point-prevalence study of 100 feedlots in the USA, *E. coli* O157:H7 was isolated on 63% of the feedlots and, overall, from 1.8% of 11,881 faecal samples (Hancock *et al.*, 1997c). Prevalence rates between feedlots and between pens within feedlots were highly variable, with highest rates for pens holding cattle recently entering the feedlots (32–53%). Recent information from the USA, discussed by Hancock *et al.* (1998a), suggests that *E. coli* O157:H7 probably occurs in most herds as one of many transient *E. coli* of cattle. In longitudinal studies, several herds were culture-negative for several months, but had periods of a few weeks when 10–26% of cattle shed the organism (Hancock *et al.*, 1997a). A similar pattern was evident in a dairy farm in the UK, where the peak rates of shedding ranged from 40 to 68% (Mechie *et al.*, 1997). Infection was not associated with clinical disease in either study. These findings are generally consistent with the fact that *E. coli* O157:H7 is not a bovine pathogen in naturally reared cattle (Cray and Moon, 1995) and is shed for 1–2 months following natural exposure (Wells *et al.*, 1991; Besser *et al.*, 1997; Rahn *et al.*, 1997). There are, however, herds in which *E. coli* O157:H7 was isolated more frequently over time (Faith *et al.*, 1996; Hancock *et al.*, 1997a; Shere *et al.*, 1998), possibly due to continuing exposure to the organism in water, feed or other environmental sources or to management factors.

Serological studies provide further evidence that *E. coli* O157:H7 is widespread in cattle. In a study of cattle on 80 dairy farms (Wilson *et al.*, 1996), over 85% of 885 adult dairy cattle and 49% of 589 calves less than 3 months old had antibodies reactive with the O157 lipopolysaccharide (LPS). Calves 9–13 weeks old had the lowest rate of seropositivity (37%) to this antigen (R.P. Johnson *et al.*, unpublished data). However, the high rates of seropositivity to the O157 LPS should be interpreted with awareness of the occurrence of non-VTEC of serogroup O157 in cattle, as well as potential cross-reactions due to antibodies to other organisms (Johnson *et al.*, 1996b).

All VTEC in cattle

Several microbiological surveys employing methods to detect all VTEC have confirmed that VTEC of many serotypes are widespread in cattle (Montenegro *et al.*, 1990; Wilson *et al.*, 1992; Beutin *et al.*, 1993; Butler and Clarke, 1994). For example, in a survey of faecal samples from cattle on 80 dairy farms in Ontario, Canada, all farms, 36% of lactating cows and 57% of calves had evidence of VTEC infection (Wilson *et al.*, 1994). In contrast, *E. coli* O157:H7 was isolated from only 0.45% of cattle on 5% of the farms, reflecting the low prevalence of this serotype relative to all other bovine VTEC. Prevalence rates of all VTEC and *E. coli* O157:H7 were highest among newly weaned calves and in the summer months, as noted above for *E. coli* O157:H7.

Serological studies indicate that VTEC infections occur in cattle at an even higher frequency than suggested by point prevalence studies using microbiological methods. Antibodies to verocytotoxin 1 (VT1) were found in 71–90% of cattle in Canada, Germany and Italy (Borman-Eby *et al.*, 1993; Conedera *et al.*, 1994; Pirro *et al.*, 1995). Antibodies to VT2 were present in less than 15% of cattle, despite the frequent occurrence of VT2-producing *E. coli* in cattle, suggesting a low rate of seroconversion to VT2.

Non-O157 VTEC isolated from cattle belong to over 100 serotypes (Aleksic, 1994; Clarke *et al.*, 1994). Although many of these serotypes have not been isolated from humans, numerous others are associated with disease in humans. Moreover, several of the serotypes often associated with serious human disease are common in cattle or cattle products. Of the 20 most frequently isolated serotypes of bovine VTEC in our collection, 18 have been isolated from humans, and 11 of these are serotypes associated with BD and/or HUS (Johnson *et al.*, 1996a). Comparisons of human and bovine isolates generally indicate that bovine and human VTEC of the same serotype are similar with respect to the presence of known virulence-associated properties (Barrett *et al.*, 1992; Willshaw *et al.*, 1992; Sandhu *et al.*, 1996; Gyles *et al.*, 1998). Also, differences between human and bovine isolates in the distributions of VT1 and VT2 and of the protease, EspP, and in adherence properties suggest that VTEC isolated from humans form a subset of those in the bovine population (Boerlin *et al.*, 1998).

VTEC in other animals

Domestic ruminants other than cattle also harbour VTEC (Beutin *et al.*, 1993; Kudva *et al.*, 1997; Sidjabat-Tambunan and Bensink, 1997; Robins-Browne *et al.*, 1998). Prevalence rates of all VTEC were higher in sheep (66%) and goats (56%) than in cattle (21%) in Germany (Beutin *et al.*, 1993). Also, 43% of 400 sheep and 51.1% of 262 goats tested in Italy had antibodies to VT1 (Conedera *et al.*, 1994). While the serotypes of VTEC isolated from these species differ somewhat from those in cattle, several are common to cattle, sheep and goats, and include serotypes associated with BD and/or HUS in humans (Beutin *et al.*, 1993). Although not isolated from German sheep or goats (Beutin *et al.*, 1993), *E. coli* O157:H7 was present in 1–4% of sheep surveyed at abattoirs in Australia, UK, The Netherlands and USA (Chapman *et al.*, 1997; Heuvelink *et al.*, 1998; Robins-Browne *et al.*, 1998; B. McCluskey, 1997, Fort Collins, Colorado, unpublished data). *E. coli* O157:H7 has also been isolated from deer at prevalences similar to those in cattle

(Chapman and Ackroyd, 1997; Rice *et al.*, 1998), indicating that deer and perhaps other wild ruminants are significant hosts of VTEC. Commercial poultry do not harbour *E. coli* O157:H7 or other VTEC (Read *et al.*, 1990; Smith *et al.*, 1991; Beutin *et al.*, 1993; Chapman *et al.*, 1997).

Other animals, including horses, birds, dogs, cats, wildlife, flies and, of course, humans, are potential hosts of *E. coli* O157:H7 and other VTEC in farm environments (Wilson *et al.*, 1996; Rahn *et al.*, 1997; Wallace *et al.*, 1997; Hancock *et al.*, 1998a; Shere *et al.*, 1998). Although wild animals and birds are potentially important to the epidemiology of VTEC in farm animals, the risk of human exposure from these species is probably lower than from cattle, sheep and goats, because of infrequent contact and lower faecal outputs. In contrast, horses, dogs and cats are potentially more important sources of human exposure, due to their frequent and close contact with humans during care, grooming and petting. These animals may carry VTEC from other sources on their coats or hides, as well as in their own faeces.

VTEC in the farm environment

The farm environment presents an array of possible non-animal habitats for VTEC, including manure heaps or ponds, dams and wells, barns, calf hutches and other buildings, straw and other bedding, feed and feed troughs, water and water troughs, farm equipment, ground and pasture, and watercourses. On dairy farms, milking parlours and equipment, as well as milk, are additional locations. Contamination of these sites with VTEC is most likely to occur from faeces shed by animal hosts, particularly ruminants, which produce large quantities of manure. Oral secretions of ruminants are another possible source, since *E. coli* O157:H7 has been isolated from the tonsils and from the rumen, reticulum and abomasum of infected cattle (Cray and Moon, 1995). Organisms in the forestomachs may be regurgitated during rumination. Once present in the environment, contaminated material may be disseminated to other sites by rainwater, hosing, wind and removal and spreading of manure and be carried by animals and humans.

Although there is no definitive information on environmental contamination with VTEC, levels of *E. coli* O157:H7 in faeces of infected cattle allow an estimate. During the first 10 days after experimental infection, calves shed between 10^4 and 10^8 colony-forming units (CFU) of *E. coli* O157:H7 g^{-1} of faeces and adult cattle shed between 10^1 and 10^7 CFU g^{-1}. Thereafter, calves and adult cattle shed up to about 10^4 and 10^2 CFU g^{-1}, respectively, for 7–20 weeks (Cray and Moon, 1995). Similar concentrations of *E. coli* O157:H7 (2×10^2–8.7×10^4 CFU g^{-1}) were present in the faeces of heifers on dairy farms with persistent *E. coli* O157:H7 infection (Shere *et al.*, 1998). Since adult cattle each excrete approximately 30–50 kg of faeces daily, the immediate environment of infected cattle is probably heavily contaminated.

Experimental models of survival of *E. coli* O157:H7 suggest that contaminated farm environments may remain sources of *E. coli* O157:H7 and possibly other VTEC for several months. *E. coli* O157:H7 survived for at least 10–12 weeks in cattle faeces (Wang *et al.*, 1996; Maule, 1997) and at least 20 weeks in soil (Maule, 1997). Recently, *E. coli* O157:H7 was recovered for up to 38 weeks from inoculated faecal material and from concrete blocks, wood and straw contaminated with the inoculated faecal material (C. Wray, 1997, Weybridge, UK, personal communication). In a study of numerous environmental sites on dairy farms, evidence of VTEC was found in composite samples of calf feeders (19%), calf-barn surfaces (18%), cow feeders (15%) cow-barn surfaces (11%) and individual milk filters (Rahn *et al.*, 1997). However, few VTEC were isolated, suggesting low numbers or poor viability of the organisms.

E. coli O157:H7 has been isolated from manure slurry, and the presence of manure on pastures and vegetable gardens has been linked to human infections with *E. coli* O157:H7 (see below). Also, grazing cattle on land recently fertilized with cattle manure was a possible factor contributing to bovine *E. coli* O157:H7 infections in two studies (Hancock *et al.*, 1994; Mechie *et al.*, 1997), but not in a subsequent study to better define this risk factor (Hancock *et al.*, 1997b). As the infectious dose required for human infection (< 100 organisms) is lower than for most cattle (Cray and Moon, 1995; Hancock *et al.*, 1998a), the risk of transmission of *E. coli* O157:H7 from manure may be greater for humans than for cattle.

E. coli O157:H7 is recoverable for up to 5 weeks from pond, river or rainwater and for up to 12 weeks from potable tap water (Porter *et al.*, 1997; C. Wray, 1997, Weybridge, UK, personal communication). There is also preliminary, though not confirmed, evidence that *E. coli* O157:H7 survives in water in a viable, non-culturable state (Kogure and Ikemoto, 1997). Water-borne transmission in cattle has been linked mostly to water troughs and other cattle waterers contaminated with *E. coli* O157:H7 from the manure or oral secretions of cattle drinking the water (Faith *et al.*, 1996; Hancock *et al.*, 1998b; Shere *et al.*, 1998). In contrast, water consumed by people in rural and farm environments is usually drawn from wells or other locally available supplies, which are more likely to be contaminated by surface water runoff containing manure from infected animals. At least one case of *E. coli* O157:H7 infection on a farm has been linked to this mode of transmission (Jackson *et al.*, 1998). *E. coli* O157:H7 has also been isolated from streams and rivers on land carrying cattle infected with *E. coli* O157:H7 (J. Sargent, 1998, Manhattan, Kansas, unpublished data) and, in another study, all three samples of river water containing non-O157 VTEC were collected after rainfall (Manandhar *et al.*, 1997). Preliminary results from a survey in our laboratory suggest that approximately 1% of private rural water-supplies in Ontario are contaminated with VTEC, although none of the isolates to date is *E. coli* O157:H7 (R.P. Johnson *et al.*, unpublished data).

TRANSMISSION OF VTEC TO HUMANS FROM ANIMALS AND RURAL ENVIRONMENTS

VTEC infection in farm residents

In view of the high prevalence of VTEC in cattle, we conducted a prospective study of 80 dairy-farm families as a model for transmission of VTEC from cattle to humans (Wilson *et al.*, 1996). Evidence of VTEC was found in stool samples of 46% of cattle on 100% of the farms, and *E. coli* O157:H7 was isolated from 0.6% of cattle on 10% of the farms. Twenty-one persons (6.3%) on 16 farms (20.8%) had evidence of VTEC in their stools, although infection was not associated with diarrhoeal illness. VTEC isolated from these persons included *E. coli* O157:H7 and eight other serotypes (O5:non-motile (NM), O7:H4, O80:NM, O91:H14, O103:H2, O119:H25, O132:NM and O146:H2), four of which were present in cattle on the same farms. Serological testing provided further evidence for VTEC infection of farm residents; 41% had antibodies to VT1 and 12.5% were seropositive to O157 LPS. In a similar study of urban residents of nearby Toronto, the corresponding rates of seropositivity were 7.7% and 4.7%, respectively (Reymond *et al.*, 1996). Among the farm family members, children less than 10 years old had the highest rates of VTEC carriage in stools and seropositivity to VT1 (Fig. 10.1), whereas seropositivity to O157 LPS was most frequent in adults 40–50 years old. The presence of a person seropositive to O157 LPS was associated with isolation of *E. coli* O157:H7 from an animal or person on the same farm.

These findings substantiate the ability of VTEC of bovine origin to infect humans in the farm environment. In particular, the serological results indicate much higher rates of exposure than estimated by stool culture, especially among children less than 10 years old. Also, the results suggest that dairy-farm residents may have higher levels of immunity to VTEC than their urban counterparts. Consequently, exposure to the farm environment may be of particular significance for urban residents visiting farms and for farm children with declining maternal immunity. In a family outbreak of VT1-producing *E. coli* O111:NM infection on a dairy farm in Ontario, all urban relatives visiting the farm developed VTEC-associated disease, while none of the family members who lived on the farm became ill (Karmali *et al.*, 1994). The possibility that exposure to the farm environment results in protective immunity should not be overinterpreted, however, in light of several reports of VTEC infections, particularly caused by *E. coli* O157:H7, in farm residents (see below).

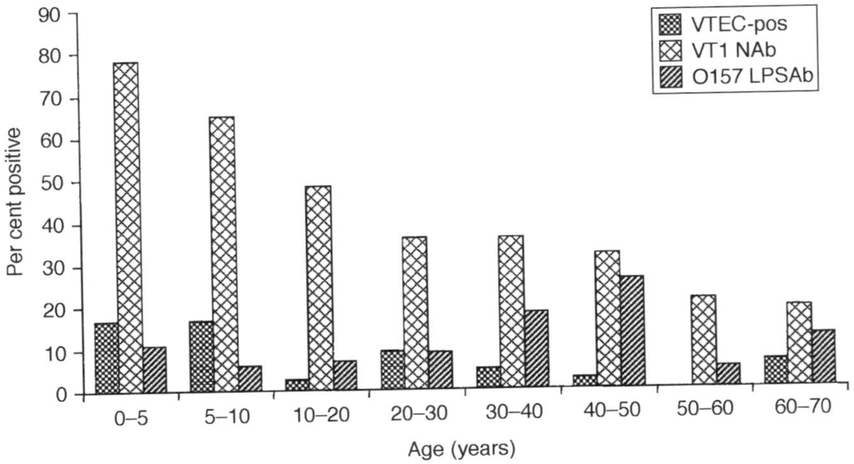

Fig. 10.1. Age-stratified frequencies of verocytotoxigenic *E. coli*-positive stool cultures (VTEC-pos), seropositivity to VT1 (VT1 NAb) and seropositivity to O157 lipopolysaccharide (O157 LPSAb) in dairy-farm family members (from Wilson *et al.*, 1996, with permission).

VTEC infection in abattoir workers

In addition to rural residents, people in other sectors may have greater risk of VTEC infection than the general population through occupational exposure. In 1995, we conducted a prospective study of beef abattoir workers and meat inspectors, who work in close contact with cattle and beef carcass products (Rahn *et al.*, 1996). VTEC were isolated from three (1.3%) of 238 healthy participants and belonged to serotypes O157:H7 and O15:NM. As in the farm-family study (Wilson *et al.*, 1996), none of the infected persons was ill. The frequency of antibodies to VT1 in the abattoir workers (19.4%, R.P. Johnson *et al.*, unpublished data) was similar to that in cattle slaughterers in Italy (15.8%) (Luzzi *et al.*, 1994) and was intermediate between the rates found in urban residents (7.7%) and farm-family members (41%) in Ontario (Reymond *et al.*, 1996). Seropositivity to O157 LPS was also more frequent in abattoir workers (12.4%, R.P. Johnson *et al.*, unpublished data) than in urban residents (4.4%) (Reymond *et al.*, 1996). These findings indicate that exposure to cattle in abattoir environments may increase the risk of VTEC infection.

DISEASE INCIDENTS LINKED TO EXPOSURE ON FARMS

Many dairy-farm residents regularly consume unpasteurized milk, a frequently implicated mode of transmission in farm-associated *E. coli*

O157:H7 infection (Martin *et al.*, 1986; Duncan *et al.*, 1987; Griffin and Tauxe, 1991). Recently however, other modes of transmission have been identified. We investigated one farm where a 13-month-old boy became ill after playing with calves in the calf barn (Renwick *et al.*, 1993). *E. coli* O157:H7 phage type (PT) 23 was isolated from the child, from one of seven calves in the barn and from the boy's older sister, who was asymptomatic. The children had not consumed unpasteurized milk or undercooked beef, suggesting that the source of infection was contact with the calves or their manure. In Scotland, one farm-related *E. coli* O157:H7 infection in a child was attributed to direct transmission from cattle, another to consumption of unpasteurized milk and a third to direct transmission or contact with dogs that roamed freely on an adjacent cattle farm (Synge *et al.*, 1993; Synge and Hopkins, 1994). Dogs were also suspected carriers of *E. coli* O157:H7 from cattle to a child at a farm-visitor centre in Wales (Parry *et al.*, 1995), and in two other farm-associated infections (Trevena *et al.*, 1996; Allison *et al.*, 1997). The organisms were possibly carried on the dogs' coats. In another incident, a pasture recently grazed by cattle was considered as a possible source of *E. coli* O157:H7 infection in campers at a music festival (Smith *et al.*, 1998).

Other ruminants have also been implicated as sources of human VTEC infection. Direct transmission of *E. coli* O157:H7 from sheep and/or cattle was suspected in a case of BD in a youth who worked with livestock in the USA (Rice *et al.*, 1996). Sheep were also implicated sources of *E. coli* O157:H7 in two of 11 farm-associated infections in Scotland (Allison *et al.*, 1997). In each of these incidents, *E. coli* O157:H7 strains with identical pulsed-field gel electrophoresis (PFGE) profiles were isolated from the patients and the implicated animals. Interestingly, both incidents in Scotland were related to lambing, when there is greater direct contact between sheep and those tending them. In addition, goats may have been a source of infection at a farm-visitor centre (Shukla *et al.*, 1995). Transmission by direct contact may also have played a role in a small outbreak of *E. coli* O157:H7 associated with home dressing and processing of a deer carcass (Keene *et al.*, 1997) and infection of a farmer handling horses (Chalmers *et al.*, 1997).

Our investigation of another farm-associated *E. coli* O157:H7 infection (Jackson *et al.*, 1998) illustrates the potential role of well water in transmission of VTEC in rural settings. A 16-month-old girl on an Ontario dairy farm developed BD due to *E. coli* O157:H7 PT 14. She had no known contact with cattle and had not consumed unpasteurized milk. *E. coli* O157:H7 of the same PT was isolated from water from the shallow well on the farm and from 63% of the cattle on the farm. The isolates from the child, the water and the cattle were identical by PFGE, except for a one-band difference in the isolate from the child. The well, which supplied water to both the farmhouse and the dairy herd, was constructed in such a manner that manure-contaminated groundwater could enter the well-head.

It is perhaps surprising that there are so few reports of human VTEC infection associated with rural water-supplies. In areas of high density of domestic and wild ruminants, the potential for contamination of rural water-supplies is undoubtedly high and, as noted above, the organisms can survive in water for several weeks. One possible explanation is that standard water testing may not detect *E. coli* O157:H7. Most methods for identification of *E. coli* in water rely on expression of β-glucuronidase activity and tolerance to temperatures of 43–44.5°C. Since *E. coli* O157:H7 lacks β-glucuronidase activity and may not grow well at these temperatures, it may not be identified as *E. coli* by standard methods, which rely on these characteristics. Where more appropriate techniques have been used, *E. coli* O157:H7 has been recovered from water likely to be contaminated with manure from cattle (Jackson *et al.*, 1998) or deer (McGowan *et al.*, 1989). Most non-O157 VTEC have β-glucuronidase activity, but testing for VTEC among other *E. coli* in water is beyond the scope of most water-testing laboratories.

Animal manure may also be a source of contamination of locally grown vegetables and other fresh produce. The first recognized outbreak of *E. coli* O157:H7 infection in the UK was associated with handling of unwashed potatoes (McGowan *et al.*, 1989). Later, Cieslak *et al.* (1993) found *E. coli* O157:H7 in soil from a vegetable garden linked to a small *E. coli* O157:H7 outbreak. The garden had been fertilized regularly with manure from cattle on the farm. In Germany, parsley from an organic garden was implicated as the vehicle in a kindergarten outbreak caused by VT-producing *Citrobacter freundii* (Tschäpe *et al.*, 1995). In addition, deer faeces were suspected as a source of contamination of dropped apples in an *E. coli* O157:H7 outbreak associated with unpasteurized apple cider (R.E. Besser, cited by Keene *et al.*, 1997).

Visitors to farms also risk exposure to VTEC from any of the above sources. Farm visits are popular among city families for holidays and family gatherings, and schools in urban areas frequently promote educational farm visits for their students. Consumption of unpasteurized milk was the probable source of *E. coli* O157:H7 infection in a 5-month-old child who visited her grandparents' dairy farm (Martin *et al.*, 1986) and in an outbreak among kindergarten children who visited a dairy farm in Ontario (Duncan *et al.*, 1987). In both incidents, *E. coli* O157:H7 was isolated from cattle on the farms. Contact with animals was the most likely mode of transmission in a small outbreak of *E. coli* O157:H7 associated with a farm-visitor centre in the UK (Shukla *et al.*, 1995). Two adults and five children developed BD after visiting the centre. *E. coli* O157:H7 isolated from four of the subjects belonged to PT 2 and were identical by restriction fragment length polymorphism (RFLP) analysis to *E. coli* O157:H7 PT 2 isolates from cattle and goats at the centre. As noted by Parry *et al.* (1995), attendance at farm-visitor centres in the UK is high and the opportunity for close contact between children and livestock at such sites heightens the risk of transmission of VTEC and other zoonoses. Also, the outcome of exposure to VTEC may be more serious for urban residents than for farm residents, because they are less likely to have immunity to VTEC (Reymond *et al.*, 1996; Wilson *et al.*, 1996).

BURDEN OF ILLNESS ASSOCIATED WITH FARMS AND RURAL ENVIRONMENTS

Since VTEC infection became nationally notifiable in Canada in 1990, the reported annual incidence of VTEC infection has fluctuated between a maximum of 5.3 per 100,000 inhabitants in 1991 and a minimum of 3.0 per 100,000 inhabitants in 1993. The incidence varies by province and by year within provinces. For the 4-year period from 1992 to 1995, the highest average annual provincial rates were noted in Prince Edward Island (10.2 per 100,000), Manitoba (7.6 per 100,000) and Alberta (7.4 per 100,000) (Spika *et al.*, 1998).

As in many other countries, surveillance in Canada identifies only a small proportion of infected persons, and the true incidence is probably substantially higher. A recent Canadian study estimated that, for every reported symptomatic case of VTEC infection, there are four to nine unreported cases (Michel, 1997). Moreover, outbreaks are more thoroughly investigated than sporadic cases, even though most infections in Canada are sporadic (Wilson *et al.*, 1997b). Under these circumstances, it is difficult to estimate the true burden of illness associated with farm and rural exposure.

In addition to the studies cited above, an association between rural exposure and VTEC-associated illness was suggested by a case-series study in Scotland, in which 20% of cases lived on or had visited a farm and 17% had been in contact with animal manure (Coia *et al.*, 1994). These findings substantiated conclusions of a smaller study in the Grampian region of Scotland, where 3.8% of the population are involved in agriculture but 13% of cases of VTEC infection occurred in people in this sector (MacDonald *et al.*, 1996). The impact of living in an agricultural area on the risk of VTEC infection was further suggested by a study comparing VTEC isolation rates of diarrhoeic patients living in urban and rural regions of Mexico (Parra *et al.*, 1991). VTEC isolation rates were higher in patients from rural regions compared with those in urban areas.

GEOGRAPHICAL INFORMATION SYSTEM (GIS) MAPPING AND MODELLING

To further investigate the risk of VTEC infection associated with living in rural as opposed to urban areas, we examined the geographical distribution of human VTEC infections in the province of Ontario, Canada, between

1990 and 1995. Although only 16% of the population of Ontario lives in rural areas (Statistics Canada, 1992), more than 19% of all VTEC infections, predominantly VTEC O157:H7, affected rural residents. Calculated annual rates of reported VTEC disease were consistently higher in rural areas (average annual rate 5.4 per 100,000) than in urban areas (average annual rate 4.4 per 100,000). These higher estimated incidence rates were substantiated by a recent study, which applied spatial-regression models and GIS methods (Michel, 1997). When disease incidence was analysed by county, the age-adjusted risk of VTEC infection was highest in counties in three southern regions of predominantly mixed agriculture (Fig. 10.2). Spatial analyses also suggested that human VTEC incidence is higher in rural regions. Furthermore, spatial analyses using animal census data (Statistics Canada, 1992) revealed that farm-animal density and, in particular, cattle density were significant predictors of the incidence of VTEC infections in many regions of Ontario.

These findings clearly identify the increased risk of VTEC infection and disease among rural populations. In addition, they may explain the high incidence of VTEC infections in the province of Prince Edward Island (Spika *et al.*, 1998). The cattle density in this province is 0.17 cattle ha^{-1}, which approximates the cattle density in the three areas of Ontario with high incidence of VTEC infection (0.2 cattle ha^{-1}).

CASE–CONTROL STUDIES

Valuable information on risk factors for sporadic VTEC infection has been obtained from case–control studies involving patients with VTEC-associated disease. The Canadian Pediatric Kidney Disease Research Centre in Ottawa has conducted a prospective study of VTEC infection in children less than 15 years of age in 18 tertiary-care paediatric hospitals across Canada. In an initial report of 34 patients with HUS and 102 controls enrolled in the study in the summer of 1990 (Rowe *et al.*, 1993), contact with a person with diarrhoea was a prominent risk factor for HUS in children. In addition, more cases than controls lived more than 25 km from the participating hospital (41% vs. 2%; $P < 0.05$), drank water from a well (44% vs. 19%, $P < 0.01$), had visited a farm (38% vs. 19%, $P < 0.01$) and had contact with cattle (26% vs. 18%, $P < 0.002$). Subsequent results from 173 patients with HUS and 512 healthy controls over 3 years substantiated contact with persons with diarrhoea and exposure to rural environments as important risk factors for sporadic HUS (Rowe *et al.*, 1994). Among children from urban areas, more cases than controls had been exposed to untreated water or well water (23% vs. 10%, odds ratio (OR) = 2.7, $P < 0.001$) or had visited a farm in the 7 days before the illness (19% vs. 9%, OR = 2.5, $P < 0.01$). Consumption of unchlorinated water was also a risk factor for sporadic *E. coli* O157:H7 disease in the USA (Slutzker *et al.*, 1998).

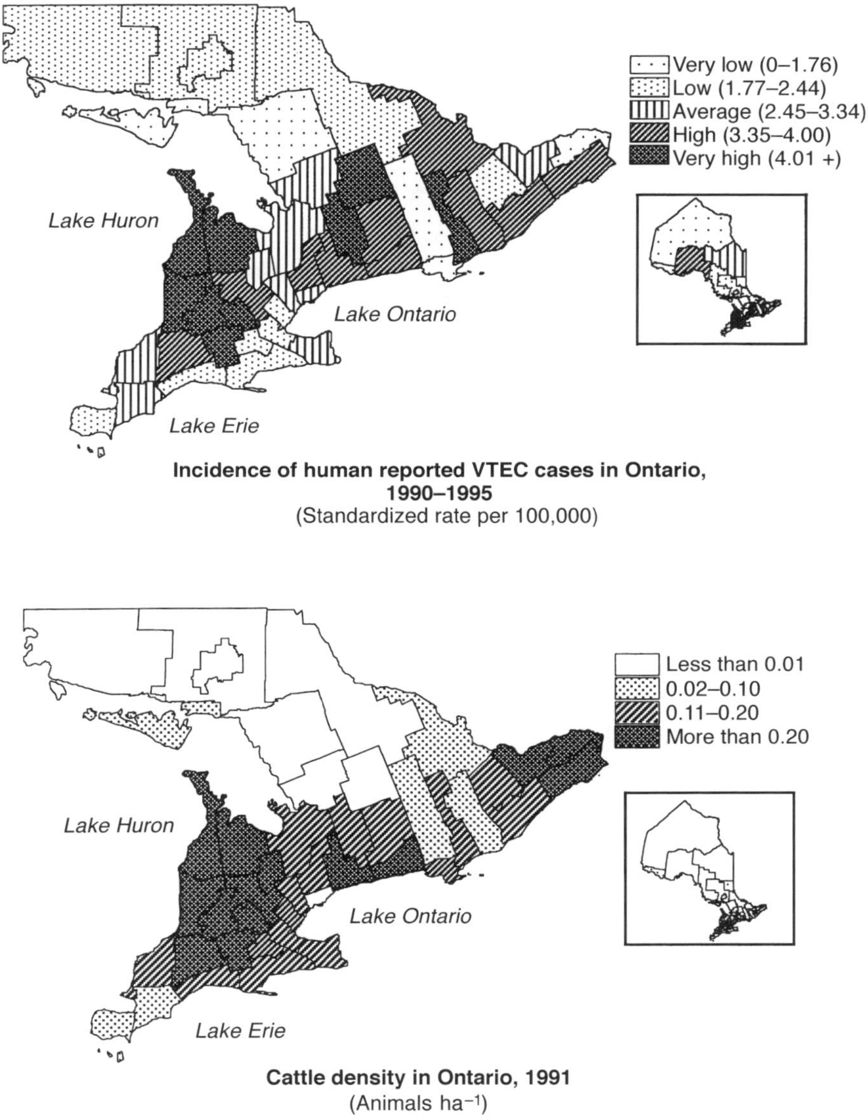

Fig. 10.2. Geographical distributions of reported human cases of verocytotoxigenic *E. coli* (VTEC)-associated disease (upper map) and cattle density (lower map) by county, in Ontario, Canada.

A timely prospective study of the association between *E. coli* O157:H7 infections and farm exposure in two counties in the UK will also provide valuable information. In a preliminary report (Trevena *et al.*, 1997), nine cases had been identified with a history of farm exposure and animal contact. *E. coli* O157:H7 was isolated from all patients and from animals on the respective farms. Isolates from six of the nine patients and from animals on the respective farms were indistinguishable, providing strong evidence for transmission from farm animals to humans.

CONCLUSIONS

The above information confirms the risk of human VTEC infection associated with farms and rural environments. This is not surprising, in view of the prevalence of VTEC in animals, the extent of contamination of farm and rural environments, including water-supplies and the survival of VTEC O157:H7 in these environments. Perhaps most importantly, it focuses attention on the increased incidence of disease linked to rural exposure, which is largely sporadic, and on the frequency of exposure and disease in children. However, apart from several established risk factors, such as consumption of unpasteurized milk, the contributions of direct transmission from animals and farm environments, contaminated water-supplies or local produce to the elevated risk for infection in these environments remain undefined.

With existing knowledge, control of exposure to VTEC in rural settings should be centred on education of public-health and health-care workers with respect to farm and rural exposure as a source of human infection. Specific strategies include reducing or eliminating consumption of unpasteurized milk by introducing home pasteurizers or purchase of pasteurized milk, reducing contact between animals and young children or old persons, testing of water-supplies and remediation, application of more stringent hygienic practices to local produce and meats and reducing exposure of farm visitors to potential risk factors.

The outcomes of several studies suggest profitable areas for future investigations. Extending the application of GIS analyses to other regions would better define the relative risks associated with different geographical regions and would identify high-risk areas. Surveillance and analytical epidemiological studies are required to identify risk factors for exposure to *E. coli* O157:H7 and other VTEC in rural areas, including regions where ruminants other than cattle are reared or are natural inhabitants. Considerably more is known about *E. coli* O157:H7 than about other VTEC. While this is appropriate for the predominant serotype associated with human disease, many non-O157 VTEC that are recognized human pathogens are harboured by animals. The recent availability of improved and economical tests for non-O157 VTEC will hopefully enable investigations of the importance of these organisms in human disease. In addition, the health outcomes and costs associated with VTEC infections acquired in rural areas need to be assessed, as does the effectiveness of education of rural residents in reducing disease incidence.

Another important need is the development of strategies to reduce the prevalence of pathogenic VTEC in animal hosts. Considerable effort has already been invested in controlling these and other pathogens in the production and processing of meats and other foods. However, controlling VTEC at the farm level will not only reduce food-borne infections but will have a substantial impact on the elevated risks associated with farms and rural environments. Several groups, including our own, have been investigating the ecology of VTEC at the farm level in an effort to identify potential control strategies. The outcomes of these and other investigations will hopefully result in cost-effective reduction of *E. coli* O157:H7 and other VTEC in rural areas and the food-chain.

REFERENCES

Aleksic, S. (1994) Annex 2: List of serotypes of SLTEC and related strains isolated from man, animals and foodstuffs. In: *Report of the WHO Working Group Meeting on Shiga-like Toxin Producing* Escherichia coli *(SLTEC), with Emphasis on Zoonotic Aspects.* WHO/CDS/VPH/94.136, World Health Organization, Bergamo, Italy, pp. 13–15.

Allison, L., Carter, P. and Thomson-Carter, F. (1997) Pinpointing human infection of *E. coli* O157 from animals. In: *VTEC 97, Abstracts of the 3rd International Symposium and Workshop on Shiga Toxin (Verocytotoxin)-producing* Escherichia coli *Infections*, Baltimore, 22–26 June, 1997, Abstract V84/I, p. 10.

Barrett, T.J., Kaper, J.B., Jerse, A.E. and Wachsmuth, I.K. (1992) Virulence factors in Shiga-like toxin-producing *Escherichia coli* isolated from humans and cattle. *Journal of Infectious Diseases* 165, 979–980.

Besser, T.E., Hancock, D.D., Pritchett, L.C., McRae, E.M., Rice, D.H. and Tarr, P.I. (1997) Duration of detection of fecal excretion of *Escherichia coli* O157:H7 in cattle. *Journal of Infectious Diseases* 175, 726–727.

Beutin, L., Geier, D., Steinrück, H., Zimmermann, S. and Scheutz, F. (1993) Prevalence and some properties of verotoxin (Shiga-like toxin)-producing *Escherichia coli* in seven different species of healthy domestic animals. *Journal of Clinical Microbiology* 31, 2483–2488.

Boerlin, P., McEwen, S.A., Boerlin-Petzold, F., Wilson, J.B., Johnson, R.P. and Gyles, C.L. (1998) Associations between virulence factors of Shiga toxin-producing *Escherichia coli* and disease in humans. *Journal of Clinical Microbiology* 37, 497–503.

Borczyk, A.A., Karmali, M.A., Lior, H. and Duncan, L.M. (1987) Bovine reservoir for verotoxin-producing *Escherichia coli* O157:H7. *Lancet* i, 98.

Borman-Eby, H.C., McEwen, S.A., Clarke, R.C., McNab, W.B., Rahn, K. and Valdivieso-Garcia, A. (1993) The seroprevalence of verocytotoxin-producing *Escherichia coli* in Ontario dairy cows and associations with production and management. *Preventive Veterinary Medicine* 15, 261–274.

Butler, D.G. and Clarke, R.C. (1994) Diarrhoea and dysentery in calves. In: Gyles, C.L. (ed.) Escherichia coli *in Domestic Animals and Humans.* CAB International, Wallingford, pp. 91–116.

Chalmers, R.M., Salmon, R.L., Willshaw, G.A., Cheasty, T., Looker, N., Davies, I. and Wray, C. (1997) Vero cytotoxin-producing *Escherichia coli* in a farmer handling horses. *Lancet* 349, 1816.

Chapman, P.A. and Ackroyd, H.J. (1997) Farmed deer as a potential source of verocytotoxin-producing *Escherichia coli* O157. *Veterinary Record* 141, 314–315.

Chapman, P.A., Wright, D.G. and Normal, P. (1989) Verotoxin-producing *Escherichia coli* infections in Sheffield: cattle as a possible source. *Epidemiology and Infection* 102, 439–445.

Chapman, P.A., Siddons, C.A., Cerdan Malo, A.T. and Harkin, M.A. (1997) A 1-year study of *Escherichia coli* O157 in cattle, sheep, pigs and poultry. *Epidemiology and Infection* 119, 245–250.

Cieslak, P.R., Barrett, T.J., Griffin, P.M., Gensheimer, G.A., Beckett, G., Buffington, J. and Smith, M.G. (1993) *Escherichia coli* O157:H7 infection from a manured garden. *Lancet* 342, 367.

Clarke, R.C., Wilson, J.B., Read, S.C., Renwick, S., Rahn, K., Johnson, R.P., Alves, D., Karmali, M.A., Lior, H., McEwen, S.A., Spika, J. and Gyles, C.L. (1994) Verocytotoxin-producing *Escherichia coli* (VTEC) in the food chain: preharvest and processing perspectives. In: Karmali, M.A. and Goglio, A.G. (eds) *Recent Advances in Verocytotoxin-producing* Escherichia coli *Infections.* Elsevier Science BV, Amsterdam, pp. 17–24.

Coia, J.E., Sharp, J.C.M., Curnow, J. and Reilly, W.J. (1994) Ten years experience of *Escherichia coli* O157 in Scotland (1984–1993). In: Karmali, M.A. and Goglio, A.G. (eds) *Recent Advances in Verocytotoxin-producing* Escherichia coli *Infections.* Elsevier Science BV, Amsterdam, pp. 41–44.

Conedera, G., Zuin, A. and Marangon, S. (1994) Seroprevalence of neutralizing antibodies to *Escherichia coli* verocytotoxins in domestic and wild animals in Italy. In: Karmali, M.A. and Goglio, A.G. (eds) *Recent Advances in Verocytotoxin-producing* Escherichia coli *Infections.* Elsevier Science BV, Amsterdam, pp. 81–84.

Cray, W.C., Jr and Moon, H.W. (1995) Experimental infection of calves and adult cattle with *Escherichia coli* O157:H7. *Applied and Environmental Microbiology* 61, 1586–1590.

Duncan, L., Mai, V., Carter, A., Carlson, J.A.K., Borczyk, A. and Karmali, M.A. (1987) Outbreak of gastrointestinal disease – Ontario. *Canada Disease Weekly Report* 13, 5–8.

Faith, N.G., Shere, J.A., Brosch, R., Arnold, K.W., Ansay, S.E., Lee, M.-S., Luchansky, J.B. and Kaspar, C.W. (1996) Prevalence and clonal nature of *Escherichia coli* O157:H7 on dairy farms in Wisconsin. *Applied and Environmental Microbiology* 62, 1519–1525.

Garber, L.P., Wells, S.J., Hancock, D.D., Doyle, M.P., Tuttle, J., Shere, J.A. and Zhao, T. (1995) Risk factors for fecal shedding of *Escherichia coli* O157:H7 in dairy calves. *Journal of the American Veterinary Medical Association* 207, 46–49.

Griffin, P.M. (1998) Epidemiology of Shiga toxin-producing *Escherichia coli* infections in the United States. In: Kaper, J.B. and O'Brien, A.D. (eds) Escherichia coli *O157:H7 and Other Shiga Toxin-producing* E. coli *Strains.* ASM Press, Washington, DC, pp. 15–22.

Griffin, P.M. and Tauxe, R.V. (1991) The epidemiology of infections caused by *Escherichia coli* O157:H7, other enterohemorrhagic *E. coli*, and the associated hemolytic uremic syndrome. *Epidemiological Reviews* 13, 60–98.

Gyles, C.L., Johnson, R.P., Gao, A., Ziebell, K., Pierard, D., Aleksic, S. and Boerlin, P. (1998) Association of enterohemorrhagic *Escherichia coli* hemolysin with serotypes of Shiga-like toxin-producing *Escherichia coli* of human and bovine origins. *Applied and Environmental Microbiology* 64, 4134–4141.

Hancock, D.D., Besser, T.E., Kinsel, M.L., Tarr, P.I., Rice, D.H. and Paros, M.G. (1994) The prevalence of *Escherichia coli* O157:H7 in dairy and beef cattle in Washington State. *Epidemiology and Infection* 113, 199–207.

Hancock, D.D., Besser, T.E., Rice, D.H., Herriott, D.E. and Tarr, P.I. (1997a) Longitudinal study of *Escherichi coli* O157 in fourteen cattle herds. *Epidemiology and Infection* 118, 193–195.

Hancock, D.D., Rice, D.H., Herriott, D.E., Besser, T.E., Ebel, E.D. and Carpenter, L.V. (1997b) Effects of farm manure handling practices on *Escherichia coli* O157 prevalence in cattle. *Journal of Food Protection* 60, 363–366.

Hancock, D.D., Rice, D.H., Thomas, L.A., Dargatz, D.A. and Besser, T.E. (1997c) Epidemiology of *Escherichia coli* O157 in feedlot cattle. *Journal of Food Protection* 60, 462–465.

Hancock, D.D., Besser, T.E. and Rice, D.H. (1998a) Ecology of *Escherichia coli* O157:H7 in cattle and impact of management practices. In: Kaper, J.B. and O'Brien, A.D. (eds) Escherichia coli *O157:H7 and Other Shiga Toxin-producing* E. coli *Strains.* ASM Press, Washington, DC, pp. 85–91.

Hancock, D.D., Besser, T.E., Rice, D.H., Ebel, E.D., Herriott, D.E. and Carpenter, L.V. (1998b) Multiple sources of *Escherichia coli* O157 in feedlots and dairy farms in the Northwestern USA. *Preventive Veterinary Medicine* 35, 11–19.

Heuvelink, A.E., van den Biggelaar, F.L.A.M., de Boer, E., Herbes, R.G., Melchers, W.J.G., Huis in 't Veld, J.H.J. and Monnens, L.A.H. (1998) Isolation and characterization of verocytotoxin-producing *Escherichia coli* O157 strains from Dutch cattle and sheep. *Journal of Clinical Microbiology* 36, 878–882.

Jackson, S.G., Goodbrand, B.R., Johnson, R.P., Odorico, V.G., Alves, D., Rahn, K., Wilson, J.B., Welch, M.K. and Khakhria, R. (1998) *Escherichia coli* O157:H7 diarrhoea associated with well water and infected cattle on an Ontario dairy farm. *Epidemiology and Infection* 120, 17–20.

Johnson, R.P., Clarke, R.C., Wilson, J.B., Read, S.C., Rahn, K., Renwick, S.A., Sandhu, K., Alves, D., Karmali, M.A., Lior, H., McEwen, S.A., Spika, J.S. and Gyles, C.L. (1996a) Growing concerns and recent outbreaks involving non-O157 serotypes of verotoxigenic *Escherichia coli. Journal of Food Protection* 59, 1112–1122.

Johnson, R.P., Cray, W.C., Jr and Johnson, S.T. (1996b) Serological responses of cattle following experimental infection with *Escherichia coli* O157:H7. *Infection and Immunity* 64, 1879–1883.

Johnson, W.M., Lior, H. and Bezanson, G.S. (1983) Cytotoxigenic *Escherichia coli* O157:H7 associated with haemorrhagic colitis in Canada. *Lancet* i, 76.

Karmali, M.A. (1989) Infection by verocytotoxin-producing *Escherichia coli. Clinical and Microbiological Reviews* 2, 15–38.

Karmali, M.A., Petric, M., Winkler, M., Bielaszewská, M., Brunton, J., Van de Kar, N., Morooka, T., Balakrishna Nair, G., Richardson, S.E. and Arbus, G.S. (1994) Enzyme-linked immunosorbent assay for detection of immunoglobulin G antibodies to *Escherichia coli* Vero cytotoxin 1. *Journal of Clinical Microbiology* 32, 1457–1463.

Keene, W.E., Sazie, E., Kok, J., Rice, D.H., Hancock, D.D., Balan, V.K., Zhao, T. and Doyle, M.P. (1997) An outbreak of *Escherichia coli* O157:H7 infections traced to jerky made from deer meat. *Journal of the American Medical Association* 277, 1229–1231.

Kogure, K. and Ikemoto, E. (1997) Wide occurrence of enterohemorrhagic *Escherichia coli* O157 in natural freshwater environment. *Nippon Saikingaku Zasshi* 52, 601–607.

Kudva, I.T., Hatfield, P.G. and Hovde, C.J. (1997) Characterization of *Escherichia coli* O157:H7 and other Shiga-like toxin-producing *E. coli* serotypes isolated from sheep. *Journal of Clinical Microbiology* 35, 892–899.

Le Saux, N., Spika, J.S., Friesen, B., Johnson, I., Melnychuck, D., Anderson, C., Dion, R., Rahman, M. and Tostowaryk, W. (1993) Ground beef consumption in non-commercial settings is a risk factor for sporadic *Escherichia coli* O157:H7 infection in Canada. *Journal of Infectious Diseases* 167, 500–502.

Luzzi, I., Farina, C., Goglio, A.A., Scardellato, U., Pizzoccaro, P., Benedetti, I., Minelli, F. and Caprioli, A. (1994) Seroprevalence of neutralizing antibodies to *Escherichia coli* verotoxins in the population of two Italian regions. In: Karmali, M.A. and Goglio, A.G. (eds) *Recent Advances in Verocytotoxin-producing* Escherichia coli *Infections*. Elsevier Science BV, Amsterdam, pp. 85–88.

MacDonald, I.A.R., Gould, I.M. and Curnow, J. (1996) Epidemiology of infection due to *Escherichia coli* O157: a 3-year prospective study. *Epidemiology and Infection* 116, 279–284.

McGowan, K.L., Wickersham, E. and Strockbine, N.A. (1989) *Escherichia coli* O157:H7 from water. *Lancet* i, 967–968.

Manandhar, R., Bettiol, S.S., Bettelheim, K.A. and Goldsmid, J.M. (1997) Isolation of verotoxigenic *Escherichia coli* from the Tasmanian environment. *Comparative Immunology, Microbiology and Infectious Disease* 20, 271–279.

Martin, M.L., Shipman, L., Wells, J.G., Potter, M.E., Hedberg, K., Wachsmuth, I.K., Tauxe, R.V., Davis, J.P., Arnoldi, J. and Tilleli, J. (1986) Isolation of *Escherichia coli* O157:H7 from dairy cattle associated with two cases of haemolytic uraemic syndrome. *Lancet* ii, 1043.

Maule, A. (1997) The survival of *Escherichia coli* O157 in model ecosystems and on surfaces. In: *VTEC 97, Abstracts of the 3rd International Symposium and Workshop on Shiga Toxin (Verocytotoxin)-producing* Escherichia coli *Infections*, Baltimore, 22–26 June, 1997, Abstract V182/II, p. 38.

Mechie, S.C., Chapman, P.A. and Siddons, C.A. (1997) A fifteen month study of *Escherichia coli* O157:H7 in a dairy herd. *Epidemiology and Infection* 118, 17–25.

Michel, P. (1997) An epidemiologic study of human cases of verocytotoxigenic *Escherichia coli* infection reported in Ontario, Canada. PhD thesis, University of Guelph.

Montenegro, M.A., Bülte, M., Trumpf, T., Aleksic, S., Reuter, G., Bulling, E. and Helmuth, R. (1990) Detection and characterization of fecal verotoxin-producing *Escherichia coli* from healthy cattle. *Journal of Clinical Microbiology* 28, 1417–1421.

Parra, M.N., Torres, L.J., Camorlinga, P.M., Giono, C.S.G.A.S. and Munoz, H.O. (1991) Frequency of identification of cytotoxigenic strains of *Escherichia coli* in cases of diarrhea from rural and urban communities. *Archives of Investigative Medicine (Mexico)* 22, 217–222.

Parry, S.M., Salmon, R.L., Willshaw, G.A., Cheasty, T., Lund, L.J., Weardon, P., Quoraishi, A.H. and Fitzgerald, T. (1995) Haemorrhagic colitis in child after visit to farm visitor centre. *Lancet* 346, 572.

Parry, S.M., Salmon, R.L., Willshaw, G.A. and Cheasty, T. (1998) Risk factors for and prevention of sporadic infections with vero cytotoxin (shiga toxin) producing *Escherichia coli* O157. *Lancet* 351, 1019–1022.

Pirro, F., Wieler, L.H., Failing, K., Bauerfeind, R. and Baljer, G. (1995) Neutralizing antibodies against Shiga-like toxins from *Escherichia coli* in colostra and sera of cattle. *Veterinary Microbiology* 43, 131–141.

Porter, J., Mobbs, K., Saunders, J.R., Pickup, R.W. and Edwards, C. (1997) Detection, distribution and probable fate of *Escherichia coli* O157 from asymptomatic cattle on a dairy farm. *Journal of Applied Bacteriology* 83, 297–306.

Rahn, K., Johnson, R.P., Wilson, J.B., Stewart, B.A., Clarke, R.C., Odomeru, J., Alves, D., Clark, C.G., Karmali, M.A., McEwen, S.A. and Spika, J. (1996) Occupational exposure of abattoir workers to verotoxigenic *Escherichia coli, Salmonella* spp. and *Campylobacter* spp. In: *Abstracts, 96th Annual Meeting of the American Society for Microbiology, New Orleans, USA, 19–23 May, 1996*, p. 370.

Rahn, K., Renwick, S.A., Johnson, R.P., Wilson, J.B., Clarke, R.C., Alves, D., McEwen, S.A., Lior, H. and Spika, J.S. (1997) Persistence of *Escherichia coli* O157:H7 in dairy cattle and the dairy farm environment. *Epidemiology and Infection* 119, 251–259.

Read, S.C., Gyles, C.L., Clarke, R.C., Lior, H. and McEwen, S. (1990) Prevalence of verocytotoxigenic *Escherichia coli* in ground beef, pork, and chicken in southwestern Ontario. *Epidemiology and Infection* 105, 11–20.

Renwick, S.A., Wilson, J.B., Clarke, R.C., Lior, H., Borczyk, A.A., Spika, J., Rahn, K., McFadden, K., Brouwer, A., Copps, A., Anderson, N.G., Alves, D. and Karmali, M.A. (1993) Evidence of direct transmission of *Escherichia coli* O157: H7 infection between calves and a human. *Journal of Infectious Diseases* 168, 792–793.

Reymond, D., Johnson, R.P., Karmali, M.A., Petric, M., Winkler, M., Johnson, S., Rahn, K., Renwick, S., Wilson, J., Clarke, R.C. and Spika, J. (1996) Neutralizing antibodies to *Escherichia coli* Vero cytotoxin 1 and antibodies to O157 lipopolysaccharide in healthy farm family members and urban residents. *Journal of Clinical Microbiology* 34, 2053–2057.

Rice, D.H., Hancock, D.D., Vettor, R.L. and Besser, T.E. (1996) *Escherichia coli* O157 infection in a human linked to exposure to infected livestock. *Veterinary Record* 138, 311.

Rice, D.H., Hancock, D.D. and Besser, T.E. (1998) Verotoxigenic *E. coli* O157 colonization of wild deer and range cattle. *Veterinary Record* 137, 524.

Riley, L.W., Remis, R.S., Helgerson, S.D., McGee, H.B., Wells, J.G., Davis, B.R., Hebert, R.J., Olcott, E.S., Johnson, L.M., Hargrett, N.T., Blake, P.A. and Cohen, M.L. (1983) Hemorrhagic colitis associated with a rare *Escherichia coli* serotype. *New England Journal of Medicine* 308, 681–685.

Robins-Browne, R., Elliott, E. and Desmarchelier, P. (1998) Shiga toxin-producing *Escherichia coli* in Australia. In: Kaper, J.B. and O'Brien, A.D. (eds) Escherichia coli *O157:H7 and Other Shiga Toxin-producing* E. coli *Strains.* ASM Press, Washington, DC, pp. 66–72.

Rowe, P.C., Orrbine, E., Lior, H., Wells, G.A., McLaine, P.N. and the CPKDRC Co-investigators (1993) Diarrhoea in close contacts as a risk factor for childhood haemolytic uraemic syndrome. *Epidemiology and Infection* 110, 1–7.

Rowe, P.C., Orrbine, E., Lior, H., Wells, G.A., McLaine, P.N. and the CPKDRC Co-investigators (1994) Diarrhoea among close contacts is an important risk factor for childhood hemolytic uremic syndrome. In: *VTEC 94: Abstracts of the 2nd International Symposium and Workshop on Verocytotoxin-producing* Escherichia coli *Infections, Bergamo, Italy, 27–30 June 1994*, Abstract P4.2, p. 78.

Sandhu, K.S., Clarke, R.C., McFadden, K., Brouwer, A., Louie, M., Wilson, J., Lior, H. and Gyles, C.L. (1996) Prevalence of the *eaeA* gene in verotoxigenic *Escherichia coli* strains from dairy cattle in southern Ontario. *Epidemiology and Infection* 116, 1–7.

Shere, J.A., Bartlett, K.J. and Kaspar, C.W. (1998) Longitudinal study of *Escherichia coli* O157:H7 dissemination on four dairy farms in Wisconsin. *Applied and Environmental Microbiology* 64, 1390–1399.

Shukla, R., Slack, R., George, A., Cheasty, T., Rowe, B. and Scotter, J. (1995) *Escherichia coli* infection associated with a farm visitor centre. *Communicable Disease Report* 6, R144–R146.

Sidjabat-Tambunan, H. and Bensink, J.C. (1997) Verotoxin-producing *Escherichia coli* from the faeces of sheep, calves and pigs. *Australian Veterinary Journal* 75, 292–293.

Slutzker, L., Ries, A.A., Maloney, K., Wells, J.G., Greene, K.D. and Griffin, P.M. (1998) A nationwide case–control study of *Escherichia coli* O157:H7 infection in the United States. *Journal of Infectious Diseases* 177, 962–966.

Smith, H.R., Cheasty, T., Roberts, D., Thomas, A. and Rowe, B. (1991) Examination of retail chickens and sausages in Britain for Vero cytotoxin-producing *Escherichia coli*. *Applied and Environmental Microbiology* 57, 2091–2093.

Smith, H.R., Rowe, B., Adak, G.K. and Reilly, W.J. (1998) Shiga toxin (verocytotoxin)-producing *Escherichia coli* in the United Kingdom. In: Kaper, J.B. and O'Brien, A.D. (eds) Escherichia coli *O157:H7 and Other Shiga Toxin-producing* E. coli *Strains*. ASM Press, Washington, DC, pp. 49–58.

Spika, J.S., Khakhria, R., Michel, P., Milley, D., Wilson, J. and Waters, J. (1998) Shiga toxin-producing *Escherichia coli* infections in Canada. In: Kaper, J.B. and O'Brien, A.D. (eds) Escherichia coli *O157:H7 and Other Shiga Toxin-producing* E. coli *Strains*. ASM Press, Washington, DC, pp. 23–29.

Statistics Canada. Agricultural Profile of Ontario – Part 1. Ottawa: Statistics Canada, 1992. 1991 Census of Agriculture. Catalogue Number 95-336D.

Statistics Canada. Profile of Census Divisions and Census Subdivisions – Part A. Ottawa: Supply and Services Canada, 1992. 1991 Census of Canada. Service Number 846-031.

Strockbine, N.A., Wells, J.G., Bopp, C.A. and Barrett, T.J. (1998) Overview of detection and subtyping methods. In: Kaper, J.B. and O'Brien, A.D. (eds) Escherichia coli *O157 and Other Shiga Toxin-producing* E. coli *Strains*. ASM Press, Washington, DC, pp. 331–356.

Synge, B.A. and Hopkins, G.F. (1992) Verotoxigenic *Escherichia coli* O157 in Scottish calves. *Veterinary Record* 130, 583.

Synge, B.A. and Hopkins, G.F. (1994) Studies of verotoxigenic *Escherichia coli* O157 in cattle in Scotland and association with human cases. In: Karmali, M.A. and Goglio, A.G. (eds) *Recent Advances in Verocytotoxin-producing* Escherichia coli *Infections*. Elsevier Science BV, Amsterdam, pp. 65–68.

Synge, B.A., Hopkins, G.F., Reilly, W.J. and Sharp, J.C.M. (1993) Possible link between cattle and *E. coli* O157 infection in a human. *Veterinary Record* 133, 507.

Trevena, W.B., Willshaw, G.A., Cheasty, T., Wray, C. and Gallagher, J. (1996) Vero cytotoxin-producing *E. coli* O157 infection associated with farms. *Lancet* 347, 60–61.

Trevena, W.B., Willshaw, G.A., Cheasty, T. and Wray, C. (1997) Associations between human infection with Vero cytotoxin-producing *E. coli* O157 and farm animal contact. In: *VTEC 97, Abstracts of the 3rd International Symposium and Workshop on Shiga Toxin (Verocytotoxin)-producing* Escherichia coli *Infections, Baltimore, 22–26 June, 1997*, Abstract V28/I, p. 3.

Tschäpe, H., Prager, R., Streckel, W., Fruth, A., Tietze, E. and Böhme, G. (1995) Verotoxinogenic *Citrobacter freundii* associated with severe gastroenteritis and cases of haemolytic uraemic syndrome in a nursery school: green butter as the infection source. *Epidemiology and Infection* 114, 441–450.

Wallace, J.S., Cheasty, T. and Rowe, B. (1997) Isolation of Vero cytotoxin-producing *Escherichia coli* O157 from wild birds. *Journal of Applied Microbiology* 82, 399–404.

Wang, G., Zhao, T. and Doyle, M.P. (1996) Fate of enterohemorrhagic *Escherichia coli* O157:H7 in bovine feces. *Applied and Environmental Microbiology* 62, 2567–2570.

Wells, J.G., Davis, B.R., Wachsmuth, I.K., Riley, L.W., Remis, R.S., Sokolow, R. and Morris, G.K. (1983) Laboratory investigation of hemorrhagic colitis outbreaks associated with a rare *Escherichia coli* serotype. *Journal of Clinical Microbiology* 18, 512–520.

Wells, J.G., Shipman, L.D., Greene, K.D., Sowers, E.G., Green, J.H., Cameron, D.N., Downes, F.P., Martin, M.L., Griffin, P.M., Ostroff, S.M., Potter, M.E., Tauxe, R.V. and Wachsmuth, I.K. (1991) Isolation of *Escherichia coli* serotype O157:H7 and other shiga-like-toxin-producing *E. coli* from dairy cattle. *Journal of Clinical Microbiology* 29, 985–989.

Willshaw, G.A., Scotland, S.M., Smith, H.R. and Rowe, B. (1992) Properties of vero cytotoxin-producing *Escherichia coli* of human origin of O serogroups other than O157. *Journal of Infectious Diseases* 166, 797–802.

Wilson, J.B., McEwen, S.A., Clarke, R.C., Leslie, K.E., Wilson, R.A., Waltner-Toews, D. and Gyles, C.L. (1992) Distribution and characteristics of verocytotoxigenic *Escherichia coli* isolated from Ontario dairy cattle. *Epidemiology and Infection* 108, 423–439.

Wilson, J.B., Clarke, R.C., Renwick, S., Rahn, K., Johnson, R.P., Alves, D., Karmali, M.A., Lior, H., McEwen, S.A. and Spika, J. (1994) Verocytotoxigenic *Escherichia coli* infections on dairy farms in southern Ontario. In: Karmali, M.A. and Goglio, A.G. (eds) *Recent Advances in Verocytotoxin-producing* Escherichia coli *Infections*. Elsevier Science BV, Amsterdam, pp. 61–64.

Wilson, J.B., Clarke, R.C., Renwick, S.A., Rahn, K., Johnson, R.P., Karmali, M.A., Lior, H., Alves, D., Gyles, C.L., Sandhu, K.S., McEwen, S.A. and Spika, J.S. (1996) Verocytotoxigenic *Escherichia coli* infections in dairy farm families. *Journal of Infectious Diseases* 174, 1021–1027.

Wilson, J.B., Johnson, R.P., Clarke, R.C., Rahn, K., Renwick, S.A., Alves, D., Karmali, M.A., Michel, P., Orrbine, E. and Spika, J. (1997a) Canadian perspectives on verocytotoxin-producing *Escherichia coli* infections. *Journal of Food Protection* 60, 1451–1453.

Wilson, J.B., Johnson, R.P., Clarke, R.C., Rahn, K., Renwick, S., Michel, P., Johnson, W., Khakhria, R., Todd, E. and Spika, J. (1997b) Working paper on current trends and activities related to verocytotoxigenic *Escherichia coli* (VTEC) infection in Canada. In: *World Health Organization Consultation on the Prevention and Control of Enterohaemorrhagic* Escherichia coli *(EHEC) Infections, Geneva, Switzerland, 28 April–1 May, 1997*, World Health Organization Publication FSF/FOS/97.6, Geneva, pp. 4–5.

Zhao, T., Doyle, M.P., Shere, J. and Garber, L. (1995) Prevalence of enterohemorrhagic *Escherichia coli* O157:H7 in a survey of dairy herds. *Applied and Environmental Microbiology* 61, 1290–1293.

11

Control of *Escherichia coli* O157:H7 at Slaughter

V.P.J. Gannon

Food Directorate, Health Canada, c/o Animal Disease Research Institute, Lethbridge, Alberta, Canada

INTRODUCTION

It can be reasonably assumed that some level of microbial contamination of beef carcasses will occur at slaughter and that, at best, this can be minimized through fastidious control of hygiene and the product temperature. It is felt by many, including authorities in government, industry and academia, that this can be best accomplished by the use of a quality-control system, such as hazard analysis and critical control points (National Advisory Committee on Microbiological Criteria for Foods, 1998). However, it is clear that *Escherichia coli* O157:H7 presents a unique challenge to the beef industry and, indeed, to the entire food industry, in that it not only has a very low infectious dose, but is also able to withstand low pH (Abdul-Raouf *et al.*, 1993; Weagant *et al.*, 1994; Arnold and Kaspar, 1995; Uljas and Ingham, 1998). This implies not only that low levels of product contamination may result in a disease risk but also that new or altered processing procedures are required to ensure product safety. Fortunately, several intervention strategies have been identified which should decrease the risk of *E. coli* O157:H7 infection associated with consuming beef. The most promising of these methods include: (i) a combined whole-carcass treatment, consisting of hot water or pressurized steam, followed by a wash using a hot lactic or acetic acid solution (Nutsch *et al.*, 1997; Phebus *et al.*, 1997; Dorsa *et al.*, 1998b); and (ii) low- to medium-dose irradiation of packaged beef products (Thayer and Boyd, 1993; Roberts and Weese, 1998; Lopez-Gonzalez *et al.*, 1999). Despite these advances, it is generally felt that control strategies for this and other food-borne pathogens must extend along the food-production continuum (from 'gate to plate') and include not only slaughter and processing steps but also measures to control the pathogen in cattle populations. At the other end of this continuum, steps can be taken to limit growth and survival of *E. coli* O157:H7 during transport, storage and retail display and to provide effective decontamination and cooking procedures.

EPIDEMIOLOGY OF *E. COLI* O157:H7 IN CATTLE

The isolation of *E. coli* O157:H7 from cattle faeces in many countries worldwide, the seasonal and animal-to-animal variations in this process and the links to human disease have been widely reported (Chapman *et al.*, 1993) and are reviewed in the companion chapters in this publication. Recently, van Donkersgoed *et al.* (1999) reported the isolation of *E. coli* O157:H7 from 12.4% of yearling beef cattle, with 33.6% of the slaughter process lots (usually a single shipment from one feedlot) testing positive. Given that only five animals were sampled per process lot, it suggests that many positive feedlots exist. In contrast, only 2.0% of culled adult cattle were found to shed the organism in their faeces. A seasonal trend was also noted in this Canadian study, with the organism isolated from the faeces of 0.75% of all cattle at slaughter in the winter (December–February) and from 19.7% of all cattle in the summer (June–August).

Unfortunately, most of these epidemiological studies have concentrated on the number of cattle shedding the organism in their faeces. With the advent of more sensitive isolation methods, the number of faecal-positive animals in studies has increased. Selective culture of faeces in broth media followed by immunomagnetic separation (IMS) and subculture on to selective and differential media, such as cefixime tellurite sorbitol MacConkey agar (CT-SMAC) is now favoured by a number of workers (Chapman *et al.*, 1997; Chapman, Chapter 8, this volume). Where side-by-side comparisons have been made between direct faecal culture on CT-SMAC and IMS methods, increases in the number of positive samples by as much as sevenfold have been reported over direct culture (Heuvelink *et al.*, 1998). However, the number of *E. coli* O157:H7 shed per gram of faeces at slaughter is likely to be the most important factor in determining the extent and level of carcass contamination. Zhao *et al.* (1995) reported that 16/31 dairy calves from which the organism was isolated had populations ranging from 10^3 to 10^5 colony-forming units (CFU) g^{-1} of faeces. Shere *et al.* (1998) reported that, in a 15-month study of a Wisconsin dairy herd, heifers shed *E. coli* O157:H7 in their faeces at levels ranging from 2.0×10^2 to 8.7×10^4 CFU g^{-1}. The IMS enrichment techniques are claimed to detect as few as 1 CFU *E. coli* O157:H7 g^{-1}. If the minimal infectious dose (MID) of *E. coli* O157:H7 for humans is, indeed, close to 10 CFU (Griffin and Tauxe, 1991), 1 g of faeces from an animal shedding 10^5 CFU g^{-1} would represent about 10^4 MIDs, or enough MIDs to produce 10,000 potentially infectious 100 g hamburger patties. Improper cooking of just one of these 10,000 patties could be responsible for human infection and systematic improper cooking of these patties could result in an outbreak, such as the one observed in a Washington State fast-food restaurant in 1993 (Bell *et al.*, 1994). In contrast, 10 g of faeces would be required to deliver 1 MID from an animal shedding 1 CFU *E. coli* O157:H7 g^{-1}. Clearly, the level of faecal shedding is an important determinant of risk and deserves more detailed study. This component of risk is enhanced if subsequent processing steps allow the growth of the organism.

A limited number of studies have provided evidence of the direct causal linkage between faecal shedding of *E. coli* O157:H7 by cattle and carcass contamination. Chapman *et al.* (1993) reported contamination of 30% (7/23) of carcasses from *E. coli* O157:H7 rectal swab-culture-positive cattle, compared with 8% (2/25) of carcasses from rectal swab-culture-negative cattle. Richards *et al.* (1998) reported isolation of *E. coli* O157:H7 from 0.47% of neck-muscle samples taken from cattle at slaughter in 210 abattoirs in the UK and reported a tendency for positive samples to be found in the same abattoir on the same day.

DNA fingerprinting studies, with methods such as pulsed-field gel electrophoresis (PFGE), suggest that single, relatively stable, *E. coli* O157:H7 subtypes occur in certain herds of cattle (Shere *et al.*, 1998), while as many as five subtypes of the organism have been reported to exist in other herds (Besser *et al.*, 1997). Most human outbreaks of *E. coli* O157:H7 infection have been associated with single subtypes or clusters of single subtypes (Barrett *et al.*, 1994; Bender *et al.*, 1997; Izumiya *et al.*, 1997). However, *E. coli* O157:H7 subtypes vary from outbreak to outbreak and many *E. coli* O157:H7 subtypes have been associated with sporadic cases of human infection. It is therefore reasonable to hypothesize that spikes of contamination from cattle (one or more individuals in a lot) which are shedding high levels of a particular *E. coli* O157:H7 subtype in their faeces may be responsible for contaminating relatively large lots of product and causing disease. While there are many interpretations of the data and alternative hypotheses are plausible, accepting this hypothesis provides a rationale for testing the adequacies of intervention steps and 'good manufacturing' processes. It would suggest that spikes of 'significant' contamination occur in a random fashion, rather than that product contamination is a constant low-level event that is entirely process-dependent. This suggests that many representative samples would have to be taken from a product from each process lot to determine if they are free from *E. coli* O157:H7. In the case of large-scale ground-beef manufacture, this might result in the analysis of several samples from each day's production. Baseline data would be required over time to determine the precise sampling plan necessary to adequately monitor ground-beef production to ensure freedom from this pathogen.

Alternatively, the slaughter process and subsequent steps in production of ground beef would need to be sufficiently robust to prevent growth and preferably to eliminate a suitable indicator organism representative of faecal contaminants. The most obvious candidate in this regard is biotype 1 *E. coli*, also referred to as 'generic' *E. coli*. While *E. coli* O157:H7 may be more acid-resistant than many other *E. coli* (Arnold and Kaspar, 1995), growth-temperature and thermal-inactivation profiles are not very different from *E. coli* O157:H7 (Doyle and Schoeni, 1984). The implicit assumption is made that, on rare occasions, during spikes of product contamination with *E. coli* O157:H7, *E. coli* counts will be equivalent to *E. coli* O157:H7 counts. While much progress has been made in lowering generic *E. coli* counts in beef and ground beef, the ultimate goal of elimination has not yet been achieved.

CATTLE SLAUGHTER AND *E. COLI* O157:H7 CONTAMINATION

The processing line

In modern high-speed slaughter plants, over 300 cattle may be killed per hour on one processing line. This allows a 12 s gap between animals, and a plant operating at 400 animals h^{-1} has a 9 s gap between animals and so on. This animal disassembly line is very efficient in producing red meat at low cost but limits the manner in which safety can be 'built into the product'. This stated, carcasses from modern high-speed slaughter plants are no dirtier, in terms of visual contamination, nor do they carry greater microbial populations than those from facilities where the pace of killing and processing is lower (Jericho *et al.*, 1994). However, the line speed and volume of animals processed places constraints on decontamination procedures, particularly if their effectiveness is time-dependent. Many of the heat and chemical treatments described below are in fact time-dependent and in many cases may not work well if contact time is brief.

Controlling sources of carcass contamination

The principal sources of contamination of carcasses following slaughter are associated with hide removal and include: faeces, hide contact, aerosols and sprays, contact with workers' hands, gloves and other equipment and accidental spillage of body fluids during skinning and evisceration. Contamination of the carcass can take a number of forms.

1. Accidental, random, visible contamination of carcasses, e.g. when faeces or intestinal contents contaminate a carcass following a knife puncture.
2. Systematic visible contamination, e.g. defined areas or zones of the carcass shown to have higher visible demerit scores than others (Jericho *et al.*, 1993, 1994). This contamination usually consists of small quantities of faeces, ingesta, hairs or 'specks' (material of unknown origin).

3. Accidental or random invisible contamination from aerosols, dusts and sprays.
4. Systematic invisible contamination from contact, smears, aerosols, dusts and sprays. Just as areas of the carcass have been shown to have high and low visible demerit scores, carcasses also have areas with characteristically high and low bacterial populations (Jericho *et al.*, 1993; Gill *et al.*, 1996). Studies have shown that bacterial contamination of these areas is relatively predictable and, to a large extent, reflects the nature of the slaughter process.

Unfortunately, there is a relatively low correlation between visible demerit scores on a particular carcass and bacterial counts on the carcass (Jericho *et al.*, 1993). Therefore, limiting cleaning to areas of carcasses with visual demerits is not likely to result in carcasses with significantly reduced bacterial populations.

It is thought that much of the bacterial contamination of the carcass occurs during removal of the hide (Gill *et al.*, 1998). Some of these organisms are likely to come directly from faeces in the anal region and this may explain why the rump is one of the locations with has the highest *E. coli* and coliform counts (Gill *et al.*, 1996, 1998). Attempts have been made to minimize faecal contamination of this area by enclosing the anus and adjacent portion of the rectum or 'bung' in a plastic bag and binding this to the outer wall of the rectum. Hudson *et al.* (1998) reported that this procedure reduced but did not entirely prevent carcass contamination by an *E. coli* K-12 nalidixic acid-resistant marker strain, which was inoculated into the anal region before the hide was removed.

The neck, the brisket and legs are also areas of high contamination with *E. coli* (Bell, 1997). This is presumably related to contact between these areas of the carcass and the outside surface of the hide during skinning. Bell (1997) reported that points on the carcass which were touched by the inside of the hide typically had *E. coli* counts $< 2 \log_{10}$ CFU cm^{-2}. In contrast, sites in direct contact with the outer surface of the hide had *E. coli* counts $> 2 \log_{10}$ CFU cm^{-2}. Castillo *et al.* (1998b) examined the effects of chemical dehairing of hides that had been contaminated with bovine faeces containing *E. coli* O157:H7. Counts of this pathogen on hides were reduced from $> 5 \log_{10}$ CFU cm^{-2} to $< 0.5 \log_{10}$ CFU cm^{-2} after chemical dehairing. However, Schnell *et al.* (1995) reported that there were no significant differences in *E. coli* and coliform counts between samples from the carcasses of chemically dehaired cattle and those from cattle with their hair intact. Similarly, van Donkersgoed *et al.* (1998) found little difference in *E. coli* counts on the carcasses from cattle slaughtered with high hide 'tag' (caked faeces and mud adherent to the hair of the hide) scores and cattle with low hide tag scores. Not surprisingly, chemical dehaired carcasses had few visible specks and fewer total carcass defects than did carcasses of conventionally slaughtered animals (Schnell *et al.*, 1995). It would appear, that 'clean' hides may be more important in terms of meeting visual inspection requirements and preventing the dulling of cutting equipment than in relation to the bacteriological safety of the product.

Contact of workers' hands or glove and knives with faeces and material on hides, with subsequent contact of carcass surfaces, is also likely to be an important source of contamination. Cleaning of hands and aprons and 'pasteurization' of knives between carcasses have been reported to reduce *E. coli* counts on sheep carcasses (Bell and Hathaway, 1996). These workers also reported that a 44°C water rinse significantly reduced the amount of bacterial contamination of workers' hands in a sheep slaughter-house, but that even rinsed hands had aerobic bacterial plate counts of > 4 $\log_{10}$ CFU cm^{-2}. They also reported that a 44°C rinse of knives, followed by an 82°C water dip, reduced the contamination on knife blades to < 3 $\log_{10}$ CFU cm^{-2}. Given the high line speeds of modern beef plants, adequately cleaning hands, protective clothing and equipment between each carcass is exceedingly difficult. However, more rapid and effective methods of decontamination of certain equipment may be possible. For example, Snijders *et al.* (1985) reported that 'pasteurization' of knives at 82°C was difficult if fat and protein were adherent; however, a pressurized lactic acid sprayer effectively removed this material and provided increased bactericidal activity.

In some cases, the process can be altered to reduce this systematic contamination of the carcass region, e.g. to prevent rubbing of carcasses against a piece of equipment; however, in other cases, this may be more difficult, e.g. in leg skinning and tying off the rectum (Gill *et al.*, 1998).

Cleaning contaminated carcasses

Fratamico *et al.* (1996) reported that *E. coli* O157:H7 binds to beef surfaces within 1 min of application in liquid media and that the numbers of organisms that attach are proportional to their concentration in the media. However, these investigators also noted that, while *E. coli* O157:H7 appeared to be heavily piliated, there was no significant difference between levels of this organism that attached to beef surfaces when compared with a laboratory *E. coli* K-12 strain. Scanning electron photomicrographs of meat tissue with adherent *E. coli* O157:H7 suggested that the bacteria attach primarily to collagen and elastin fibres.

In recent years, various procedures have been developed by the industry to spot-clean visible areas of contamination on beef carcasses. The push for this has, at least partially, been made to meet the recent requirements set out by the Food Safety Inspection Service of the US Department of Agriculture (USDA) for 'zero tolerance' for visible contamination of beef carcasses (described by Dorsa, 1997). Under this directive, any area of contamination by hair, faeces, ingesta or milk on carcasses which is less than 2.5 cm in its greatest dimension is to be removed either by knife trimming or by steam vacuum. In addition, any faecal material on carcasses with dimensions larger than 2.5 cm, in addition to abscesses, bruises, parasites and parasitic lesions and udders from lactating animals, are to be trimmed away with a knife. Prasai *et al.* (1995) reported a 0.3 $\log_{10}$ CFU cm^{-2} reduction in aerobic plate counts of bacteria on beef carcasses following washing with water, compared to a reduction from 3.5 to 0.5 $\log_{10}$ CFU cm^{-2} in aerobic plate counts by knife trimming of surface layers of carcasses. Hardin *et al.* (1995) reported that knife trimming reduced 5 $\log_{10}$ CFU cm^{-2} of *E. coli* O157:H7 to mean levels ranging from 1.8 and 0.6 $\log_{10}$ CFU cm^{-2} on four cuts from beef carcasses which had been artificially contaminated with faeces containing the organism. A central criticism of these studies is that the trimming was conducted with clean instruments by trained staff on defined carcass areas where the contamination was readily apparent. This would certainly not be the case in many commercial slaughterhouses.

Another simple way to reduce visible contamination is to wash carcass surfaces with either cold or warm (32–35°C) water. This can be done for the whole carcass or at selected spots where contamination is apparent. Hudson *et al.* (1998) found no difference in the number of an *E. coli* K-12 nalidixic acid-resistant marker strain on carcasses following cold-water washing. Studies done in commercial slaughter facilities have likewise found little or no effect on microbial populations from simple carcass washing procedures (Jericho *et al.*, 1995; Prasai *et al.*, 1995). However, cold-water washing seems to be effective in decreasing microbial contamination which may follow hide removal (such as during evisceration and splitting), by decreasing the ability of bacteria to adhere to the carcass surface (Prasai *et al.*, 1995).

Both knife trimming and washing are effective in decreasing visible defects on carcass surfaces. They also appear to reduce but not eliminate bacterial populations at the site of contamination. Thus, Prasai *et al.* (1995) reported a 0.9 $\log_{10}$ CFU cm^{-2} reduction in aerobic plate counts of bacteria on beef carcasses following washing with water. However, washing and trimming may also cause the bacteria from these sites to be redistributed to other regions of the carcass (Jericho *et al.*, 1995; Gill *et al.*, 1996; Bell, 1997; Castillo *et al.*, 1998b). Again, while the aesthetic objective is accomplished, very little is accomplished in terms of the microbial 'load' of the carcass. Jericho *et al.* (1993) found a weak correlation between 'visual demerit' scores (specks, hair, staining by faeces and ingesta) and bacterial numbers at particular carcass sites.

Somewhat better results can be achieved if hot water is applied to areas of carcass contamination. Castillo *et al.* (1998a) reported that beef carcasses inoculated with *E. coli* O157:H7 at a concentration of 5 $\log_{10}$ CFU cm^{-2} were reduced by 3.7 $\log_{10}$ CFU cm^{-2} following spray washing with cold water, followed by a warm-water whole-carcass wash at 35°C and finally by a hot (95°C) water spray of faecally contaminated regions of carcasses for 5 s. However, they also found that the efficacy of hot-water treatments was affected by the region of the carcass that was involved. Time is required to apply the spray to affected areas, a skilled operator is needed and sprays of very hot water may present a danger to workers.

Recently, hot-water and steam-vacuum systems have been developed that allow the operator to 'spot-clean' and decontaminate specific areas of the carcass surface (Dorsa, 1997). Kochevar *et al.* (1997a) reported that steam-vacuuming of faecally soiled carcass surfaces reduced aerobic plate and coliform counts by about 2 $\log_{10}$ CFU cm^{-2}. This was comparable to knife trimming, which reduced aerobic plate and coliform counts by approximately 1.6 and 1.7 $\log_{10}$ CFU cm^{-2}, respectively. Dorsa *et al.* (1996) reported that beef-carcass 'short plates' inoculated with faeces containing 7.6 $\log_{10}$ CFU cm^{-2} of *E. coli* O157:H7 yielded an average residual level of *E. coli* O157:H7 of 2 $\log_{10}$ CFU cm^{-2} after steam-vacuum treatments. Kochevar *et al.* (1997a) reported that steam-vacuum systems on uninoculated beef carcasses also achieved modest reductions in average aerobic plate (*c.* 0.7 $\log_{10}$ CFU cm^{-2}) and coliform (*c.* 0.3 $\log_{10}$ CFU cm^{-2}) counts and reduced visible signs of contamination.

Decontamination procedures that rely entirely on operator skill, such as those described above, should be discouraged as part of hazard analysis and critical control point (HACCP) systems. This is partially because of the time element and variation in skill between operators, which makes this step difficult to standardize and control, but, more importantly, because much of the microbial contamination is invisible. While there is no reason to discourage spot-cleaning and trimming treatments, it is clear we cannot rely on these procedures alone to ensure safe red meat. Whole-carcass decontamination procedures have been shown to do a better job than spot treatments (Nutsch *et al.*, 1997; Phebus *et al.*, 1997).

The use of hot water and steam to reduce carcass contamination

Whole-carcass decontamination procedures must be sufficiently robust to decrease high levels of the pathogen at all points on the carcass surface. One simple way to achieve this is by heat treatment. This can be best accomplished by hot-water washes or steam treatment, performed in cabinets and sealed chambers, respectively. The objective is to raise the temperature of the carcass surface (inside and out) as well as the interior of cuts, crevices, cracks and fissures, to a temperature of 80–82°C (Smith, 1992; Castillo *et al.*, 1998a). This temperature treatment should be sufficient to kill *E. coli* O157:H7, as well as most other pathogens and spoilage organisms. One concern about surface heat treatment is consumers' reaction to the change of colour (from raw red to cooked brown) that accompanies surface heating. Happily, this colour change is temporary if heat treatment is brief and has been reported to diminish on cold storage, with a return to the colour more commonly associated with the raw product. It has been suggested that the initial colour change may also be helpful as a step in monitoring the thoroughness and distribution of the heat treatment of each carcass (Smith, 1992).

At present, two technologies appear to be vying for this heat-decontamination niche in the market, namely those based on hot water and those based on pressurized steam. Hot-water and steam treatments of whole carcasses appear to be equally effective in reducing levels of bacterial contamination. Smith (1992) reported that 6.3 $\log_{10}$ CFU cm^{-2} of *E. coli* O157:H7 in a mixed faecal suspension that was inoculated on to beef surfaces were reduced to populations of 3.6 and 3.3 $\log_{10}$ CFU cm^{-2} after the application of water at 80°C for 10 and 20 s, respectively. Nutsch *et al.* (1997) evaluated the effects of steam treatment (8 s steam exposure) on bacterial counts of 140 beef carcasses. They found that the mean aerobic plate counts were reduced from 2.2 $\log_{10}$ CFU cm^{-2} before treatment to 0.8 $\log_{10}$ CFU cm^{-2} immediately after treatment. Before steam treatment, generic *E. coli* was isolated from 6.4% of carcasses, at levels ranging from 0.6 to 1.5 $\log_{10}$ CFU cm^{-2}. After this treatment, generic *E. coli* was not isolated from any of the carcasses. Coliforms were isolated from 37.9% and 1.4% of the carcasses before and after steam treatment, respectively. Nutsch *et al.* (1998) also reported that steam treatment (82.5°C for 5–6 s) significantly reduced the number of carcass samples from which generic *E. coli* could be isolated – 68% of all carcasses before and 15% of carcasses after steam treatment. The highest number of generic *E. coli* detected after steam treatment on any one carcass was 0.25 CFU cm^{-2}.

Chemical treatments to reduce carcass contamination

A variety of chemical agents have been added to wash water to improve tissue cleaning and provide a level of disinfection for contaminated carcass sites. Gorman *et al.* (1995) compared treatment of carcasses with various chemical solutions, including 5% hydrogen peroxide, 0.5% ozone, 12% trisodium phosphate, 2% acetic acid and a 0.3% solution of a commercial sanitizer in spray-washing of beef tissues contaminated with faeces containing *E. coli* American Type Culture Collection (ATCC) 11370. The best results were obtained with two washes rather than one and the most important factor appeared to be the temperature of the water of the first wash rather than the chemical constituents of the second wash. A water wash at 74°C caused reductions in counts exceeding 3.0 $\log_{10}$ CFU cm^{-2} and, when followed by a second (16°C) wash with either water or any one of the antimicrobial solutions tested, this treatment achieved superior reductions to those obtained with a combination of knife-trimming followed by spray-washing with the antimicrobial solutions. In this study, hydrogen peroxide and ozonated water were more effective than were trisodium phosphate (TSP), acetic acid and a commercial sanitizer when applied after a first wash with plain hot water. Kochevar *et al.* (1997b) also concluded that the temperature of the solution, rather than the pressure of the spray or the nature of the antimicrobial compound in the solution, was the most important parameter in reducing aerobic plate counts on lamb adipose tissues contaminated with faeces. Optimal reductions (3.8 $\log_{10}$ CFU cm^{-2}) in bacterial counts were obtained with knife-trimming followed by spraying with 2.0% acetic acid at a temperature of 74°C for 18 s. Other solutions tested in the study included 12% TSP, 5% hydrogen peroxide and water with 0.003% available chlorine.

Podolak *et al.* (1996) tested the ability of solutions containing fumaric, acetic or lactic acids to sanitize lean beef surfaces inoculated with 5 $\log_{10}$ CFU cm^{-2} *E. coli* O157:H7. These workers reported that fumaric acid at a concentration of 1% (v/v) at 55°C for 5 s was the most effective of these organic acids in reducing levels of *E. coli* O157:H7 (1.3 $\log_{10}$ units). Bell *et al.* (1997) reported that a combination wash of acetic acid/3% hydrogen peroxide resulted in reductions of 4.0 and 3.7 $\log_{10}$ CFU cm^{-2} for *E. coli* on lean and adipose tissue, respectively.

Fratamico *et al.* (1996) reported that the numbers of bacteria removed from tenderloin tissue following rinses of 10% TSP, 2% acetic acid and phosphate-buffered saline (PBS) did not differ considerably. However, when beef tissues were stored at 4°C for 18 h, the TSP rinse treatments reduced the numbers of *E. coli* K-12 and *E. coli* O157:H7 attached to adipose tissue up to 3.4 and 2.7 $\log_{10}$ units, respectively, compared with rinsing with PBS.

Combined treatments

Phebus *et al.* (1997) reported that combinations of carcass-cleaning procedures provided superior results to any one treatment alone. They found that combination treatments involving: (i) trimming and a warm-water wash; (ii) trimming, a warm-water wash and steam pasteurization; (iii) a warm-water wash and steam pasteurization; (iv) trimming, a warm-water wash, a hot lactic acid wash and steam pasteurization; and (v) a steam vacuum, a warm-water wash, a hot lactic acid wash and steam pasteurization were equally effective in reducing *E. coli* O157:H7 levels from 4.2 to 5.3 $\log_{10}$ CFU cm^{-2}. Used alone, trimming, steam-vacuuming and steam pasteurization resulted in reductions ranging from 2.5 to 3.7 $\log_{10}$ CFU cm^{-2}, with steam pasteurization resulting in greater reductions in *E. coli* O157:H7 than trimming or vacuuming alone.

Similarly, Castillo *et al.* (1998c) reported that water-washing and carcass knife-trimming, while effective for cleaning up contaminated sites, also spread bacterial contamination to other areas of the carcass surface. However, the relocated contamination could effectively be reduced by washing with hot water and then applying a lactic acid spray. This combined treatment yielded 0% positive samples for *E. coli* O157:H7 in areas outside the inoculated areas, whereas the percentage of positive samples after applying other combined treatments ranged from 0 to 44%. They noted that, following an initial cleaning procedure involving water-washing or knife-trimming, reductions of counts of *E. coli* O157:H7 inoculated on to carcass surfaces with a hot-water wash ranged from 4.0 to > 4.8 $\log_{10}$ CFU cm^{-2}, with a lactic acid spray from 4.6 to > 4.9 $\log_{10}$ CFU cm^{-2}, with hot water followed by lactic acid spray from 4.5 to > 4.9 $\log_{10}$ CFU cm^{-2} and with lactic acid spray followed by a hot-water wash from 4.4 to > 4.6 $\log_{10}$ CFU cm^{-2}.

A central problem in many of the studies mentioned above is that the culture media employed to enumerate both generic *E. coli* and *E. coli* O157:H7 may not be suitable for growth of these bacteria sublethally injured by heat or other physical or chemical agents (Bromberg *et al.*, 1998). Selective ingredients in these media as well as exposure to oxygen may be lethal to injured *E. coli* cells and cause overestimates of population declines and the effectiveness of a given treatment. It has been shown that injured bacteria have the ability to repair themselves under the proper conditions. In addition, recontamination of the beef by *E. coli* from dirty equipment may occur during cutting and grinding. Dorsa *et al.* (1998a) have noted that growth of *E. coli* O157:H7 short plates prepared from beef from carcasses treated with lactic acid or acetic acid and ground beef prepared from beef treated with these organic acids (Dorsa *et al.*, 1998c) were better able to suppress the growth of this pathogen than was beef from carcasses simply treated with hot water or steam. These studies argue strongly not only for the use of multiple carcass treatment steps but also for the use of chemical agents, such as organic acids, with residual bactericidal activity.

In addition to thermal and chemical methods, research is also being conducted on a number of other promising bactericidal technologies, including treatment of meat to high hydrostatic pressure (Kalchayanand *et al.*, 1998), high-intensity white-light and ultraviolet-light emissions (MacGregor *et al.*, 1998; Wong *et al.*, 1998) and pulsed-power electricity (Tinney *et al.*, 1997). So far, among the alternative physical methods, ionizing radiation has been the best studied and appears the most effective in eliminating bacterial pathogens, such as *E. coli* O157:H7, from ground beef and extending product shelf-life (Roberts and Weese, 1998).

IRRADIATION AND *E. COLI* O157:H7

The commonly used source of ionizing irradiation consists of gamma rays generated by the decay of cobalt-60 or caesium-137; however, electron beams and X-rays may also be used for this purpose (Newsome, 1987). *E.*

coli O157:H7 and other bacterial food-borne pathogens, as well as other Gram-negative food-spoilage organisms, such as pseudomonads, are sensitive to relatively low doses of ionizing radiation (Monk *et al.*, 1995; Farkas, 1998). Accordingly, it may be possible to produce red meats free of *E. coli* O157:H7, other bacterial pathogens and metazoan parasites, as well as possessing extended product shelf-life. For this reason, irradiation has been referred to as 'cold pasteurization'. Since the procedure can be performed after the meat is packaged, recontamination of the product is also less of a concern.

Thayer and Boyd (1993) reported that D_{10} (the radiation dose required to eliminate 90%, or 1 $\log_{10}$ cycle, of the bacterial population) values for *E. coli* O157:H7 in mechanically deboned chicken ranged from 0.27 to 0.42 kilogray (kGy). This is similar to the D_{10} value of 0.24 to 0.31 kGy reported by Clavero *et al.* (1994) for the organism in ground beef. Log-phase cells are reported to be somewhat more sensitive to irradiation than stationary-phase cells (Thayer and Boyd, 1993; Byun *et al.*, 1998) and minor differences in irradiation sensitivity have been noted in poultry versus ground lean beef (Thayer and Boyd, 1993) and in 0.85% saline solution versus a chicken-breast suspension (Dion *et al.*, 1994).

The fat content of ground beef has little effect on D_{10} values for *E. coli* O157:H7 (Clavero *et al.*, 1994). Fielding *et al.* (1997) noted sharp increases in the sensitivity of the organism to electron-beam irradiation at pH < 4.1 and have reported that a synergistic effect in the killing of this pathogen is achieved with acetic acid in concentrations between 0.02% and 0.1%, combined with irradiation treatment. The most dramatic increase in irradiation resistance of the organism is observed at temperatures below 0°C (Thayer and Boyd, 1993; Clavero *et al.*, 1994; Byun *et al.*, 1998), with the resistance increasing between 0°C and about −15°C (Thayer and Boyd, 1993). It has been suggested that the lethal effect of irradiation may be related to the generation of radicals, such as hydroxyl (OH), resulting from the hydrolysis of water (Billen, 1987), that fewer of these radicals are formed at low temperature and that ice may impede the movement of these molecules (Thayer and Boyd, 1993).

Thayer and Boyd (1993) reported that a dose of 1.5 kGy produced a 6.7 $\log_{10}$ reduction of *E. coli* O157:H7 in broth media and eliminated $10^{4.8}$ CFU g^{-1} of *E. coli* O157:H7 inoculated into ground beef. Clavero *et al.* (1994) calculated that an applied dose of 2.5 kGy would be sufficient to kill $10^{8.1}$ CFU of *E. coli* O157:H7 g^{-1} in ground beef. Fu *et al.* (1995) reported that the organism could not be detected in beef steaks and ground beef that had been inoculated with *E. coli* O157:H7, irradiated at 1.5 to 2.0 kGy and storage at 7°C for 7 days. These doses are well below those recently approved by the Food and Drug Administration of the USA (4.5 kGy for fresh and 7 kGy for frozen products).

Public apprehension, regulatory approval and cost have limited the widespread use of irradiation of red meats. Changes in taste and other sensory attributes, minor losses of certain vitamins and the generation of small amounts of substances such as benzene and formaldehyde are cited as problems with the use of this technology. However, greater losses of vitamins occur during cooking, canning and even cold storage of foods and many natural foods contain higher levels of benzene than found in irradiated products (Thayer, 1994; WHO, 1994; FDA, 1997). In addition, studies on several generations of laboratory animals and on human volunteers fed irradiated diets have shown no greater rates of malignancy or incidence of genetic diseases than found in their counterparts fed non-irradiated foods (WHO, 1994; FDA, 1997).

Irradiation of foods such as red meats is supported by a number of international and national professional health, scientific, consumers and food-industry organizations (Lagunas-Solar, 1995; Monk *et al.*, 1995; Farkas, 1998). The World Health Organization and the Food and Agricultural Organization of the United Nations have long supported irradiation of foods, and currently over 40 countries allow its restricted use for the preservation or decontamination of specific food products (WHO, 1994). Despite the widespread endorsement of irradiation of foods as a sound practice, its use for certain foods is prohibited in many jurisdictions and there is keen interest in the development of methods for the detection of irradiated foods to restrict their importation and sale (Schreiber *et al.*, 1994).

THE EFFECTS OF COOKING TEMPERATURE

Numerous outbreaks of infection with *E. coli* O157:H7 are thought to have resulted from the consumption of hamburgers and other beef products which were inadequately cooked. However, in other beef-associated outbreaks, contamination of the meat dish after cooking or of other food items by contact with juices from raw beef has been suspected. In one survey of beef in Columbia (Mattar and Vasquez, 1998), *E. coli* O157:H7 has been isolated from 'cooked' beef patties; however, no details of the cooking methods were given. In several cases, the organism has been isolated from the raw product and it is assumed that a sufficient number of organisms survived cooking to cause human illness. However, in most cases, there is no direct evidence that organisms survived the cooking process, but rather epidemiological evidence which show associations between the food consumed and illness. For example, in the multistate outbreak in the Pacific North-West of the USA in 1993, Bell *et al.* (1994) reported that, of 501 cases investigated, 398 (86%) reported eating at a specific Washington State restaurant and 92% of the people affected reported eating 'regular' hamburgers. Subsequent investigation revealed that 10/16 (63%) of regular hamburgers cooked according to this restaurant's policy had internal temperatures below 60°C. Bryant *et al.* (1989) in Canada and Parry *et al.* (1998) have reported that sporadic cases of infection with this pathogen were also associated with eating undercooked meat. Recent results of a larger American study (Slutsker *et al.*, 1998) of sporadic cases of *E. coli* O157:H7 infection also suggest that eating undercooked ground beef is associated with illness.

It is postulated that certain cooking temperatures may have allowed survival of the pathogen and that the low infectious dose of *E. coli* O157:H7 results in human disease. Accordingly, cooking procedures have been modified to address the 'worst case' scenario – that is, they have been designed to eliminate high populations (5 D_{10}) of the organism from beef. The current target, as with other processes, such as in ready-to-eat meats (sausages, salami, etc.) and irradiation, is a 5 D_{10} reduction – that is, to decrease bacterial populations by 99.999%. Clavero *et al.* (1998) and Juneja *et al.* (1997) suggest that cooking ground-beef patties to an internal temperature of 68.3°C for 40 s should inactivate at least 99.99% (4 D_{10}) of *E. coli* O157:H7 cells. Therefore, the current recommendation for home cooking is an internal temperature of 71.1°C (160°F), with no holding time specified (Clavero *et al.*, 1998). It has been shown that the previous advice to 'wait until the juices run clear' may not always be valid. This parameter appears to vary considerably, depending on the storage conditions of the ground beef. The use of a quick-reading thermometer to assess internal temperature is now recommended in the USA. USDA regulations concerning proper cooking of beef products in commercial settings have set minimum time and temperature requirements, with as many as 16 possible time–temperature combinations for cooking or roasting beef (Orta-Ramirez *et al.*, 1997), and manufacturers of cooked ground-beef patties are allowed to use as many as seven time and temperature combinations, ranging from 66.1°C for 41 s to 69.4°C or above for 10 s. An alternative to the rigid time-and-temperature approach is a recommendation that the cooking process achieve the desired 5 D_{10} reductions in the number of *E. coli* O157:H7. The use of the 5 D_{10} limit increases the number of possible cooking methods and time and temperature combinations, but necessitates that each of the processes be verified either by following bacterial killing or by the use of a suitable indirect indicator of killing. Veeramuthu *et al.* (1998) have suggested that triose phosphate isomerase may be a suitable indicator, because this heat-labile enzyme has thermal inactivation characteristics that closely parallel the thermal death parameters of *Salmonella senftenberg* and *E. coli* O157:H7.

Thermal inertia, or the time taken to bring the product up to the desired internal temperature, increases with the mass of the meat, in the case of roasting, or the thickness, in the case of grilling or frying ground-beef patties. If the product temperature is low, as in the case of frozen ground-beef patties, more resistance to heating will be encountered. Heat penetration in a ground-beef patty is thought to result from steam-vapour flow rather than from simple conduction and, once a given temperature is achieved, thermal inertia tends to maintain the temperature for several seconds. As a consequence, a sufficiently high internal temperature may achieve optimal kill and stipulating holding times may not be necessary.

Several reports suggest that the greater the percentage of fat, the greater the thermal resistance. However, the increase in heat resistance is minor and one study found no increase in heat resistance to the killing of *E. coli* O157:H7 with increased fat content of the product (Kotrola and Conner, 1997). There is also concern that survival and subsequent regrowth of organisms sublethally injured during the cooking process may occur. Therefore it is important to calculate D_{10} (time and temperature combinations) values using media that will support growth of organisms injured by thermal treatment (McCarthy *et al.*, 1998). Clavero *et al.* (1998) reported that modified eosin methylene-blue agar is a better recovery medium than sorbitol MacConkey agar for thermally injured *E. coli* O157:H7. This conclusion was based on the fact that in their study significantly greater periods of time were required at all temperatures examined to obtain D_{10} population reductions if bacterial numbers were measured with modified eosin methylene-blue agar rather than with sorbitol MacConkey-based agar.

CHARACTERISTICS OF *E. COLI* O157:H7 RELEVANT TO SURVIVAL IN MEAT AND HUMAN INFECTION

The minimal infectious dose

Determination of the appropriate dose–response is important in predicting the outcome of ingesting specific pathogens, such as *E. coli* O157:H7, present in ground beef. From this exposure assessment, a probability distribution of outcomes can be determined for the population or subpopulation in question. These outcomes include factors such as frequency and severity of illness, number of deaths and associated costs. In addition, these data can be used in setting maximum safety or, at least, target levels for pathogen contamination (CFU g^{-1}) in a given food, i.e. those levels which would be expected to minimize disease levels to 'acceptable' levels or, put another way, 'tolerable' safety limits (Mossel *et al.*, 1998). The decision as to what is 'acceptable' or 'tolerable' has not, to the author's knowledge, been defined; however, there is an implicit assumption that this refers to levels achievable with current technology, using processes which are acceptable to consumers and provided at a reasonable cost.

The concept of 'minimal infectious dose' suggests that a critical threshold dose of molecules is necessary to cause death or illness in a proportion (usually 50%) of the population (Coleman and Marks, 1998). In contrast to chemical toxins, bacteria reproduce. It is therefore theoretically possible for a single bacterium to cause severe illness. However, in order to do this, it would first need to survive the journey into the appropriate location in the gastrointestinal tract and to overcome host defence mechanisms, such as the low pH of the stomach and intestinal immunity. The rate and level of bacterial proliferation are likely to have an influence on the time of onset and the severity of disease. However, in the case of *E. coli* O157:H7, while the damage done to the host would in part be determined by virulence properties of the bacteria, such as the potency and level of toxins produced, the degree to which toxins would be absorbed into the bloodstream from the intestine, antitoxin immunity and the presence or absence of toxin receptors on target cells would also be expected to have a profound influence on the outcome of infection. Identification of particularly susceptible segments of the population, such as young children and the elderly, are important in targeting strategies for these groups, such as avoidance of certain high-risk foods and/or enhanced vigilance in food preparation. However, efforts may also be made to enhance host immunity through vaccination or to target specific therapies, such as oral administration of toxin-receptor analogues (Ling *et al.*, 1998) to children with diarrhoea.

In the risk-assessment model for *E. coli* O157:H7 in ground-beef hamburgers described by Cassin *et al.* (1998), calculation of the level of exposure includes a probability distribution of number of burgers consumed, as well as the probability distribution of the thoroughness to which beef hamburgers are cooked. Logically, the greater consumption of underdone hamburgers by a susceptible population, the greater the chance of illness. Several epidemiological studies (Bryant *et al.*, 1989; Bell *et al.*, 1994; Parry *et al.*, 1998; Slutsker *et al.*, 1998) support the observation that eating undercooked ground beef is indeed associated with *E. coli* O157:H7 infection.

Factors affecting infectious dose

Small and Gordon (1993) suggested that acid-tolerant organisms are more likely to have a low infectious dose. The infectious dose of *E. coli* O157:H7 for humans is thought to be low. The value of 10 CFU has often been cited (Griffin and Tauxe, 1991). This infectious dose is based on quantification of the numbers of *E. coli* O157:H7 isolated from foods associated with human illness and the fact that, in many cases, such as suspected cases of water-borne infections, no organisms could be isolated (Keene *et al.*, 1994; Ackman *et al.*, 1997). No human volunteer studies have been conducted or are likely to be conducted using *E. coli* O157:H7, due to the severity of its effects. Data from studies on feeding of *Shigella dysenteriae* to human volunteers suggests an infective dose again as low as 10 CFU (Levine *et al.*, 1973). Similar low infectious-dose values have also been reported for *Shigella flexneri* (DuPont *et al.*, 1989). In contrast, the infectious dose for non-typhoid *Salmonella* is thought to be in the range of 10^5–10^8 CFU (Blaser and Newman, 1982). Small and Gordon (1993) reported that a number of *Shigella* strains, as well as pathogenic and non-pathogenic *E. coli* strains, survived for 2 h in artificial gastric fluid with a pH of 2.5; in contrast, none of the 11 strains of *Salmonella*, representing five different species, survived this treatment.

Lin *et al.* (1995) reported that at least three acid-resistance mechanisms could be found in acid-resistant *E. coli* strains. This includes an oxidative system, which is controlled by *rpo*S, which produces an alternative sigma factor involved in initiation of the transcription of as many as 30–50 stress genes (Lin *et al.*, 1996; Loewen *et al.*, 1998). This acid-tolerant state has been shown to be induced in stationary-phase cultures, and by salt or starvation of log-phase cells (see also Booth *et al.*, Chapter 2, this volume). As would be expected with any process relying on protein synthesis, resistance to acid does not develop at low temperature and is diminished in the presence of chloramphenicol. According to Cheng and Kaspar (1998), this *rpo*S-dependent acid tolerance of *E. coli* O157:H7 is decreased at low growth temperature (15°C versus 37°C). However, acid tolerance at stationary phase (16 h) appears to be equivalent for both anaerobic and aerobic cultures of the organism. Cheville *et al.* (1996) reported that an *E. coli* O157:H7 strain which they generated with an *rpo*S mutation was less heat- and salt-tolerant than the wild-type *E. coli* O157:H7 strain. Furthermore, populations of this mutant declined in numbers much more rapidly in dry-fermented salami than did the wild type. It appears that, once the stress proteins are synthesized and incorporated into the cell wall, the acid-resistance phenotype is retained at low storage temperatures. This observation contradicts conventional wisdom that cool (zero growth < 8°C) temperatures must be maintained throughout the grinding and storage process. Cheng and Kaspar (1998) reported that acid tolerance was lost in *E. coli* O157:H7 which was inoculated into irradiated ground beef and held at 15°C for 4 h before storage at 4°C or −20°C. In contrast, acid tolerance was maintained in *E. coli* O157:H7 held at these storage temperatures if the 15°C holding time was omitted. Clearly, there would be little opportunity for growth during the slaughter process, and acid-tolerant organisms from the animal's faeces may enter the product and be resistant to bactericidal steps in processing. In addition, it is thought that this phenotype may allow passage of the organism through the extremely low pH environment of the stomach and present an increased risk for humans. In addition to conferring acid resistance, resistance to high salt concentration and thermal inactivation have also been reported with this *E. coli* phenotype. Temporary elevation of temperature may initiate bacterial growth in a substrate such as ground beef or tissue films and increase the susceptibility of the organism to killing by acids and other cell-damaging agents.

Two other acid-protective systems involving amino acids have also been reported in *E. coli*. In these systems, it is thought that, when arginine and glutamine, respectively, are cleaved within the cell, their products elevate intracellular pH and prevent acid-mediated cell damage (Lin *et al.*, 1995). It is thought that these systems are activated at low to medium pH and are not regulated by the *rpoS* gene product. It has been suggested that the glutamine and arginine systems function to protect the bacteria against weaker acids, such as volatile fatty acids, found in the small and large intestine. Interestingly, *E. coli* O157:H7 strains were found to have a more potent arginine-based system than other acid-resistant *E. coli* strains examined (Lin *et al.*, 1996).

Waterman and Small (1998) have suggested that the acid-resistant phenotype of *S. flexneri* is associated with faecal–oral and water-borne transmission, as well as food-borne transmission. The same rationale may be applied to *E. coli* O157:H7. It has been suggested that a significant number of cases (Rowe *et al.*, 1993; Bell *et al.*, 1994) can be attributed to secondary transmission from asymptomatic contacts which shed the pathogen in their faeces. Similarly, water-borne transmission of *E. coli* O157:H7 is well documented (Wallace, Chapter 12, this volume). This underlines the point that *E. coli* O157:H7 infection of individuals from food sources may result in asymptomatic shedding of the organism. This enhanced ability to survive in the environment implies a significantly greater possibility (risk) of cross-contamination of foods and recontamination of product in the processing environment and in the kitchen and fits in well with data from outbreak investigations.

Together, this information argues for very low target levels for *E. coli* O157:H7 in beef products. The USDA-based zero tolerance seems reasonable in this respect; however, in practical terms, an intensive sampling would be required to meet this noble objective. Despite the steady march of technology, the ability to accept or reject lots of ground beef based on the presence of *E. coli* O157:H7 seems unlikely and largely unnecessary, provided that intervention procedures are used which can consistently bring about 5 D_{10} (worst-case scenario) reductions in the numbers of the *E. coli* O157:H7 in beef products prior to delivery to the retail outlet or home. This may be the most cost-effective way of minimizing risk, and it justifies changes in slaughter processes to provide additional hurdles to prevent survival of the organism. Low infectious-dose attributes may also contribute to the survival of this bacterium in the farm environment and the gastrointestinal tracts of cattle.

Finally, the age distribution in the human population of affected individuals (Griffin and Tauxe, 1991; Rowe *et al.*, 1991; Waters *et al.*, 1994) argues that disease is a function of susceptibility and not dose. Therefore, strategies to decrease host susceptibility through vaccination may be a cost-effective strategy to reduce illness and the horizontal spread of the pathogen.

REFERENCES

Abdul-Raouf, U.M., Beuchat, L.R. and Ammar, M.S. (1993) Survival and growth of *Escherichia coli* O157:H7 in ground, roasted beef as affected by pH, acidulants, and temperature. *Applied and Environmental Microbiology* 59, 2364–2368.

Ackman, D., Marks, S., Mack, P., Caldwell, M., Root, T. and Birkhead, G. (1997) Swimming-associated haemorrhagic colitis due to *Escherichia coli* O157:H7 infection: evidence of prolonged contamination of a fresh water lake. *Epidemiology and Infection* 119, 1–8.

Arnold, K.W. and Kaspar, C.W. (1995) Starvation- and stationary-phase-induced acid tolerance in *Escherichia coli* O157:H7. *Applied and Environmental Microbiology* 61, 2037–2039.

Barrett, T.J., Lior, H., Green, J.H., Khakhria, R., Wells, J.G., Bell, B.P., Greene, K.D., Lewis, J. and Griffin, P.M. (1994) Laboratory investigation of a multistate food-borne outbreak of *Escherichia coli* O157:H7 by using pulsed-field gel electrophoresis and phage typing. *Journal of Clinical Microbiology* 32, 3013–3017.

Bell, B.P., Goldoft, M., Griffin, P.M., Davis, M.A., Gordon, D.C., Tarr, P.I., Bartleson, C.A., Lewis, J.H., Barrett, T.J. and Wells, J.G. (1994) A multistate outbreak of *Escherichia coli* O157:H7-associated bloody diarrhea and hemolytic uremic syndrome from hamburgers. The Washington experience. *Journal of the American Medical Association* 272, 1349–1353.

Bell, K.Y., Cutter, C.N. and Sumner, S.S. (1997) Reduction of food borne micro-organisms on beef carcass tissue using acetic acid, sodium bicarbonate, and hydrogen peroxide spray washes. *Food Microbiology* 14, 439–448.

Bell, R.G. (1997) Distribution and sources of microbial contamination on beef carcasses. *Journal of Applied Microbiology* 82, 292–300.

Bell, R.G. and Hathaway, S.C. (1996) The hygienic efficiency of conventional and inverted lamb dressing systems. *Journal of Applied Bacteriology* 81, 225–234.

Bender, J.B., Hedberg, C.W., Besser, J.M., Boxrud, D.J., MacDonald, K.L. and Osterholm, M.T. (1997) Surveillance by molecular subtype for *Escherichia coli* O157:H7 infections in Minnesota by molecular subtyping. *New England Journal of Medicine* 337, 388–394.

Besser, T.E., Hancock, D.D., Pritchett, L.C., McRae, E.M., Rice, D.H., Tarr, P.I., Cieslak, P.R., Noble, S.J., Maxson, D.J., Empey, L.C., Ravenholt, O., Legarza, G., Tuttle, J., Doyle, M.P., Barrett, T.J., Wells, J.G., McNamara, A.M. and Griffin, P.M. (1997) Duration of detection of fecal excretion of *Escherichia coli* O157:H7 in cattle. Hamburger-associated *Escherichia coli* O157:H7 infection in Las Vegas: a hidden epidemic. *American Journal of Public Health* 87, 176–180.

Billen, D. (1987) Free radical scavenging and the expression of potentially lethal damage in X-irradiated repair-deficient *Escherichia coli*. *Radiation Research* 111, 354–360.

Blaser, M.J. and Newman, L.S. (1982) A review of human salmonellosis: I. Infective dose. *Reviews in Infectious Diseases* 4, 1096–1106.

Bromberg, R., George, S.M. and Peck, M.W. (1998) Oxygen sensitivity of heated cells of *Escherichia coli* O157:H7. *Journal of Applied Microbiology* 85, 231–237.

Bryant, H.E., Athar, M.A. and Pai, C.H. (1989) Risk factors for *Escherichia coli* O157:H7 infection in an urban community. *Journal of Infectious Diseases* 160, 858–864.

Byun, M.W., Kwon, O.J., Yook, H.S. and Kim, K.S. (1998) Gamma irradiation and ozone treatment for inactivation of *Escherichia coli* O157:H7 in culture media. *Journal of Food Protection* 61, 728–730.

Cassin, M.H., Lammerding, A.M., Todd, E.C., Ross, W. and McColl, R.S. (1998) Quantitative risk assessment for *Escherichia coli* O157:H7 in ground beef hamburgers. *International Journal of Food Microbiology* 41, 21–44.

Castillo, A., Lucia, L.M., Goodson, K.J., Savell, J.W. and Acuff, G.R. (1998a) Use of hot water for beef carcass decontamination. *Journal of Food Protection* 61, 19–25.

Castillo, A., Dickson, J.S., Clayton, R.P., Lucia, L.M. and Acuff, G.R. (1998b) Chemical dehairing of bovine skin to reduce pathogenic bacteria and bacteria of fecal origin. *Journal of Food Protection* 61, 623–625.

Castillo, A., Lucia, L.M., Goodson, K.J., Savell, J.W. and Acuff, G.R. (1998c) Comparison of water wash, trimming, and combined hot water and lactic acid treatments for reducing bacteria of fecal origin on beef carcasses. *Journal of Food Protection* 61, 823–828.

Chapman, P.A., Wright, D.J., Norman, P., Fox, J. and Crick, E. (1993) Cattle as a possible source of verocytotoxin-producing *Escherichia coli*-O157 infections in man. *Epidemiology and Infection* 111, 439–447.

Chapman, P.A., Malo, A.T., Siddons, C.A. and Harkin, M. (1997) Use of commercial enzyme immunoassays and immunomagnetic separation systems for detecting *Escherichia coli* O157 in bovine fecal samples. *Applied and Environmental Microbiology* 63, 2549–2553.

Cheng, C.M. and Kaspar, C.W. (1998) Growth and processing conditions affecting acid tolerance in *Escherichia coli* O157:H7. *Food Microbiology* 15, 157–166.

Cheville, A.M., Arnold, K.W., Buchrieser, C., Cheng, C.M. and Kaspar, C.W. (1996) rpoS regulation of acid, heat, and salt tolerance in *Escherichia coli* O157:H7. *Applied and Environmental Microbiology* 62, 1822–1824.

Clavero, M.R., Monk, J.D., Beuchat, L.R., Doyle, M.P. and Brackett, R.E. (1994) Inactivation of *Escherichia coli* O157:H7, salmonellae, and *Campylobacter jejuni* in raw ground beef by gamma irradiation. *Applied and Environmental Microbiology* 60, 2069–2075.

Clavero, M.R., Beuchat, L.R. and Doyle, M.P. (1998) Thermal inactivation of *Escherichia coli* O157:H7 isolated from ground beef and bovine feces, and suitability of media for enumeration. *Journal of Food Protection* 61, 285–289.

Coleman, M.E. and Marks, H.M. (1998) Topics in dose–response modelling. *Journal of Food Protection* 61, 1550–1559.

Dion, P., Charboneau, G. and Thibault, C. (1994) Effect of ionizing dose rate on the radioresistance of some food pathogenic bacteria. *Canadian Journal of Microbiology* 40, 369–374.

Dorsa, W.J. (1997) New and established carcass decontamination procedures commonly used in the beef-processing industry. *Journal of Food Protection* 60, 1146–1151.

Dorsa, W.J., Cutter, C.N. and Siragusa, G.R. (1996) Effectiveness of a steam-vacuum sanitizer for reducing *Escherichia coli* O157:H7 inoculated to beef carcass surface tissue. *Letters in Applied Microbiology* 23, 61–63.

Dorsa, W.J., Cutter, C.N. and Siragusa, G.R. (1998a) Long-term effect of alkaline, organic acid, or hot water washes on the microbial profile of refrigerated beef contaminated with bacterial pathogens after washing. *Journal of Food Protection* 61, 300–306.

Dorsa, W.J., Cutter, C.N. and Siragusa, G.R. (1998b) Bacterial profile of ground beef made from carcass tissue experimentally contaminated with pathogenic and spoilage bacteria before being washed with hot water, alkaline solution, or organic acid and then stored at 4 or 12 degrees C. *Journal of Food Protection* 61, 1109–1118.

Dorsa, W.J., Cutter, C.N. and Siragusa, G.R. (1998c) Long-term bacterial profile of refrigerated ground beef made from carcass tissue, experimentally contaminated with pathogens and spoilage bacteria after hot water, alkaline, or organic acid washes. *Journal of Food Protection* 61, 1615–1622.

Doyle, M.P. and Schoeni, J.L. (1984) Survival and growth characteristics of *Escherichia coli* associated with hemorrhagic colitis. *Applied and Environmental Microbiology* 48, 855–856.

DuPont, H.L., Levine, M.M., Hornick, R.B. and Formal, S.B. (1989) Inoculum size in shigellosis and implications for expected mode of transmission. *Journal of Infectious Diseases* 159, 1126–1128.

Farkas, J. (1998) Irradiation as a method for decontaminating food: a review. *International Journal of Food Microbiology* 44, 189–204.

FDA (1997) Irradiation in the production, processing and handling of food. US Food and Drug Administration. *Federal Register* 62, 64102–64121.

Fielding, L.M., Cook, P.E. and Grandison, A.S. (1997) The effect of electron beam irradiation, combined with acetic acid, on the survival and recovery of *Escherichia coli* and *Lactobacillus curvatus. International Journal of Food Microbiology* 35, 259–265.

Fratamico, P.M., Schultz, F.J., Benedict, R.C., Buchanan, R.L. and Cooke, P.H. (1996) Factors influencing attachment of *Escherichia coli* O157:H7 to beef tissues and removal using selected sanitizing rinses. *Journal of Food Protection* 59, 453–459.

Fu, A.H., Sebranek, J.G. and Murano, E.A. (1995) Survival of *Listeria monocytogenes, Yersinia enterocolitica* and *Escherichia coli* O157:H7 and quality changes after irradiation of beef steaks and ground beef. *Journal of Food Science* 60, 972–977.

Gill, C.O., McGinnis, J.C. and Badoni, M. (1996) Use of total of *Escherichia coli* counts to assess the hygienic characteristics of a beef carcass dressing process. *International Journal of Food Microbiology* 31, 181–196.

Gill, C.O., McGinnis, J.C. and Bryant, J. (1998) Microbial contamination of meat during the skinning of beef carcass hindquarters at three slaughtering plants. *International Journal of Food Microbiology* 42, 175–184.

Gorman, B.M., Sofos, J.N., Morgan, J.B., Schmidt, G.R. and Smith, G.C. (1995) Evaluation of hand-trimming, various sanitizing agents, and hot water spray-washing as decontamination interventions for beef brisket adipose tissue. *Journal of Food Protection* 58, 899–907.

Griffin, P.M. and Tauxe, R.V. (1991) The epidemiology of infections caused by *Escherichia coli* O157: H7, other enterohemorrhagic *E. coli*, and the associated hemolytic uremic syndrome. *Epidemiology Review* 13, 60–98.

Hardin, M.D., Acuff, G.R., Lucia, L.M., Osman, J.S. and Savell, J.W. (1995) Comparison of methods for decontamination from beef carcass surfaces. *Journal of Food Protection* 58, 368–374.

Heuvelink, A.E., van den Biggelaar, F.L., de Boer, E., Herbes, R.G., Melchers, W.J., Huis in 't Veld, J.H. and Monnens, L.A. (1998) Isolation and characterization of verocytotoxin-producing *Escherichia coli* O157 strains from Dutch cattle and sheep. *Journal of Clinical Microbiology* 36, 878–882.

Hudson, W.R., Mead, G.C. and Hinton, M.H. (1998) Assessing abattoir hygiene with a marker organism. *Veterinary Record* 142, 545–547.

Izumiya, H., Terajima, J., Wada, A., Inagaki, Y., Itoh, K.I., Tamura, K. and Watanabe, H. (1997) Molecular typing of enterohemorrhagic *Escherichia coli* O157:H7 isolates in Japan by using pulsed-field gel electrophoresis. *Journal of Clinical Microbiology* 35, 1675–1680.

Jericho, K.W.F., Bradley, J.A., Gannon, V.P. and Kozub, G.C. (1993) Visual demerit and microbiology evaluation of beef carcasses: methodology. *Journal of Food Protection* 56, 114–119.

Jericho, K.W., Bradley, J.A. and Kozub, G.C. (1994) Bacteriological evaluation of groups of beef carcasses before the wash at six Alberta abattoirs. *Journal of Applied Bacteriology* 77, 631–634.

Jericho, K.W., Bradley, J.A. and Kozub, G.C. (1995) Microbiologic evaluation of carcasses before and after washing in a beef slaughter plant. *Journal of the American Veterinary Medical Association* 206, 452–455.

Juneja, V.K., Snyder, O.P., Williams, A.C. and Marmer, B.S. (1997) Thermal destruction of *Escherichia coli* O157:H7 in hamburger. *Journal of Food Protection* 60, 1163–1166.

Kalchayanand, N., Sikes, A., Dunne, C.P. and Ray, B. (1998) Factors influencing death and injury of food borne pathogens by hydrostatic pressure. *Food Microbiology* 15, 207–208.

Keene, W.E., McAnulty, J.M., Hoesly, F.C., Williams, L.P.J., Hedberg, K., Oxman, G.L., Barrett, T.J., Pfaller, M.A., Fleming, D.W. and Williams, L.P., Jr (1994) A swimming-associated outbreak of hemorrhagic colitis caused by *Escherichia coli* O157:H7 and *Shigella sonnei*. *New England Journal of Medicine* 331, 579–584.

Kochevar, S.L., Sofos, J.N., Bolin, R.R., Reagan, J.O. and Smith, G.C. (1997a) Steam vacuuming as a pre-evisceration intervention to decontaminate beef carcasses. *Journal of Food Protection* 60, 107–113.

Kochevar, S.L., Sofos, J.N., Levalley, S.B. and Smith, G.C. (1997b) Effect of water temperature, pressure and chemical solution on removal of fecal material and bacteria from lamb adipose tissue by spray-washing. *Meat Science* 45, 377–388.

Kotrola, J.S. and Conner, D.E. (1997) Heat inactivation of *Escherichia coli* O157:H7 in turkey meat as affected by sodium chloride, sodium lactate, polyphosphate, and fat content. *Journal of Food Protection* 60, 898–902.

Lagunas-Solar, M.C. (1995) Radiation processing of foods: an overview of scientific principles and current status. *Journal of Food Protection* 58, 186–192.

Levine, M.M., DuPont, H.L., Formal, S.B., Hornick, R.B., Takeuchi, A., Gangarosa, E.J., Snyder, M.J. and Libonati, J.P. (1973) Pathogenesis of *Shigella dysenteriae* 1 (Shiga) dysentery. *Journal of Infectious Diseases* 127, 261–270.

Lin, J., Lee, I.S., Slonczewski, J.L. and Foster, J.W. (1995) Comparative analysis of extreme acid survival in *Salmonella typhimurium*, *Shigella flexneri*, and *Escherichia coli*. *Journal of Bacteriology* 177, 4097–4104.

Lin, J., Smith, M.P., Chapin, K.C., Baik, H.S., Bennett, G.N. and Foster, J.W. (1996) Mechanisms of acid resistance in enterohemorrhagic *Escherichia coli*. *Applied and Environmental Microbiology* 62, 3094–3100.

Ling, H., Boodhoo, A., Hazes, B., Cummings, M.D., Armstrong, G.D., Brunton, J.L. and Read, R.J. (1998) Structure of the shiga-like toxin I B-pentamer complexed with an analogue of its receptor Gb3. *Biochemistry* 37, 1777–1788.

Loewen, P.C., Hu, B., Strutinsky, J. and Sparling, R. (1998) Regulation in the *rpo*S regulon of *Escherichia coli*. *Canadian Journal of Microbiology* 44, 707–717.

Lopez-Gonzalez, V., Murano, P.S., Brennan, R.E. and Murano, E.A. (1999) Influence of various commercial packaging conditions on survival of *Escherichia coli* O157:H7 to irradiation by electron beam versus gamma rays. *Journal of Food Protection* 62, 10–15.

McCarthy, J., Holbrook, R. and Stephens, P.J. (1998) An improved direct plate method for the enumeration of stressed *Escherichia coli* O157:H7 from food. *Journal of Food Protection* 61, 1093–1097.

MacGregor, S.J., Rowan, N.J., Mcllvaney, L., Anderson, J.G., Fouracre, R.A. and Farish, O. (1998) Light inactivation of food-related pathogenic bacteria using a pulsed power source. *Letters in Applied Microbiology* 27, 67–70.

Mattar, S. and Vasquez, E. (1998) *Escherichia coli* O157:H7 infection in Colombia [letter]. *Emerging Infectious Diseases* 4, 126–127.

Monk, J.D., Beuchat, L.R. and Doyle, M.P. (1995) Irradiation inactivation of food-borne microorganisms. *Journal of Food Protection* 58, 197–208.

Mossel, D.A., Weenk, G.H., Morris, G.P. and Struijk, C.B. (1998) Identification, assessment and management of food-related microbiological hazards: historical, fundamental and psycho-social essentials. *International Journal of Food Microbiology* 40, 211–243.

National Advisory Committee on Microbiological Criteria for Foods (1998) Hazard analysis and critical control points principles and applications. *Journal of Food Protection* 61, 762–775.

Newsome, R.L. (1987) Perspective on food irradiation. *Food Technology* 12, 100–101.

Nutsch, A.L., Phebus, R.K., Riemann, M.J., Schafer, D.E., Boyer, J.E., Wilson, R.C., Leising, J.D. and Kastner, C.L. (1997) Evaluation of a steam pasteurization process in a commercial beef processing facility. *Journal of Food Protection* 60, 485–492.

Nutsch, A.L., Phebus, R.K., Riemann, M.J., Kotrola, J.S., Wilson, R.C., Boyer, J.E., Jr and Brown, T.L. (1998) Steam pasteurization of commercially slaughtered beef carcasses: evaluation of bacterial populations at five anatomical locations. *Journal of Food Protection* 61, 571–577.

Orta-Ramirez, A., Price, J.F., Hsu, Y.C., Veeramuthu, G.J., Cherrymerritt, J.S. and Smith, D.M. (1997) Thermal inactivation of *Escherichia coli* O157:H7, *Salmonella senftenberg*, and enzymes with potential as time–temperature indicators in ground beef. *Journal of Food Protection* 60, 471–475.

Parry, S.M., Salmon, R.L., Willshaw, G.A. and Cheasty, T. (1998) Risk factors for and prevention of sporadic infections with vero cytotoxin (shiga toxin) producing *Escherichia coli* 0157. *Lancet* 351, 1019–1022.

Phebus, R.K., Nutsch, A.L., Schafer, D.E., Wilson, R.C., Riemann, M.J., Leising, J.D., Kastner, C.L., Wolf, J.R. and Prasai, R.K. (1997) Comparison of steam pasteurization and other methods for reduction of pathogens on surfaces of freshly slaughtered beef. *Journal of Food Protection* 60, 476–484.

Podolak, R.K., Zayas, J.F., Kastner, C.L. and Fung, D.Y.C. (1996) Inhibition of *Listeria monocytogenes* and *Escherichia coli* O157: H7 on beef by application of organic acids. *Journal of Food Protection* 59, 370–373.

Prasai, R.K., Phebus, R.K., Zepeda, C.M., Kastner, C.L., Boyle, A.E. and Fung, D.Y.C. (1995) Effectiveness of trimming and/or washing on microbiological quality of beef carcasses. *Journal of Food Protection* 58, 1114–1117.

Richards, M.S., Corkish, J.D., Sayers, A.R., McLaren, I.M., Evans, S.J. and Wray, C. (1998) Studies of the presence of verocytotoxic *Escherichia coli* O157 in bovine faeces submitted for diagnostic purposes in England and Wales and on beef carcases in abattoirs in the United Kingdom. *Epidemiology and Infection* 120, 187–192.

Roberts, W.T. and Weese, J.O. (1998) Shelf life of ground beef patties treated by gamma radiation. *Journal of Food Protection* 61, 1387–1389.

Rowe, P., Orrbine, E., Wells, G. and McLaine, P. (1991) Epidemiology of hemolytic–uremic syndrome in Canadian children from 1986 to 1988. The Canadian Pediatric Kidney Disease Reference Centre. *Journal of Pediatrics* 119, 218–224.

Rowe, P.C., Orrbine, E., Loir, H., Wells, G.A., McLaine, P.N. and CPKDRC (1993) Diarrhoea in close contacts as a risk factors for childhood haemolytic uraemic syndrome. *Epidemiology and Infection* 110, 9–16.

Schnell, T.D., Sofos, J.N., Littlefield, V.G., Morgan, J.B., Gorman, B.M., Clayton, R.P. and Smith, G.C. (1995) Effects of postexsanguination dehairing on the microbial load and visual cleanliness of beef carcasses. *Journal of Food Protection* 58, 1297–1302.

Schreiber, G.A., Schulzki, G., Spiegelberg, A., Helle, N. and Bogl, K.W. (1994) Evaluation of a gas chromatographic method to identify irradiated chicken, pork, and beef by detection of volatile hydrocarbons. *Journal of the Association of Analytical Chemistry International* 77, 1202–1217.

Shere, J.A., Bartlett, K.J. and Kaspar, C.W. (1998) Longitudinal study of *Escherichia coli* O157:H7 dissemination on four dairy farms in Wisconsin. *Applied and Environmental Microbiology* 64, 1390–1399.

Slutsker, L., Ries, A.A., Maloney, K., Wells, J.G., Greene, K.D. and Griffin, P.M. (1998) A nationwide case-control study of *Escherichia coli* O157:H7 infection in the United States. *Journal of Infectious Diseases* 177, 962–966.

Small, P.L.C. and Gordon, J. (1993) Acid resistance in enteric bacteria. *Infection and Immunity* 61, 364–367.

Smith, M.G. (1992) Destruction of bacteria on fresh meat by hot water. *Epidemiology and Infection* 109, 491–496.

Snijders, J.M., Janssen, M.H., Corstiaensen, G.P. and Gerats, G.E. (1985) Cleaning and disinfection of knives in the meat industry. *Zentralblatt für Bakteriologie, Mikrobiologie und Hygiene [B]* 181, 121–131.

Thayer, D.W. (1994) Wholesomeness of irradiated foods. *Food Technology* 48, 132–135.

Thayer, D.W. and Boyd, G. (1993) Elimination of *Escherichia coli* O157:H7 in meats by gamma irradiation. *Applied and Environmental Microbiology* 59, 1030–1034.

Tinney, K.S., Miller, M.F., Ramsey, C.N., Thompson, L.E. and Carr, M.A. (1997) Reduction of microorganisms on beef surfaces with electricity and acetic acid. *Journal of Food Protection* 60, 625–628.

Uljas, H.E. and Ingham, S.C. (1998) Survival of *Escherichia coli* O157:H7 in synthetic gastric fluid after cold and acid habituation in apple juice or trypticase soy broth acidified with hydrochloric acid or organic acids. *Journal of Food Protection* 61, 939–947.

Van Donkersgoed, J., Jericho, K.W.F., Grogan, H. and Thorlakson, B. (1998) Preslaughter hide status of cattle and the microbiology of carcasses. *Journal of Food Protection* 60, 1502–1508.

Van Donkersgoed, J., Graham, T. and Gannon, V. (1999) The prevalence of verotoxins, *Escherichia coli* 0157:H7 and *Salmonella* in the faeces and rumen of cattle at processing. *Canadian Veterinary Journal* 40, 332–338.

Veeramuthu, G.J., Price, J.F., Davis, C.E., Booren, A.M. and Smith, D.M. (1998) Thermal inactivation of *Escherichia coli* 0157:H7, *Salmonella senftenberg*, and enzymes with potential as time–temperature indicators in ground turkey thigh meat. *Journal of Food Protection* 61, 171–175.

Waterman, S.R. and Small, P.L.C. (1998) Acid-sensitive enteric pathogens are protected from killing under extremely acidic conditions of pH 2.5 when they are inoculated onto certain solid foods. *Applied and Environmental Microbiology* 64, 3882–3886.

Waters, J.R., Sharp, J.C. and Dev, V.J. (1994) Infection caused by *Escherichia coli* O157:H7 in Alberta, Canada, and in Scotland: a five-year review, 1987–1991. *Clinical Infectious Diseases* 19, 834–843.

Weagant, S.D., Bryant, J.L. and Park, D.H. (1994) Survival of *Escherichia coli* O157:H7 in mayonnaise and mayonnaise-based sauces at room and refrigerated temperatures. *Journal of Food Protection* 57, 629–631.

WHO (1994) *Safety and Nutritional Adequacy of Irradiated Food.* World Health Organization, Geneva, 161 pp.

Wong, E., Linton, R.H. and Gerrard, D.E. (1998) Reduction of *Escherichia coli* and *Salmonella senftenberg* on pork skin and pork muscle using ultraviolet light. *Food Microbiology* 15, 415–423.

Zhao, T., Doyle, M.P., Shere, J. and Garber, L. (1995) Prevalence of enterohemorrhagic *Escherichia coli* O157:H7 in a survey of dairy herds. *Applied and Environmental Microbiology* 61, 1290–1293.

12

The Ecological Cycle of *Escherichia coli* O157:H7

J.S. Wallace

Department of Life Sciences, University of East London, London, UK

INTRODUCTION

Escherichia coli O157:H7 is an emerging pathogen, which was first recognized as the cause of human infection in 1982 (Riley *et al.*, 1983). Since this time, the incidence of infection has escalated, as a consequence of the proliferation of the organism as a human pathogen, concurrently with increased clinical/laboratory awareness and surveillance (Sharp *et al.*, 1994; Anon., 1995; Easton, 1997).

Beef and dairy cattle are perceived to be the major reservoirs of *E. coli* O157:H7 (Chapman *et al.*, 1993; Hancock *et al.*, 1994; Zhao *et al.*, 1995). Outbreaks of infection have been directly associated with the consumption of foods of bovine origin, especially beefburgers (Padhye and Doyle, 1992; Synge *et al.*, 1993; Willshaw *et al.*, 1994), faecal contamination of other food products (Morgan *et al.*, 1988; Cieslak *et al.*, 1993) and direct contact with infected animals (Renwick *et al.*, 1993; Shukla *et al.*, 1995).

Numerous surveys have been conducted to establish reservoirs and vehicles of infection. Recent evidence suggests that sheep may also be a natural reservoir of this organism, although there are no documented epidemiological case-studies implicating lamb products as the source of human infection (Kudva *et al.*, 1996; Chapman *et al.*, 1997). Similarly, while there have been no microbiologically confirmed cases of *E. coli* O157:H7 infection from a poultry source, two case–control studies have statistically linked poultry meat as a possible risk factor for infection (Salmon *et al.*, 1989; Salmon and Smith, 1994). Similarly, Doyle and Schoeni (1987) isolated *E. coli* O157:H7 from 1.5% of poultry samples, while Abdul-Raouf *et al.* (1996) isolated the organism from 4% of chicken samples. In both instances, cross-contamination from other meat products may have occurred. Other surveys have failed to isolate the organism from poultry products, indicating a prevalence of less than 0.25% (Smith *et al.*, 1991; Chapman *et al.*, 1997).

Other animals that have been either shown to carry *E. coli* O157:H7 or epidemiologically implicated in transmission include dogs (Synge *et al.*, 1993), deer (Rice *et al.*, 1995; Chapman and Ackroyd, 1997), goats (Synge *et al.*, 1993; Shukla *et al.*, 1995), orang-utan (Beutin *et al.*, 1996) and wild birds (Wallace *et al.*, 1997b). *E. coli* O157 has also been isolated from the faeces of apparently healthy pigs and piglets; however, the strains isolated were non-verotoxigenic and were serotypes other than H7 (Linggood and Thompson, 1987; Gannon *et al.*, 1988).

While cattle, and possibly sheep, are important in the maintenance of *E. coli* O157:H7 within the farm environment, they form only one link in the ecological cycle of the organism (Fig. 12.1). The ability of the organism to survive in the environment and carriage by other vectors will also influence maintenance and transmission. It has been suggested that the use of intervention strategies on the farm, to prevent entry into the food-chain, is the way forward in controlling this pathogen (Wuethrich, 1994). Thorough understanding of how the organism enters and is maintained in the farm environment is essential before such strategies can be implemented. The following reviews current knowledge on this subject.

FAECAL SHEDDING BY BOVINE AND OVINE RESERVOIRS

Cattle, and possibly sheep, are currently recognized as the principal reservoirs responsible for the proliferation of *E. coli* O157:H7 on the farm.

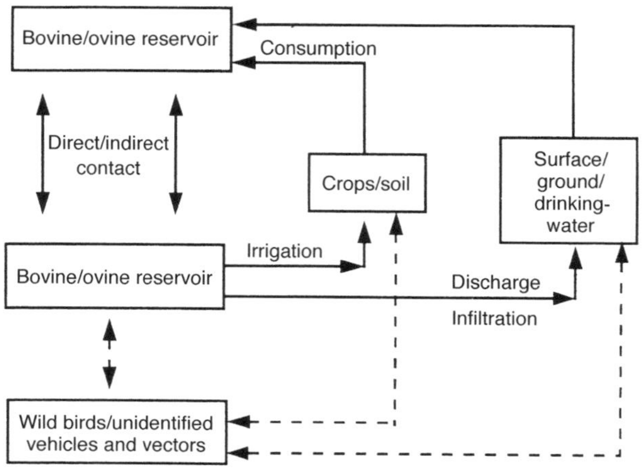

Fig. 12.1. The ecological cycle of *E. coli* O157:H7 in the farm environment.

Since infection occurs via the faecal–oral route, the numbers shed in faeces and the susceptibility of the host (see below) will ultimately determine transmission of this organism.

Numbers shed

Cattle and sheep account for approximately 90% of the total of 200 million tonnes of livestock waste produced in England and Wales each year (Mawdsley *et al.*, 1995). Although carriage of *E. coli* O157:H7 among cattle and sheep is not universal, the sheer volume of waste produced by these animals indicates their phenomenal ability to disseminate *E. coli* O157:H7 into the environment. The majority of studies that state the quantities of *E. coli* O157:H7 shed in faeces have been conducted using animals inoculated orogastrically with artificially high doses of *E. coli* O157:H7. Although these animals generally shed higher numbers of the organism and for longer intervals than naturally infected animals, they provide important information regarding the potential extent of environmental contamination.

Cray and Moon (1995) reported average shedding levels of 1.0×10^5 per gram of faeces (range 1.5×10^2–1.3×10^7) in adult cattle, fed an oral dose of 10^{10} organisms, when examined 2–4 days postinoculation. In the same study, calves were demonstrated to shed larger numbers of the organism, the average faecal count 3 days postinoculation being 6.3×10^6 (range 5×10^6–1.0×10^7), indicating the importance of calves in dissemination into the environment (Cray and Moon, 1995). Sanderson *et al.* (1995) artificially inoculated week-old calves with a milk meal containing 5×10^8 colony-forming units (CFU), and demonstrated shedding of the organism in the range < 1000 to $\geq 1{,}000{,}000$ CFU per gram of faeces. Naturally infected cattle have been reported to shed at levels of greater than 10^2 CFU g^{-1} to $\geq 10^6$ (Zhao *et al.*, 1995). Similar data regarding the numbers shed by infected sheep have not yet been published.

Intermittent shedding

Following colonization, periods of faecal shedding of *E. coli* O157:H7 are intermittent and generally brief. In cattle, the duration of shedding varies widely among animals of the same age-group but persists longer in calves than in adults (Cray and Moon, 1995). Naturally infected animals generally shed for shorter periods than animals artificially inoculated with high doses. The maximum period of shedding reported by Mechie *et al.* (1997) in a dairy herd was 4 weeks by one naturally infected calf. Other studies have shown the duration of shedding by naturally infected animals to be less than 2 months (Rahn *et al.*, 1997). Similarly, in a study by Shukla *et al.* (1995), six out of seven naturally infected goats ceased shedding the organism within

6 weeks. Using artificially infected animals, the oral dose of *E. coli* O157:H7 administered has been shown to influence shedding patterns, with higher doses resulting in extended shedding. An oral inoculum of 10^{10} organisms induced shedding by calves for 7 weeks postinoculation (Cray and Moon, 1995), while a lower dose resulted in shedding by week-old calves for an average of 32 days (range 24–43 days) (Sanderson *et al.*, 1995). In the study by Cray and Moon (1995), one animal remained culture-positive for at least 27 weeks. Faecal shedding by sheep appears to be shorter. Studies with lambs have shown that, when dosed with 10^9 CFU, the animals became positive approximately 2 weeks earlier than those dosed with 10^5 CFU. The average duration of shedding by animals administered the higher dose was 6 days, while those dosed with 10^5 shed, on average, for 2 days. The maximum period of shedding in one sheep was 50 days (Kudva *et al.*, 1995).

Suggestions as to why intermittent shedding occurs include: the effects of dietary changes (Kudva *et al.*, 1995, 1997a); the age of the animals (Mechie *et al.*, 1997); sensitivity of detection methods (Cray and Moon, 1995; Garber *et al.*, 1995; Zhao *et al.*, 1995); prevalence in the population below sample size limitations (Garber *et al.*, 1995); and that the animals become reinfected after the initial infection (Zhao *et al.*, 1995). The latter proposal is supported by evidence suggesting that infection with *E. coli* O157:H7 does not confer protection against re-infection (Cray and Moon, 1995; Johnson *et al.*, 1996).

Seasonality

The human incidence of *E. coli* O157:H7 infection peaks during the warmest months of the year in Canada (Cahoon and Thompson, 1987; Pai *et al.*, 1988), the UK (Chapman *et al.*, 1989, 1990; Anon., 1995), the USA (Karmali, 1989; Ostroff *et al.*, 1989) and Belgium (Pierard *et al.*, 1990).

Although still under debate, the evidence that faecal shedding of *E. coli* O157:H7 by animals also occurs in a seasonal fashion is mounting, with times of maximum numbers of culture-positive animals occurring at times coinciding with peaks in human infection (Hancock *et al.*, 1994; Kudva *et al.*, 1996, 1997b; Mechie *et al.*, 1997).

Kudva *et al.* (1997b) showed that shedding by sheep occurred in the summer (June) of two successive years and August of one. *E. coli* O157:H7 was not isolated from the flock at any other time of the year. Mechie *et al.* (1997) reported seasonal shedding in a dairy herd, with maximal shedding occurring in spring and November. In accord with the results of Kudva *et al.* (1997b), no evidence was found of excretion during the interval November–May, despite close confinement within housing. Factors such as changes in diet, environment and copasturage with wild animals that may serve as *E. coli* O157:H7 reservoirs were hypothesized to have influenced seasonal shedding in sheep (Kudva *et al.*, 1997b). In cattle, seasonality was thought to have occurred as a consequence of the movement of non-lactating cows and heifers into a lactating herd at calving and also due to close contact between calving cows and their calves (Mechie *et al.*, 1997). Seasonal variation in the numbers of *E. coli* O157:H7 isolated from rectal swabs of cattle after slaughter has also been reported, being highest during the spring (April–May) and late summer (September) (Chapman *et al.*, 1997). In the same survey, seasonality was not demonstrated in sheep, due to the limited number of isolates recovered; however, 17 of the 22 isolates were isolated in summer (June–September) (Chapman *et al.*, 1997).

Seasonal influences on the carriage of bacterial pathogens by domestic animals and poultry is not an uncommon phenomenon. Seasonal trends in the numbers of thermophilic campylobacters has been reported. Statistical analyses of data recorded over a 2-year interval revealed significant evidence for seasonal periodicity in the number of campylobacters shed by dairy herds, each herd having two peaks per year, in approximately spring and autumn (Stanley *et al.*, 1998b). Lambs also showed periodicity in the populations of campylobacters in the small intestine at slaughter; however, no statistical correlation was found with environmental factors, such as temperature, rainfall or sunshine hours (Stanley *et al.*, 1998a).

Seasonal peaks in the carriage of thermophilic campylobacters by poultry has also been reported (Genigeorgis *et al.*, 1986; Kapperud *et al.*, 1993; Jacobs-Reitsma *et al.*, 1994; Wallace *et al.*, 1997a). Direct factors, including temperature and humidity, have been proposed to explain the reported seasonal fluctuations (Doyle, 1984; Willis *et al.*, 1991; Wallace *et al.*, 1997a). Jacobs-Reitsma *et al.* (1994) hypothesized that indirect temperature-dependent factors, such as the activities of migratory birds, rodents or darkling beetles, may also influence the seasonal fluctuation in carriage rates.

Changing strains with time

Molecular characterization and phage typing of isolates taken from sheep and cattle have shown that animals are capable of harbouring more than one strain of *E. coli* O157:H7 simultaneously and that the strains isolated change with time (Synge and Hopkins, 1994; Zhao *et al.*, 1995; Faith *et al.*, 1996; Kudva *et al.*, 1997b; Rahn *et al.*, 1997). Strain-to-strain variation with time implies either that animals acquire new strains of *E. coli* O157:H7 from the environment or that mutations occurred during growth within the gastrointestinal tract. Genetic instability of *E. coli* O157:H7 has been shown (Tzipori *et al.*, 1986; Dorn and Angrick, 1991; Chapman *et al.*, 1997). Karch *et al.* (1995) reported restriction enzyme digest profile (REDP) changes in sequential isolates obtained from patients infected with *E. coli* O157 and proposed that genetic change(s) or clonal turnover was the likely cause. In contrast, strain stability has been reported in an ovine model for periods up to 60 days (Kudva *et al.*, 1995, 1997b). Strain stability within the ovine population supports the view of others that there is more than one source of *E. coli* O157:H7 in the farm environment (Faith *et al.*, 1996).

VEHICLES AND VECTORS WITHIN THE FARM ENVIRONMENT

Research to date has focused on determining herd status and relatively few studies have been conducted to identify environmental sources of *E. coli* O157:H7.

Farm surveys

Rahn *et al.* (1997) investigated the persistence of *E. coli* O157:H7 on farms with previously culture-positive cattle. Samples were taken from rodents, cats, wild birds, flies, water and farm surfaces. None of the environmental samples were culture-positive for *E. coli* O157, although some – calf mangers, calf water-bowls, calf barn surfaces and composite fly samples – were positive for verocytotoxigenic *E. coli* (VTEC), as assessed by polymerase chain reaction (PCR) of the verocytotoxin (VT) genes and a Vero cell cytotoxicity assay. In a similar study, Faith *et al.* (1996) examined 302 environmental samples. These included 101 water samples and samples from non-bovine faeces (i.e. cat, dog, racoon, pig, rabbit), grain, silage, bedding, buildings and manure pits. Of these, *E. coli* O157:H7 was only isolated from three water samples. One isolate was identical to the strain found in five out of the six positive animals on the same farm and it was concluded that horizontal transmission via water is important in the maintenance and dissemination of *E. coli* O157:H7 within a herd. Kudva *et al.* (1997a) also proposed that water is important in the dissemination of *E. coli* O157:H7 in the farm environment. The remaining two isolates, from a different farm, were distinct from that isolated from the only culture-positive animal identified. The lack of similarity inferred that they were separate clones and probably originated from different sources (Faith *et al.*, 1996). The lack of isolation from the farm environment reflects the presence of the target organisms in much lower numbers than other flora, a problem which is compounded by the limitations of the cultural procedures employed to detect sublethally injured populations (see below).

Wild birds as vectors

The increased incidence of *E. coli* O157:H7 infection in south Cumbria (UK) between 1992 and 1995 prompted an investigation into the extent to which

E. coli O157:H7 was found in dairy herds in that area. Four dairy herds were sampled and one was found to be culture-positive for *E. coli* O157:H7 (Wallace and Jones, 1996). It was noted that large numbers of birds visited the farm each day and were frequently seen foraging on the pasture-land used by the dairy herd.

The major roosting sites of birds in the vicinity of the farm were Morecambe Bay at low tide and the local landfill site (Lancaster Waste Services, Ltd., Salt Ayre, Lancaster, UK). In Morecambe Bay, there are tens of thousands of gulls (Wilson, 1988). One hundred freshly voided faecal samples were collected from each site on four separate occasions. Faecal samples from shore birds were predominantly from herring gulls, *Larus argentatus*, black-headed gulls, *Larus ridibundus*, common gull, *Larus canus*, and lapwings, *Vanellus vanellus*. At the landfill site, the main birds were herring gulls, black-headed gulls and common gulls. A small number of crows, *Corvus corone corone*, and jackdaws, *Corvus monedula*, were also present. Samples were amalgamated and tested for the presence of *E. coli* O157:H7. The organism was isolated intermittently from faecal samples at both sites, indicating that a proportion of these birds were carriers. All of the isolates contained the VT1 and VT2 genes and were phage type 4. Although not the most commonly isolated, phage type 4 constituted 18% of a total of 17 different phage types isolated from cattle in a 1-year survey (Chapman *et al.*, 1997). Phage type 4 also constituted 6.2% of the *E. coli* O157:H7 isolates sent to the Laboratory of Enteric Pathogens, Central Public Health Laboratory, London, UK, in the interval 1992–1994 (Thomas *et al.*, 1996). The isolation of the organism from wild birds, the phage type and the presence of VT genes provide circumstantial evidence of the importance of wild birds in the environmental dissemination of *E. coli* O157:H7. This finding is supported by the work of Smith *et al.* (1997), who, in a later study, isolated the organism from the faeces of wild birds at the same landfill site, and also by the isolation of the organism from geese (B.A. Synge, 1998, Caithness, personal communication). Others have failed to isolate *E. coli* O157:H7 from wild birds (Synge and Hopkins, 1992). The isolation of *E. coli* O157:H7 from wild birds is not entirely surprising, since wild birds have been shown to carry a multitude of bacterial pathogens that cause infection in humans (Table 12.1).

Role of birds in disease dissemination

Wild birds may be of particular importance to the spread of *E. coli* O157:H7 in the UK, due to the sheer numbers of birds that visit the country each year and also due to the increase in populations of certain native species that have managed to take advantage of human adaptation of the environment (Chabrzyk and Coulson, 1976; Monaghan and Coulson, 1977; Houston, 1993). Due to their great mobility, wild birds may function as effective

Table 12.1. Bacterial pathogens isolated from wild birds.

Bird	Bacterial species isolated	Author
Pigeons	*Candida albicans*, *Campylobacter coli*, *Listeria* spp., *Shigella* spp., *Salmonella* spp., *Yersinia intermedia*	Casanovas *et al.*, 1995; Grunder, 1996
Crow, gulls, common tern, puffin, Ural owl, herring gull, gull, rook, pigeon, blackbird, starling, sparrow, lapwing, redshank, oyster-catcher, turnstone	*Campylobacter jejuni*	Skirrow and Benjamin, 1980; Fenlon, 1981; Kapperud and Rosef, 1983; Fricker and Metcalfe, 1984; Glunder *et al.*, 1992
Reed bunting, black-headed gull, common tern	*Yersinia* spp.	Kapperud and Rosef, 1983
Black-headed gull, common gull, great black-backed gull, herring gull	*Salmonella* spp.	Jones *et al.*, 1978; Fricker, 1984; Girdwood *et al.*, 1985; Monaghan *et al.*, 1985
Ring-billed gull	*Salmonella* spp., *Campylobacter* spp., *Listeria monocytogenes*, *Salmonella* spp., *Aeromonas* spp.	Quessy and Messier, 1992; Levesque *et al.*, 1993
Seagulls	*Shigella* spp., *Salmonella* spp.	Karaguzel *et al.*, 1993
Rooks and gulls	*Listeria* spp.	Fenlon, 1985
Aquatic birds	*Vibrio cholerae*	Lee *et al.*, 1982; Ogg *et al.*, 1989

disseminators of disease, especially migrating birds, which are able to spread pathogens across phenomenal areas as they commute each year between breeding and wintering grounds. The UK plays an important role in the life cycles of a vast array of avian species, occupying a key geographical position in the east Atlantic flyway, which birds from diverse locations, such as north-east Canada and central Siberia, use during their migratory periods (Prys-Jones *et al.*, 1994). Britain is estimated to have a migratory bird population of 75 million pairs (Nice, 1994).

Human influence on feeding and roosting habits

Human activity has influenced the feeding habits and roosting sites of certain birds. In addition to their traditional coastal haunts, *Larus* gulls now feed at refuse tips and sewage outfalls, roost at night at inland water reservoirs and by day on pasture-land, and nest on inhabited buildings. This brings them into contact with the pathogens of humans and domestic animals and also their foodstuffs and water-supplies (Monaghan *et al.*, 1985). Proliferation of certain bird species, especially *Larus* gulls, in the UK between 1940 and the early 1970s prompted speculation regarding their role in the dissemination of disease. While certain authors have implicated wild birds in the transmission of bacterial infection to humans and domestic animals (Jones *et al.*, 1978; Reilly *et al.*, 1981; Coulson *et al.*, 1983a, b; Sacks *et al.*, 1986), others have negated their importance as a direct source of infection (Whelan *et al.*, 1988; Quessy and Messier, 1992). A notable exception to the latter is the transmission of *Campylobacter* spp. to humans via contamination of milk by birds, e.g. magpies, crows and jackdaws, during the nesting season (Southern *et al.*, 1990; Hudson *et al.*, 1991; Lighton *et al.*, 1991; Stuart *et al.*, 1997).

Tucker (1992) tentatively associated the use of cultivated fields by invertebrate-feeding birds with high frequencies of farmyard-manure application. Lapwing, starling, fieldfare and redwing foraged on frequently manured grass fields. Foraging of pasture-land by magpies and jackdaws was positively associated with the frequency of sheep grazing, while foraging by the plover and lapwing was associated with cattle grazing. Increased foraging following manure application is a consequence of increased invertebrate activity and density. Curry (1976) found a 43% increase in earthworm density following the application of cattle slurry, while Scullian and Ramshaw (1987) demonstrated increased earthworm surface activity, and therefore availability to birds, following the application of poultry manure to grass fields. Preferential foraging on contaminated land provides further credence to the hypothesis that birds are involved in the ecology of *E. coli* O157:H7.

Factors influencing carriage of bacterial pathogens by wild birds

The problem of pathogen carriage by birds is exacerbated in areas of high population densities, such as occur at roosting sites. Several authors have indicated the hazard posed to public health by pollution of water-storage reservoirs in the vicinity of roosting sites (Fennel *et al.*, 1974; Benton *et al.*, 1983; Monaghan *et al.*, 1985; Smith *et al.*, 1993). Carriage of bacterial pathogens by birds is not universal (Hill and Grimes, 1984). It is influenced by factors including: feeding habits (Whelan *et al.*, 1988); season (Jones *et al.*, 1978; Fricker and Girdwood, 1984; Fenlon, 1985; Whelan *et al.*, 1988); age, young birds being more prone to be carriers (Ogg *et al.*, 1989; Glunder *et al.*, 1992), although Monaghan *et al.* (1985) found no significant age-associated difference with respect to *Salmonella* carriage by gulls; levels of environmental contamination, areas of high human population being correlated with high carriage rates (Girdwood *et al.*, 1985; Whelan *et al.*, 1988); and avian population density (Casanovas *et al.*, 1995). Differences that exist within the literature regarding the carrier status of birds also reflect the isolation methods employed and the source of the sample analysed, e.g. gut contents, faeces or cloacal swab (Leuchtefeld *et al.*, 1980; Fricker and Metcalf, 1984). Thus, the lack of isolation of *E. coli* O157:H7 from any of 113 birds examined by Synge and Hopkins (1992) may be a consequence of the lack of sensitivity of the direct plating technique employed. Others have demonstrated that enrichment culture is essential for the isolation of *E. coli* O157:H7 (Sanderson *et al.*, 1995; Kudva *et al.*, 1996; Wallace and Jones, 1996; Wallace *et al.*, 1997b). Methods used for the detection and culture of *E. coli* O157:H7 have been reviewed elsewhere (Smith and Scotland, 1993; Vernozy-Rozand, 1997).

Completing the cycle to domestic animals

Following the colonization of birds, bacteria complete the cycle back to domestic animals by being deposited on to grazing land and into troughs and streams used by domestic animals. Jones *et al.* (1978) hypothesized that it is unlikely that animals imbibing water faecally contaminated by birds will consume an infective dose, unless faecal contamination has been recent and extensive. The pathogens present may, however, without causing infection, be passaged and excreted on to pasture in more concentrated numbers and in a more viable state. Passaging acts as a means of resuscitation, and infective dose levels may be attained in contact animals (Jones *et al.*, 1978). Recovery via passaging is supported by studies that have shown *in vitro* and *in vivo* repair and recovery of chlorine-injured cells of enterotoxigenic *E. coli* with retention of virulence (Singh and McFeters, 1986; Singh *et al.*, 1986; Walsh and Bissonnette, 1987). Nice (1994) reviewed the evidence linking the carriage of *Salmonella* by birds with infection in cattle and sheep and concluded that, although the numbers of *Salmonella* shed in gull faeces are much lower than the infective dose for healthy cattle and sheep, starving or stressed animals might be infected by lower doses and pass infection on to other, healthy, livestock. Carriage of *E. coli* O157:H7 by wild birds may be responsible for the limited farm-to-farm transmission demonstrated by the isolation of strains with the same REDP (Faith *et al.*, 1996) and the same phage types (Rahn *et al.*, 1997) on different farms.

Studies on poultry

Further evidence which corroborates the importance of wild birds in the transmission of *E. coli* O157:H7 can be gleaned from studies investigating the carriage of the organism in artificially inoculated animals.

Infective dose

The number of organisms required to establish infection in orally inoculated animals is shown in Table 12.2. Cattle have been frequently cited as the major reservoir of *E. coli* O157; however, the infective dose for a normal adult animal is surprisingly high, being greater than 10^4 and probably greater than or equal to 10^7 CFU of an organism grown *in vitro* (Cray and Moon, 1995). The comparatively high infective dose of cattle (Cray and Moon, 1995; Sanderson *et al.*, 1995), in contrast to that of chickens (Beery *et al.*, 1985; Stavric *et al.*, 1992, 1993; Schoeni and Doyle, 1994) and sheep (Kudva *et al.*, 1995), casts doubt on the hypothesis that cattle are more susceptible to infection than other animals, although strain-to-strain variability in pathogenicity may have influenced the outcomes of these studies.

Table 12.2. The number of organisms required to cause infection in domestic animals.

	Age	Dose	% infected	Author
Chickens				
Broilers and layers	1 day	10^5–10^9	100	Stavric *et al.*, 1993
Broilers	1 day : 3 days	10^9	85–100	
Layers	1 day : 3 days	10^9	63–90	
Chicks	1 day	1.6×10^9	100	Beery *et al.*, 1985
Chicks	1 day	2.6×10^1– 2.6×10^5 2.6×10^1	50–83	Schoeni and Doyle, 1994
Sheep				
Lambs	14 days ± 0.5	10^9	100	Kudva *et al.*, 1995
		10^5	67	
Adult ram	Adult	10^9	100[a]	
		10^5	100[a]	
Ewes	1 year	10^{10}	100	Kudva *et al.*, 1997a
Cattle				
Calves	7 days	5×10^9	79[b]	Sanderson *et al.*, 1995
Cattle	1–3 years	10^4	0	Cray and Moon, 1995
		10^7	40	
		10^{10}	100	
Calves	3–14 weeks	10^{10}	100	

[a] Only one animal challenged.
[b] 79% of faecal samples tested were culture-positive.

Duration of shedding in poultry

Studies on artificially inoculated chickens have further shown that chickens shed the organism in faeces at higher numbers and for a longer duration than cattle or sheep. The ability of *E. coli* O157:H7 to adhere to and penetrate the epithelia of the caeca is postulated to be the mechanism for prolonged faecal shedding of the bacterium (Beery *et al.*, 1985). Colonization and shedding of *E. coli* O157:H7 by poultry have also been shown to be influenced by factors including the following: challenge dose, higher doses resulting in greater numbers per gram of caecal tissue (Stavric *et al.*, 1993); age, a significantly greater percentage being colonized at 1 day of age than at 2 or 3 days of age (Stavric *et al.*, 1993); breed, broilers (White Rock × Cornish) being more susceptible to colonization than layers (Leghorn) (Stavric *et al.*, 1993); and gender – hens shed larger numbers of *E. coli* O157:H7 and the caeca were colonized faster than was the case in roosters (Schoeni and Doyle, 1994).

As with sheep and cattle, faecal shedding of *E. coli* O157:H7 by birds, especially when using low challenge doses, is frequently intermittent. Schoeni and Doyle (1994) showed that, although the organism was not detected in the faeces of chicks 3 months postchallenge with 2.6×10^1 organisms, when examined, two out of six of the birds carried 10^3–10^4 organisms per gram of caecal tissue.

As reported for sheep and cattle (see above), faecal shedding of *E. coli* O157:H7 by poultry is seasonal. In a 10-month study, shedding by poultry was maximal in July, when the birds were 4 months old, coinciding with the seasonal peak in human infections (Schoeni and Doyle, 1994).

ENVIRONMENTAL CONTAMINATION

Farm management practices and intensification

Management practices introduced in the 1980s may have created the niche in which *E. coli* O157:H7 can survive within the farm environment (Garber *et al.*, 1995). Intensification of farming, i.e. increased herd sizes and the number of housed animals and concurrent modifications of husbandry practices, has resulted in increased quantities of livestock waste that must be managed and a concomitant alteration in the methods used to treat these wastes. Several associations have been made between herd status and husbandry practices. Hancock *et al.* (1994) found that culture-positive herds were less likely to have been fed whole cottonseed and were more likely to use automated computer feeders. Herd size was also associated with status, with smaller herds tending to be positive. Others have also reported an association between diet and shedding of *E. coli* O157:H7 (Garber *et al.*, 1995; Kudva *et al.*, 1995, 1997a). Further associations with herd status include the grouping and housing of calves prior to weaning. This practice increases animal contact, induces stress and may serve to concentrate the bacterium (Garber *et al.*, 1995). Stress has previously been associated with increased shedding of *Salmonella* in cattle (Corrier *et al.*, 1990).

Changes in the management of livestock waste also influence the dissemination of *E. coli* O157:H7, and other pathogens, into the farm environment. The housing of cattle between October/November and May results in the generation of large amounts of slurry, which requires storage before application to land. Prior to agricultural intensification, livestock wastes were managed as farmyard manure and contained large amounts of bedding. The process of aerobic composting destroyed the majority of pathogens. As a consequence of intensification, slurry is now frequently stored in such a way that conditions become anaerobic and the destruction of pathogens is reduced (Mawdsley *et al.*, 1995). Due to pressures on storage space, caused by the housing of animals, farmers are more likely to put untreated slurry on land in winter, during brief intervals of good weather, than in summer (Stanley *et al.*, 1999c). Such practices no doubt influence the cycling of bacterial pathogens in the environment. Intensification has also resulted in significant increases in the quantities of manure deposited directly on to the land at times when animals are not housed.

Association between slurry management and herd status

An association between slurry management practices and herd status was first reported by Hancock *et al.* (1994), who noted that, among the herds where slurry was placed on to crops and pasture, herds that were culture-positive for *E. coli* O157:H7 tended to have a shorter interval between application and grazing. Mechie *et al.* (1997) also made a tentative association between slurry management and herd status. The highest excretion rate in heifers during a 15-month survey was observed 3 days after the animals entered a silage field recently treated with slurry. In contrast, Garber *et al.* (1995) found no association between faecal shedding and manure-handling methods. Avian feeding habits have been shown to be influenced by farming practices.

SURVIVAL IN THE FARM ENVIRONMENT

To be successful, bacterial pathogens must be capable of surviving the stresses imposed within the host and those occurring in the environment to which they are voided before the cycle back to the host is completed. The escalating incidence of *E. coli* O157:H7 clearly indicates that it is a successful pathogen. Although microbiologists have seldom cultured the organism from environmental samples, this is not prima facie evidence that the organism is either dead or absent. Laboratory studies indicate that the organism is very hardy, being able to tolerate acidic conditions in food better than most food-borne pathogens (Zhao *et al.*, 1993; Leyer *et al.*, 1995) and having a similar salt tolerance to other *E. coli*, which is greater than that of *Salmonella* spp. and *Campylobacter jejuni* (Conner, 1992). The literature, although limited, also indicates that *E. coli* O157:H7 has similar mechanisms to other strains of *E. coli* to facilitate survival in hostile conditions. These mechanisms include RpoS regulation of stress-response genes, which enhances the ability of organisms to withstand certain chemical and physical challenges, e.g. hydrogen peroxide (H_2O_2), acid and alkaline pH, heat and osmolarity (Murano and Pierson, 1992; Benjamin and Datta, 1995; Cheville *et al.*, 1996; Lin *et al.*, 1996). Molecular processes and survival strategies influencing the survival of *E. coli* in adverse conditions have been discussed in detail elsewhere (Dodd *et al.*, 1988; Farr and Kogoma, 1991; Loewen and Hengge-Aronis, 1994; Jones, 1997; Booth, 1998).

Factors influencing survival in the environment

Bacteria entering the environment are exposed to various types of stress, which greatly influence their longevity. These include: temperature (Gameson, 1984; Huq *et al.*, 1984); pH (Sjogren and Gibson, 1981); predation (González *et al.*, 1992; Iriberri *et al.*, 1994); heavy metals (Cenci *et al.*, 1985); salinity levels (Munro *et al.*, 1987; Bordalo, 1993); competition (Klein and Casida, 1967); lack of nutrients (Sinclair and Alexander, 1984); light (Davies and Evison, 1991; Curtis *et al.*, 1992); and oxidative stress (Christman *et al.*, 1985). Parameters known to extend the longevity of allochthonous bacteria in aquatic environments include: attachment to suspended particles (Berman *et al.*, 1988); biofilm formation (Hicks and Rowbury, 1987; Frank and Koffi, 1990; Carpentier and Cerf, 1993; Jones and Bradshaw, 1996); and ingestion, but not lysis, by protozoa (King *et al.*, 1988). Little is known regarding the influence of these factors on the longevity of *E. coli* O157:H7 in the environment.

Sublethal injury

Unless faecal contamination has been recent and massive, gut-derived pathogens in the environment are generally present in very low numbers in comparison with other microorganisms, making detection by conventional methods difficult. Problems of cultural detection of enteropathogenic bacteria are further exacerbated by entry of the organism into a sublethally injured state. Sublethal injury of bacteria is reversible and is manifested as phenotypic change, resulting in reduced ability of the organism to grow either in or on selective media, while maintaining the ability to be cultured on non-selective media (McFeters, 1997). Following repair of cellular damage, organisms should regain tolerance for growth under restrictive or selective conditions (McFeters, 1990).

Numerous authors have reported the inadequacy of commonly used selective media, as opposed to non-selective media, for the isolation of *E. coli* O157:H7 following intervals of physical and chemical stress. MacConkey sorbitol agar was found inadequate for the recovery of salt- and cold-injured cells (Conner, 1992). MacConkey sorbitol agar supplemented with 4-methyl-umbelliferyl-β-D-glucuronide (MSMA) has also been shown to perform poorly in comparison with non-selective tryptic soy agar (TSA) for the recovery of cells stressed by cold, heat, acid or drying (Abdul-Raouf *et al.*, 1993; Conner and Hall, 1994; Clavero and Beuchat, 1995, 1996; McCleery and Rowe, 1995). TSA also performed better than modified eosin methylene-blue and modified SD-39 (Clavero and Beuchat, 1995, 1996). Similarly, Pyle *et al.* (1995) demonstrated the influence of growth phase on the ability of certain selective media to isolate *E. coli* O157:H7. Growth of *E. coli* O157:H7 to logarithmic phase in low-nutrient medium caused injury, as demonstrated by a reduced ability to form colonies on selective media (MacConkey sorbitol agar, MacConkey lactose agar and tryptone lactose agar with deoxycholate), as opposed to non-selective media (R_2A and tryptone lactose agar). A smaller proportion of the population grown to stationary phase were injured when assessed in the same fashion indicating that actively growing cells are more sensitive to antimicrobial agents (Pyle *et al.*, 1995). As stated previously, sublethal injury is reversible under the correct conditions. McCleery and Rowe (1995) found that a short period of growth (2 h) on non-selective TSA, prior to overlay with MSMA, resulted in significantly higher counts, indicating recovery of injured cells. Supplementation of TSA with catalase prior to overlay further increased recovery of heat- and freeze-injured cells.

Due to the variety of stresses to which *E. coli* O157:H7 is exposed after being shed, it is likely that the organism enters a sublethally injured state. In light of this, although selective culture is necessitated, as a consequence of the presence of non-target organisms within a sample, it is hardly surprising that researchers have been unsuccessful in their attempts to isolate the organism from the environment. Pyle *et al.* (1995) proposed that direct methods of detection of *E. coli* O157:H7 may be more appropriate and sensitive than cultural procedures.

The survival of *E. coli* O157:H7 in the terrestrial environment

Although rarely detected, evidence that *E. coli* O157:H7 can survive in the environment for extended periods can be elicited from outbreak information and laboratory-based studies.

Laboratory studies

Laboratory studies using artificially inoculated samples clearly demonstrate the ability of *E. coli* O157:H7 to survive in the terrestrial environment for extended intervals. Maule (1997) reported extended survival in faecal and soil samples. Cattle faeces, cattle slurry and soil cores were inoculated with an 18 h culture and incubated at 18°C. In cattle faeces, numbers fell from 7.1×10^7 to 3.8×10^5 in 54 days. In soil cores, numbers fell from 8.1×10^7 to 8.7×10^6 in 63 days, while, in cattle slurry inoculated with 1.2×10^8 CFU ml^{-1}, the organism became undetectable by direct plating techniques within 9 days. In accord with the extended survival recorded in artificially inoculated samples, Kudva *et al.* (1995) showed that *E. coli* O157:H7 shed from inoculated sheep can survive in collective ovine faecal slurry for at least 6 weeks, which was longer than the organism was shed by the sheep in the study. Factors such as strain type, cultural methodology, temperature and inoculum size influence the ability to detect *E. coli* O157:H7 in bovine faeces (Wang *et al.*, 1996). When artificially inoculated with a five-strain mixture of *E. coli* O157:H7, strain 932 (human isolate) remained culturable for a longer interval in bovine faeces when incubated at 22°C and 37°C than strains E0122 (calf faecal isolate), C7927 (human isolate), E09 (meat isolate) and E0018 (calf faecal isolate). No discernible difference in survival was noted for strains when incubated at 5°C. Strain-to-strain variability in survival of *E. coli* O157:H7 has also been demonstrated in highly acidic conditions (Arnold and Kaspar, 1995). When incubated at 37°C and 22°C, *E. coli* O157:H7 remained detectable for 7 and 8 weeks, respectively, using enrichment procedures. The use of direct culture techniques reduced the period when the organism could be detected by 5 weeks in both instances. Incubation at 5°C extended the interval of detection to 7 and 10 weeks by direct and enrichment procedures, respectively. The use of a higher inoculum (10^5) extended detection by a further week in all instances. Strains retained the ability to produce VT1 and VT2 throughout (Wang *et al.*, 1996).

Multiplication in faeces

The importance of faecal waste for the survival of *E. coli* O157:H7 entering the environment is emphasized by evidence that the organism can multiply in this material. Wang *et al.* (1996) reported increases in the number of organisms detected after 2 and 3 days when artificially inoculated bovine faeces was incubated at 37°C and 22°C, respectively. Maule (1997) also reported increases in the number of organisms detected in cattle faeces, cattle slurry and soil cores artificially inoculated with *E. coli* O157:H7 and incubated at 18°C. Similar results have also been reported for naturally inoculated ovine faecal slurry (Kudva *et al.*, 1995).

Outbreaks associated with bovine faeces

Further evidence of the ability of *E. coli* O157:H7 to survive in the soil and faecal material can be deduced from sporadic outbreaks of human infection.

Infection of a lacto-ovo-vegetarian was linked to the consumption of vegetables fertilized with manure from a cow and calf. *E. coli* O157:H7 was not isolated from either animal, although both had high *E. coli* O157:H7 lipopolysaccharide titres; however, retrospective swab samples taken from the garden confirmed the presence of *E. coli* O157:H7 (Cieslak *et al.*, 1993). Although not confirmed microbiologically, a case–control study of a cluster of infections in East Anglia, UK, associated infection with the handling, though not consumption, of raw vegetables, especially potatoes (Morgan *et al.*, 1988). Besser *et al.* (1993) attributed an outbreak caused by the consumption of fresh-pressed apple cider to the inadequacy of washing and brushing of the fruit prior to processing. The majority of apples collected for production were windfalls and consequently may have had contact with cattle manure before collection (Besser *et al.*, 1993). *E. coli* O157:H7 was not isolated from any of the cattle tested in the vicinity or from environmental samples taken 7 weeks after the outbreak. An outbreak of *E. coli* O157:H7 at a music festival was linked to faecal contamination of the site, since no common food or water source was identified. Approximately 500 dairy cattle had grazed on the site until 1 week prior to the festival (Anon., 1997).

Survival in water

Despite the number of water-borne outbreaks attributed to *E. coli* O157:H7 (Dev *et al.*, 1991; Swerdlow *et al.*, 1992; Brewster, *et al.*, 1994; Keene *et al.*, 1994) and the implication that water may contribute to the dissemination and/or maintenance of *E. coli* O157:H7 on farms (Faith *et al.*, 1996; Kudva *et al.*, 1997a), very little is known about the survival of the bacterium in the aquatic environment.

Laboratory studies

As with the detection of *E. coli* O157:H7 in faecal samples, the outcome of laboratory-based studies will be influenced by the strains used, previous culture conditions, the type of water into which the strain is inoculated and subsequent incubation conditions. Selective culture will also limit the detection of injured organisms, and consequently the results obtained may be an underestimation of the true survival. Laboratory studies have shown that *E. coli* O157:H7 can survive in a culturable state for more than 20 days in sterile pond water when incubated at 13°C in the dark (Porter *et al.*, 1997) and for more than 35 days when incubated at 5°C and 20°C in filter-sterilized potable water (Geldreich *et al.*, 1992). The use of non-sterile water significantly reduces the period in which *E. coli* O157:H7 remains detectable. Cultures suspended in non-sterile pond water declined to non-detectable numbers within 20 days when incubated at 13°C (Porter *et al.*, 1997). Similarly, Maule (1997) showed that *E. coli* O157:H7 became non-detectable after 13 days when incubated in non-sterile river water at 18°C.

Water-borne outbreaks

The first isolation of *E. coli* O157:H7 from water was reported in 1989 (McGowan *et al.*, 1989). Samples of water were evaluated from 15 streams and reservoirs within and surrounding Philadelphia. Wildlife, especially deer, were implicated in the contamination of the water, as no dairy or cattle-raising farms were located upstream and human contamination was considered unlikely. Similarly, following a mainly water-borne outbreak in Africa, *E. coli* O157:H7 was isolated from 18.4% of 76 river-water samples and a domestic water-storage drum. Contamination of the water was thought to have occurred as a consequence of heavy rain, following a period of drought, which resulted in the flushing of contaminated cattle carcasses and manure into surface waters. This hypothesis was supported by the isolation of *E. coli* O157:H7 from 14.3% of 42 samples of cattle dung and fly-infected maize at the same time as the water samples were taken. *E. coli* O157:H7 became undetectable 2 months later, when further samples were examined (Isaacson *et al.*, 1993). An outbreak of infections associated with swimming in lake water provided tentative evidence that *E. coli* O157:H7 can survive in natural waters for periods of up to 3 weeks; however, *E. coli* O157:H7 was not isolated from the water (Keene *et al.*, 1994).

CONCLUDING SUMMARY

E. coli O157:H7 remains an enigma to microbiologists. It is clear that cattle and sheep play an important role in the epidemiology of this organism. Molecular analysis of *E. coli* O157:H7 isolates from cattle and sheep has indicated that horizontal transmission on the farm is important, that animals are capable of being reinfected with the same strain and that animals can shed more than one strain of *E. coli* O157:H7 simultaneously.

Shedding of *E. coli* O157:H7 is intermittent and there is evidence that it occurs in a seasonal fashion. Farm-management practices resulting from intensification may play an integral role in the maintenance and transmission of this organism within the farm environment. Alternative routes of transmission on to the farm remain elusive. *E. coli* O157:H7 has been isolated from the faeces of wild birds and these may serve as a vector of this organism. Evidence from artificially infected poultry corroborates the potential importance of wild birds in transmission.

After being voided from the host, the organism must survive until a new host is found. Laboratory studies indicate that *E. coli* O157:H7 can survive in the environment for extended periods. The inability of researchers to isolate the organism from the environment following faecal shedding is a consequence of the presence of the organism in low numbers in comparison with other microorganisms and the inability of the selective procedures employed to recover stressed cells.

If intervention strategies on the farm are to be successfully implemented to prevent transmission of *E. coli* O157:H7 into the food-chain, substantially more information regarding the ecology of this organism on the farm is required.

REFERENCES

Abdul-Raouf, U.M., Beuchat, L.R. and Ammar, M.S. (1993) Survival and growth of *Escherichia coli* O157:H7 in ground roasted beef as affected by pH, acidulants, and temperature. *Applied and Environmental Microbiology* 59, 2364–2368.

Abdul-Raouf, U.M., Beuchat, L.R. and Ammar, M.S. (1996) Isolation of *Escherichia coli* O157:H7 from some Egyptian foods. *International Journal of Food Microbiology* 29, 423–426.

Anon. (1995) *Report on Verocytotoxin-producing* Escherichia coli. Advisory Committee on the Microbiological Safety of Food, HMSO, London.

Anon. (1997) Two outbreaks of vero cytotoxin producing *Escherichia coli* O157 infection associated with farms: an outbreak at a music festival. *Communicable Disease Report Weekly* 30, 263.

Arnold, K.W. and Kaspar, C.W. (1995) Starvation- and stationary-phase induced acid tolerance in *Escherichia coli* O157:H7. *Applied and Environmental Microbiology* 61, 2037–2039.

Beery, J.T., Doyle, M.P. and Schoeni, J.L. (1985) Colonization of chicken cecae by *Escherichia coli* associated with hemorrhagic colitis. *Applied and Environmental Microbiology* 49, 310–315.

Benjamin, M.M. and Datta, A.R. (1995) Acid tolerance of enterohemorrhagic *Escherichia coli. Applied and Environmental Microbiology* 61, 1669–1672.

Benton, C., Khan, F., Monaghan, P., Richards, W.N. and Sheddon, C.B. (1983) The contamination of a major water supply by gulls (*Larus* sp.): a study of the problem and remedial action taken. *Water Research* 17, 789–798.

Berman, D., Rice, E.W. and Hoff, J.C. (1988) Inactivation of particle-associated coliforms by chlorine and monochloramine. *Applied and Environmental Microbiology* 54, 507–512.

Besser, R.E., Lett, S.M., Weber, J.T., Doyle, M.P., Barrett, T.J., Wells, J.G and Griffin, P.M. (1993) An outbreak of diarrhea and hemolytic uremic syndrome from *Escherichia coli* O157:H7 in fresh-pressed apple cider. *Journal of the American Medical Association* 269, 2217–2219.

Beutin, L., Knollmannschanbacher, G., Rietschel, W. and Seeger, H. (1996) Animal reservoirs of *Escherichia coli* O157:H7. *Veterinary Record* 139, 70–71.

Booth, I. (1998) The bacteria strike back. *The Biochemist* 20, 8–11.

Bordalo, A.A. (1993) Effects of salinity on bacterioplankton: field and microcosm experiments. *Journal of Applied Bacteriology* 75, 393–398.

Brewster, D.H., Brown, M.I., Robertson, D., Houghton, G.L., Bimson, J. and Sharp, J.C.M. (1994) An outbreak of *Escherichia coli* O157 associated with a children's paddling pool. *Epidemiology and Infection* 112, 441–447.

Cahoon, F.E. and Thompson, J.S. (1987) Frequency of *Escherichia coli* O157:H7 isolation from stool specimens. *Canadian Journal of Microbiology* 33, 914–915.

Carpentier, B. and Cerf, O. (1993) A review: biofilms and their consequences with particular reference to hygiene in the food industry. *Journal of Applied Bacteriology* 75, 499–511.

Casanovas, L., De Simon, M., Ferrer, M.D., Arques, J. and Monzon, G. (1995) Intestinal carriage of campylobacters, salmonellas, yersinias and listerias in pigeons in the city of Barcelona. *Journal of Applied Bacteriology* 78, 11–13.

Cenci, G., Morozzi, G. and Caldini, G. (1985) Injury by heavy metals in *Escherichia coli*. *Bulletin of Environmental Contamination and Toxicology* 34, 188–195.

Chabrzyk, G. and Coulson, J.C. (1976) Survival and recruitment in the herring gull (*Larus argentatus*). *Journal of Animal Ecology* 42, 187–203.

Chapman, P.A. and Ackroyd, H.J. (1997) Farmed deer as a potential source of verocytotoxin-producing *Escherichia coli* O157. *Veterinary Record* 141, 314–315.

Chapman, P.A. and Siddons, C.A. (1996) Sheep as a potential source of verocytotoxin-producing *Escherichia coli* O157. *Veterinary Record*, 138, 23–24.

Chapman, P.A., Wright, D.J. and Norman, P. (1989) Verotoxin-producing *Escherichia coli* infections in Sheffield: cattle as a possible source. *Epidemiology and Infection* 102, 439–445.

Chapman, P.A., Jewes, L., Siddons, C.A., Norman, P. and George, S.L. (1990) Verocytotoxin-producing *Escherichia coli* infections in Sheffield: 1985–1989. *PHLS Microbial Digest* 7, 163–166.

Chapman, P.A., Siddons, C.A., Wright, D.J., Norman, P., Fox, J. and Crick, E. (1993) Cattle as a possible source of verocytotoxin-producing *Escherichia coli* O157 infections in man. *Epidemiology and Infection* 111, 439–447.

Chapman, P.A., Siddons, C.A., Cerdan Malo, A.T. and Harkin, M.A. (1997) A 1-year study of *Escherichia coli* O157 in cattle, sheep, pigs and poultry. *Epidemiology and Infection* 119, 245–250.

Cheville, A.M., Arnold, K.W., Buchrieser, C., Cheng, C.M. and Kaspar, C.W. (1996) RpoS regulation of acid, heat, and salt tolerance in *Escherichia coli* O157:H7. *Applied and Environmental Microbiology* 62, 1822–1824.

Christman, M.F., Morgan, R.W., Jacobson, F.S. and Ames, B.A. (1985) Positive control of a regulon for defenses against oxidative stress and some heat shock proteins in *Salmonella typhimurium*. *Cell* 41, 753–762.

Cieslak, P.R., Barrett, T.J., Griffin, P.M., Gensheimer, K.F., Beckett, G., Buffington, J. and Smith, M.G. (1993) *Escherichia coli* O157:H7 infection from a manured garden. *Lancet* 342, 367.

Clavero, M.R.S. and Beuchat, L.R. (1995) Suitability of selective plating media for recovering heat- or freeze-stressed *Escherichia coli* O157:H7 from tryptic soy broth and ground beef. *Applied and Environmental Microbiology* 61, 3268–3273.

Clavero, M.R.S. and Beuchat, L.R. (1996) Survival of *Escherichia coli* O157:H7 in broth and processed salami as influenced by pH, water activity, and temperature and suitability of media for its recovery. *Applied and Environmental Microbiology* 62, 2735–2740.

Conner, D.E. (1992) Temperature and NaCl affect growth and survival of *Escherichia coli* O157:H7 in poultry-based and laboratory media. *Journal of Food Science* 57, 532–533.

Conner, D.E. and Hall, G.S. (1994) Efficacy of selected media for recovery of *Escherichia coli* O157:H7 from frozen chicken meat containing sodium chloride, sodium lactate or polyphosphate. *Food Microbiology* 11, 337–344.

Corrier, D.E., Purdy, C.W. and Deloach, J.R. (1990) Effects of marketing stress on fecal excretion of *Salmonella* spp. in feeder calves. *American Journal of Veterinary Research* 51, 866–869.

Coulson, J.C., Butterfield, J. and Thomas, C. (1983a) The herring gull (*Larus argentatus*) as a likely transmitting agent of *Salmonella montevideo* to sheep and cattle. *Journal of Hygiene, Cambridge* 91, 437–443.

Coulson, J.C., Monaghan, P., Butterfield, J., Duncan, N., Thomas, C. and Shedden, C. (1983b) Seasonal-changes in the herring gull in Britain – weight, molt and mortality. *Ardea* 71, 235–244.

Cray, W.C. and Moon, H.W. (1995) Experimental infection of calves and adult cattle with *Escherichia coli* O157:H7. *Applied and Environmental Microbiology* 61, 1586–1590.

Curry, J.P. (1976) Some effects of animal manures on earthworms in grassland. *Pedobiologia* 16, 425–438.

Curtis, T.P., Mara, D.D. and Silva, S.A. (1992) Influence of pH, oxygen, and humic substances on the ability of sunlight to damage faecal coliforms in waste stabilisation pond water. *Applied and Environmental Microbiology* 58, 1335–1343.

Davies, C.M. and Evison, L.M. (1991) Sunlight and the survival of enteric bacteria in natural waters. *Journal of Applied Bacteriology* 70, 265–274.

Dev, V.J., Main, M. and Gould, I. (1991) Waterborne outbreak of *Escherichia coli* O157. *Lancet* 337, 1412.

Dodd, C., Bloomfield, S., Booth, I. and Stewart, G. (1988) Suicide through stress: a cells response to lethal injury. *The Biochemist* 20, 12–14.

Dorn, C.R. and Angrick, E.J. (1991) Serotype O157:H7 *Escherichia coli* from bovine and meat sources. *Journal of Clinical Microbiology* 29, 1225–1231.

Doyle, M.P. (1984) Association of *Campylobacter jejuni* with laying hens and eggs. *Applied and Environmental Microbiology* 47, 533–536.

Doyle, M.P and Schoeni, J.L. (1987) Isolation of *Escherichia-coli* O157:H7 from retail fresh meats and poultry. *Applied and Environmental Microbiology* 53, 2394–2396.

Easton, L. (1997) *Escherichia coli* O157: occurrence, transmission and laboratory detection. *British Journal of Biomedical Science* 54, 57–64.

Faith, N.G., Shere, J.A., Brosch, R., Arnold, K.W., Ansay, S.E., Lee, M.S., Luchansky, J.B. and Kaspar, C.W. (1996) Prevalence and clonal nature of *Escherichia coli* O157:H7 on dairy farms in Wisconsin. *Applied and Environmental Microbiology* 62, 1519–1525.

Farr, S.B. and Kogoma, T. (1991) Oxidative stress responses in *Escherichia coli* and *Salmonella typhimurium*. *Microbiological Review* 55, 561–585.

Fenlon, D.R. (1981) Seagulls (*Larus* spp.) as vectors of salmonellae: an investigation into the range of serotypes and numbers of salmonellae in gull faeces. *Journal of Hygiene* 86, 195–202.

Fenlon, D.R. (1985) Wild birds and silage as reservoirs of *Listeria* in the agricultural environment. *Journal of Applied Bacteriology* 59, 537–543.

Fennel, H., James, D.B. and Morris, J. (1974) Pollution of a water storage reservoir by roosting gulls. *Water Treatment and Examination* 23, 5–20.

Frank, J.F. and Koffi, R.A. (1990). Surface adherent growth of *Listeria monocytogenes* is associated with increased resistance to surfactant sanitizers and heat. *Journal of Food Protection* 53, 550–554.

Fricker, C.R. (1984) A note on *Salmonella* excretion in the black headed gull (*Larus ribibundis*) feeding at sewage works. *Journal of Applied Bacteriology* 56, 499–502.

Fricker, C.R. and Girdwood, R.W.A. (1984) Dissemination of salmonellas by seagulls in Scotland – a national survey. *Journal of Applied Bacteriology* 57, R13–R14.

Fricker, C.R. and Metcalfe, N. (1984) Campylobacters in wading birds (*Charadrii*): incidence, biotypes and isolation techniques. *Zentralblatt für Bakteriologie, Mikrobiologie und Hygiene I Abteilung Originale B – Umwelthygiene Krankenhaushygiene Arbeitshygiene Praventive Medizin* 179, 469–475.

Gameson, A.L.H. (1984) Bacterial mortality. Part 1. In: *Investigations of Sewage Discharge into some British Coastal Waters.* Water Research Centre Technical Report TR201, Water Research Centre Environment, Medmenham, pp. 1–34.

Gannon, V.P.J., Gyles, C.L. and Frienship, R.W. (1988) Characteristics of verotoxigenic *Escherichia coli* from pigs. *Canadian Journal of Veterinary Research* 52, 331–337.

Garber, L.P., Wells, S.J., Hancock, D.D., Doyle, M.P., Tuttle, J., Shere, J.A. and Zhao, T. (1995) Risk factors for faecal shedding of *Escherichia coli* O157:H7 in dairy calves. *Journal of the American Veterinary Medical Association* 207, 46–49.

Geldreich, E.E., Fox, K.R., Goodrich, J.A., Rice, E.W., Clark, R.M. and Swerdlow, D.L. (1992) Searching for a water supply connection in the Cabool, Missouri disease outbreak of *Escherichia coli* O157:H7. *Water Research* 26, 1127–1137.

Genigeorgis, C., Hassuney, M. and Collins, P. (1986) *Campylobacter jejuni* infection on poultry farms and its effect on poultry meat contamination during slaughter. *Journal of Food Protection* 49, 895–903.

Girdwood, R.W.A., Fricker, C.R., Munro, D., Shedden, C.B. and Monaghan, P. (1985) The incidence and significance of *Salmonella* carriage by gulls (*Larus* spp.) in Scotland. *Journal of Hygiene* 95, 229–241.

Glunder, G., Neumann, U. and Braune, S. (1992) Occurrence of *Campylobacter* spp. in young gulls, duration of *Campylobacter* infection and reinfection by contact. *Journal of Veterinary Medicine* B 39, 119–122.

González, J.M., Iriberri, J., Egea, L. and Barcina, I. (1992) Characterization of culturability, protistan grazing, and death of enteric bacteria in aquatic ecosystems. *Applied and Environmental Microbiology* 58, 998–1004.

Grunder, P. (1996) Beware, feeding the pigeons may be hazardous to your health. *Evening Standard*, 12 August, p. 15.

Hancock, D.D., Besser, T.E., Kinsel, M.L., Tarr, P.I., Rice, D.H. and Paros, M.G. (1994) The prevalence of *Escherichia coli* O157:H7 in dairy and beef cattle in Washington state. *Epidemiology and Infection* 113, 199–207.

Hicks, S.J. and Rowbury, R.J. (1987) Bacteriophage resistance of attatched organisms is a factor in the survival of plasmid bearing strains of *Escherichia coli. Letters in Applied Microbiology* 4, 129–132 .

Hill, G.A. and Grimes, D.J. (1984) Seasonal study of a freshwater lake and migratory waterfowl for *Campylobacter jejuni. Canadian Journal of Microbiology* 30, 845–849.

Houston, D.C. (1993) Carrion and hooded crow. In: Wingfield Gibbons, D., Reid, J.B. and Chapman, R.A. (eds) *The New Atlas of Breeding Birds in Britain and Ireland: 1988–1991.* T. and A.D. Poyser, London, pp. 394–399.

Hudson, S.J., Lightfoot, N.F., Coulson, J.C., Russell, K., Sisson, P.R. and Sabo A.O. (1991) Jackdaws and magpies as vectors of milkborne human *Campylobacter* infection. *Epidemiology and Infection* 107, 36–72.

Huq, A., West, P.A., Small, E.B., Huq, M.I. and Colwell, R.R. (1984) Influence of water temperature, salinity and pH on survival and growth of toxigenic *Vibrio cholerae* serovar 01 associated with live copepods in laboratory microcosms. *Applied and Environmental Microbiology* 48, 420–424.

Iriberri, J., Ayo, B., Artolozaga, I., Barcina, I. and Egea, L. (1994) Grazing on allochthonous vs autochthonous bacteria in river waters. *Letters in Applied Microbiology* 18, 12–14 .

Isaacson, M., Canter, P.H., Effler, P., Arntzen, L., Bomans, P. and Heenan, R. (1993) Haemorrhagic colitis epidemic in Africa. *Lancet* 341, 961.

Jacobs-Reitsma, W.F., Bolder, N.M. and Mulder, R.W.A.W. (1994) Cecal carriage of *Campylobacter* and *Salmonella* in Dutch broiler flocks at slaughter – a one-year study. *Poultry Science* 73, 1260–1266.

Johnson, R.P., Cray, W.C. and Johnson, S.T. (1996) Serum antibody responses of cattle following experimental infection with *Escherichia coli* O157:H7. *Infection and Immunity* 64, 1879–1883.

Jones, F., Smith, P. and Watson, D.C. (1978) Pollution of a water supply catchment by breeding gulls and the potential environmental health implications. *Journal of the Institute of Water Engineers and Scientists* 32, 469–482.

Jones, K. (1997) Strategies for survival. In: Kay, D. and Fricker, C. (eds) *Coliforms and* E. coli*: Problem or Solution.* Athenaeum Press, Gateshead, pp. 133–144.

Jones, K. and Bradshaw, S.B. (1996) Biofilm formation by the Enterobacteriaceae – a comparison between *Salmonella enteritidis, Escherichia coli* and a nitrogen-fixing strain of *Klebsiella pneumoniae. Journal of Applied Bacteriology* 80, 458–464.

Kapperrud, G. and Rosef, O. (1983) Avian wildlife reservoir of *Campylobacter fetus* subsp. *jejuni, Yersinia* spp., and *Salmonella* spp. in Norway. *Applied and Environmental Microbiology* 45, 375–380.

Kapperud, G., Skjerve, E., Vik, L., Hauge, K., Lysaker, A., Aalmen, I., Ostroff, S.M. and Potter, M. (1993) Epidemiological investigation of risk factors for *Campylobacter* colonization in Norwegian broiler flocks. *Epidemiology and Infection* 111, 245–255.

Karaguzel, A., Koksal, I., Baki, A., Ucar, F., Gok, I. and Cirav, Z. (1993) *Salmonella* and *Shigella* carriage by gulls (*Larus* sp) on the east black-sea region of Turkey. *Microbios* 74, 77–80.

Karch, H., Russmann, H., Schmidt, H., Schwarzkopf, A. and Heesemann, J. (1995) Long-term shedding and clonal turnover of enterohemorrhagic *Escherichia coli* O157 in diarrheal diseases. *Journal of Clinical Microbiology* 33, 1602–1605.

Karmali, M.A. (1989) Infection by verocytotoxin-producing *Escherichia coli. Clinical Microbiology Reviews* 2, 15–38.

Keene, W.E., McAnulty, J.M., Hoesly, F.C., Williams, L.P., Hedberg, K., Oxman, G.L., Barrett, T.J., Pfaller, M.A. and Fleming, D.W. (1994) A swimming associated outbreak of hemorrhagic colitis caused by *Escherichia coli* O157:H7 and *Shigella sonnei. New England Journal of Medicine* 331, 579–584.

King, C.H., Shotts, E.B., Wooley, R.E. and Porter, K.G. (1988) Survival of coliforms and bacterial pathogens within protozoa during chlorination. *Applied and Environmental Microbiology* 54, 3023–3033.

Klein, D.A. and Casida, C.L. (1967) *Escherichia coli* die-out from normal soil as related to nutrient availability and indigenous microflora. *Canadian Journal of Microbiology* 13, 1461–1469.

Kudva, I.T., Hatfield, P.G. and Hovde, C.J. (1995) Effect of diet on the shedding of *Escherichia coli* O157:H7 in a sheep model. *Applied and Environmental Microbiology* 61, 1363–1370.

Kudva, I.T., Hatfield, P.G. and Hovde, C.J. (1996) *Escherichia coli* O157:H7 in microbial flora of sheep. *Journal of Clinical Microbiology* 34, 431–433.

Kudva, I.T., Hunt, C.W., Williams, C.J., Nance, U.M and Hovde, C.J. (1997a) Evaluation of dietary influences on *Escherichia coli* O157:H7 shedding by sheep. *Applied and Environmental Microbiology* 63, 3878–3886.

Kudva, I.T., Hatfield, P.G. and Hovde, C.J. (1997b) Characterization of *Escherichia coli* O157:H7 and other shiga toxin-producing *Escherichia coli* serotypes isolated from sheep. *Journal of Clinical Microbiology* 35, 892–899.

Lee, J.V., Bashford, D.J., Donovan, T.J., Furniss, A.L. and West, P.A. (1982) The incidence of *Vibrio cholerae* in water, animals and birds in Kent, England. *Journal of Applied Bacteriology* 52, 281–291.

Leuchtefeld, N.A.W., Blaser, M.J., Reller, L.B. and Wang, W.L. (1980) Isolation of *Campylobacter fetus* subsp. *jejuni* from migratory wildfowl. *Journal of Clinical Microbiology* 12, 406–408.

Levesque, B., Brousseau, P., Simard, P., DeWailly, E., Meisels, M., Ramsay, D. and Joly, J. (1993) Impact of the ring-billed gull (*Larus delawarensis*) on the microbiological quality of recreational water. *Applied and Environmental Microbiology* 59, 1228–1230.

Leyer, G.J., Wang, L.L. and Johnson, E.A. (1995) Acid adaptation of *Escherichia coli* O157:H7 increases survival in acidic foods. *Applied and Environmental Microbiology* 61, 3752–3755.

Lighton, L.L., Kaczmarski, E.B. and Jones, D.M. (1991) A study of the risk factors for *Campylobacter* infection in late spring. *Public Health* 105, 199–203.

Lin, J., Smith, M.P., Chapin, K.C., Baik, H.S., Bennett, G.N. and Foster, J.W. (1996) Mechanisms of acid resistance in enterohemorrhagic *Escherichia coli. Applied and Environmental Microbiology* 62, 3094–3100.

Linggood, M.A. and Thompson, J.M. (1987) Verotoxin production among porcine strains of *Escherichia coli* and its association with oedema disease. *Journal of Medical Microbiology* 25, 359–362.

Loewen, P.C. and Hengge-Aronis, R. (1994) The role of the sigma factor σ^s (KatF) in bacterial global regulation. *Annual Review of Microbiology* 48, 53–80.

McCleery, D.R. and Rowe, M.T. (1995) Development of a selective plating technique for the recovery of *Escherichia coli* O157:H7 after heat-stress. *Letters in Applied Microbiology* 21, 252–256.

McFeters, G.A. (1990) Enumeration, occurrence and significance of injured indicator bacteria in drinking water. In: McFeters, G.A. (ed.) *Drinking Water Microbiology: Progress and Recent Developments.* Springer-Verlag, New York, pp. 478–492.

McFeters, G.A. (1997) Effects of aquatic stress on enteric bacterial pathogens. In: Kay, D. and Fricker, C. (eds) *Coliforms and* E. coli*: Problem or Solution.* Athenaeum Press, Gateshead, pp. 235–242.

McGowan, K.L., Wickersham, E. and Strockbine, N.A. (1989) *Escherichia coli* O157:H7 from water. *Lancet* i, 967–968.

Maule, A. (1997) Survival of the verotoxigenic strain *E. coli* O157 in laboratory scale microcosms. In: Kay, D. and Fricker, C. (eds) *Coliforms and* E. coli*: Problem or Solution.* Athenaeum Press, Gateshead, pp. 61–65.

Mawdsley, J.L., Bardgett, R.D., Merry, R.J., Pain, B.F. and Theodorou, M.K. (1995) Pathogens in livestock waste, their potential for movement through soil and environmental pollution. *Applied Soil Ecology* 2, 1–15.

Mechie, S.C., Chapman, P.A. and Siddons, C.A. (1997) A fifteen month study of *Escherichia coli* O157:H7 in a dairy herd. *Epidemiology and Infection* 118, 17–25.

Monaghan, P. and Coulson, J.C. (1977) The status of large gulls nesting on buildings. *Bird Study* 24, 89–104.

Monaghan, P., Shedden, C.B., Ensor, K., Fricker, C.R. and Girdwood, R.W.A. (1985) *Salmonella* carriage by herring gulls in the Clyde area of Scotland in relation to their feeding ecology. *Journal of Applied Ecology* 22, 669–680.

Morgan, G.M., Newman, C., Palmer, S.R., Allen, J.B., Shepherd, W., Rampling, A.M., Warren, R.E., Gross, R.J., Scotland, S.M. and Smith, H.R. (1988) First recognised community outbreak of haemorrhagic colitis due to verotoxin producing *Escherichia coli* O157:H7 in the UK. *Epidemiology and Infection* 101, 83–91.

Munro, P.M., Laumond, F. and Gautier, M.J. (1987) A previous growth of enteric bacteria on a salted medium increases their survival in sea water. *Letters in Applied Microbiology* 4, 121–124.

Murano, E.S. and Pierson, M.D. (1992) Effect of heat shock and growth atmosphere on the heat resistance of *Escherichia coli* O157:H7. *Journal of Food Protection* 55, 171–175.

Nice, C.S. (1994) The dissemination of human infectious disease by birds. *Reviews in Medical Microbiology* 5, 191–198.

Ogg, J.E., Ryder, R.A. and Smith, H.L (1989) Isolation of *Vibrio cholerae* from aquatic birds in Colorado and Utah. *Applied and Environmental Microbiology* 55, 95–99.

Ostroff, S.M., Kobayashi, J.M. and Lewis, J.H. (1989) Infections with *Escherichia coli* O157:H7 in Washington State: the first year of statewide disease surveillance. *Journal of the American Medical Association* 262, 355–359.

Padhye, N.V. and Doyle, M.P. (1992) *Escherichia-coli* O157:H7: epidemiology, pathogenesis, and methods for detection in food. *Journal of Food Protection* 55, 555–565.

Pai, C.H., Ahmed, N., Lior, H., Johnson, W.M., Sims, H.V. and Woods, D.E. (1988) Epidemiology of sporadic diarrhea due to verocytotoxin-producing *Escherichia coli*: a two year prospective study. *Journal of Infectious Disease* 157, 1054–1057.

Pierard, D., Van Etterijck, R., Breynaert, J., Moriau, L. and Lauwers, S. (1990) Results of screening for verocytotoxin-producing *Escherichia coli* in faeces in Belgium. *European Journal of Clinical Microbiology and Infectious Disease* 9, 198–201.

Porter, J., Mobbs, K., Hart, C.A., Saunders, J.R., Pickup, R.W. and Edwards, C. (1997) Detection, distribution and probable fate of *Escherichia coli* O157 from asymptomatic cattle on a dairy farm. *Journal of Applied Microbiology* 83, 297–306.

Prys-Jones, R.P., Underhill, L.G. and Waters, R.J. (1994) Index numbers for waterbird populations. II. Coastal wintering waders in the United Kingdom, 1970/71–1991/91. *Journal of Applied Ecology* 31, 481–492.

Pyle, H.H., Broadaway, S.C. and McFeters, G.A. (1995) A rapid, direct method for enumerating respiring enterohemorrhagic *Escherichia coli* O157:H7 in water. *Applied and Environmental Microbiology* 61, 2614–2619.

Quessy, S. and Messier, S. (1992) *Campylobacter* spp. and *Listeria* spp. in ring-billed gulls (*Larus delawarensis*). *Journal of Wildlife Diseases* 28, 526–531.

Rahn, K., Renwick, S.A., Johnson, R.P., Wilson, J.B., Clarke, R.C., Alves, D., McEwen, S., Lior, H. and Spika, J. (1997) Persistence of *Escherichia coli* O157:H7 in dairy cattle and the dairy farm environment. *Epidemiology and Infection* 119, 251–259.

Reilly, W.J., Forbes, G.L., Paterson, G.M. and Sharp, J.C.M. (1981) Human and animal salmonellosis in Scotland associated with environmental contamination. *Veterinary Record* 108, 553–555.

Renwick, S.A., Wilson, J.B., Clarke, R.C., Lior, H., Borczyk, A.A., Spika, J., Rahn, K., McFadden, K., Brouwer, A., Copps, A., Anderson, N.G., Alves, D. and Karmali, M.A. (1993) Evidence of direct transmission of *Escherichia coli* O157:H7 infection between calves and a human. *Journal of Infectious Diseases* 168, 792–793.

Rice, D.H., Hancock, D.D. and Besser, T.E. (1995) Verotoxigenic *E. coli* O157 colonisation of wild deer and range cattle. *Veterinary Record* 137, 524.

Riley, L.W., Remis, R.S., Helgerson, S.D., McGee, H.B., Wells, J.G., Davis, B.R., Hebert, R.J., Olcott, E.S., Johnson, L.M., Hargrett, N.T., Blake, P.A. and Cohen, M.L. (1983) Hemorrhagic colitis associated with a rare *Escherichia coli* serotype. *New England Journal of Medicine* 308, 681–685.

Sacks, J.J., Lieb, S., Baldy, L.M., Berta, S., Patton, C.M., White, M.C., Bigler, W.J. and Witte, J.M. (1986) Epidemic campylobacteriosis associated with a community water supply. *American Journal of Public Health* 76, 424–428.

Salmon, R.L. and Smith, R.M.M. (1994) How common is *Escherichia coli* O157 and where is it coming from? Total population surveillance in Wales 1990–1993. In: Karmali, M.A. and Goglio, A.G. (eds) *Recent Advances in Verocytotoxin-producing* Escherichia coli *Infections.* Elsevier Science BV, Amsterdam, pp. 73–75.

Salmon, R.L., Farrell, I.D., Hutchison, J.G.P., Coleman, D.J., Gross, R.J., Fry, N.K., Rowe, B. and Palmer, S.R. (1989) A christening party outbreak of hemorrhagic colitis and hemolytic uremic syndrome associated with *Escherichia coli* O157:H7. *Epidemiology and Infection* 103, 249–254.

Sanderson, M.W., Gay, J.M., Hancock, D.D., Gay, C.C., Fox, L.K. and Besser, T.E. (1995) Sensitivity of bacteriologic culture for the detection of *Escherichia coli* O157:H7 in bovine faeces. *Journal of Clinical Microbiology* 33, 2616–2619.

Schoeni, J.L. and Doyle, M.P. (1994) Variable colonization of chickens perorally inoculated with *Escherichia coli* O157:H7 and subsequent contamination of eggs. *Applied and Environmental Microbiology* 60, 2958–2962.

Scullian, J. and Ramshaw, G.A. (1987) Effects of manurial treatments on earthworm activity in grassland. *Biological Agriculture and Horticulture* 4, 271–281.

Sharp, J.C.M., Ritchie, L.D., Curnow, J. and Reid, T.M.S. (1994) High incidence of haemorrhagic colitis due to *Escherichia coli* O157 in one Scottish town: clinical and epidemiological features. *Journal of Infection* 29, 343–350.

Shukla, R., Slack, R., George, A., Cheasty, T., Rowe, B. and Scutter, J. (1995) *Escherichia coli* O157 infection associated with a farm visitor centre. *Communicable Disease Report Review* 5, R86–R90.

Sinclair, J.L. and Alexander, M. (1984) Role of resistance to starvation in bacterial survival in sewage and lake water. *Applied and Environmental Microbiology* 48, 410–415.

Singh, A. and McFeters, G.A. (1986) Recovery, growth, and production of heat-stable enterotoxin by *Escherichia coli* after copper-induced injury. *Applied and Environmental Microbiology* 51, 738–742.

Singh, A., Yeager, R. and McFeters, G.A. (1986) Assessment of *in vivo* revival, growth, and pathogenicity of *Escherichia coli* strains after copper-induced and chlorine-induced injury. *Applied and Environmental Microbiology* 52, 832–837.

Sjogren, R.E. and Gibson, M.J. (1981) Bacterial survival in a dilute environment. *Applied and Environmental Microbiology* 41, 1331–1336 .

Skirrow, M.B. and Benjamin, J. (1980) '1001' campylobacters: cultural characteristics of intestinal campylobacters from man and animals. *Journal of Hygiene* 85, 427–442.

Smith, H.R. and Scotland, S.M. (1993) ACP Broadsheet. 135. Isolation and identification methods for *Escherichia coli* O157 and other vero cytotoxin producing strains. *Journal of Clinical Pathology* 46, 10–17.

Smith, H.R., Cheasty, T., Roberts, D., Thomas, A. and Rowe, B. (1991) Examination of retail chickens and sausages in Britain for vero cytotoxin-producing *Escherichia coli. Applied and Environmental Microbiology* 57, 2091–2093.

Smith, H.V., Brown, J., Coulson, J., Morris, G. and Girdwood, R. (1993) Occurrence of oocysts of *Cryptosporidium* sp. in *Larus* sp. gulls. *Epidemiology and Infection* 110, 135–143.

Smith, P.J., Coates, D., Illingworth, D.S., Tonkin, C., Seymoor, S. and Knap, I. (1997) An evaluation of the EIAFOSS assay for the detection of *E. coli* O157:H7 in food and environmental samples. Poster presentation, Society of Applied Bacteriology, Norwich, 11–17 July.

Southern, J.P., Smith, R.M.M. and Palmer, S.R. (1990) Bird attack on milk bottles: possible mode of transmission of *Campylobacter jejuni* to man. *Lancet* 336, 1425–1427.

Stanley, K.N., Wallace, J.S., Currie, J.E., Diggle, P.J. and Jones, K. (1998a) Seasonal variation of thermophilic campylobacter in lambs at slaughter. *Journal of Applied Microbiology* 84, 1111–1116.

Stanley, K.N., Wallace, J.S., Currie, J.E., Diggle, P.J. and Jones, K. (1998b) The seasonal variation of thermophilic campylobacters in beef cattle, dairy cattle and calves. *Journal of Applied Microbiology* 85, 472–480.

Stanley, K.N., Wallace, J.S., Currie, J.E., Diggle, P.J. and Jones, K. (1998c) A note – thermophilic campylobacters in dairy slurries on Lancashire farms: seasonal effects of storage and land application. *Journal of Applied Microbiology* 85, 405–409.

Stavric, S., Buchanan, B. and Gleeson, T.M. (1992) Competitive exclusion of *Escherichia coli* O157:H7 from chicks with anaerobic cultures of faecal microflora. *Letters in Applied Microbiology* 14, 191–193.

Stavric, S., Buchanan, B. and Gleeson, T.M. (1993) Intestinal colonisation of young chicks with *Escherichia coli* O157:H7 and other verotoxin-producing serotypes. *Journal of Applied Bacteriology* 74, 557–563.

Stuart, J., Sufi, F., McNulty, C. and Park, P. (1997) Outbreak of *Campylobacter* enteritis in a residential school associated with bird pecked bottle tops. *Communicable Disease Report Review* 7, R38–R40.

Swerdlow, D.L., Woodruff, B.A., Brady, R.C., Griffin, P.M., Tippen, S., Donnell, H.D., Geldreich, E., Payne, B.J., Meyer, A., Wells, J.G., Greene, K.D., Bright, M., Bean, N.H. and Blake, P.A. (1992) A waterborne outbreak in Missouri of *Escherichia coli* O157:H7 associated with bloody diarrhea and death. *Annals of Internal Medicine* 117, 812–819.

Synge, B.A. and Hopkins, G.F. (1992) Verotoxigenic *Escherichia coli* O157 in Scottish calves. *Veterinary Record* 130, 583.

Synge, B.A. and Hopkins, G.F. (1994) Studies of verotoxigenic *Escherichia coli* O157 in cattle in Scotland and association with human cases. In: Karmali, M.A. and Goglio, A.G. (eds) *Recent Advances in Verocytotoxin-producing* Escherichia coli *Infections.* Elsevier Science BV, Amsterdam, pp. 65–68.
Synge, B.A., Hopkins, G.F., Reilly, W.J. and Sharp, J.C.M. (1993) Possible link between cattle and *Escherichia coli* O157 infection in a human. *Veterinary Record* 133, 507.
Thomas, A., Cheasty, T., Frost, J.A., Chart, H., Smith, H.R. and Rowe, B. (1996) Vero cytotoxin-producing *Escherichia coli,* particularly serogroup O157, associated with human infections in England and Wales: 1992–4. *Epidemiology and Infection* 117, 1–10.
Tucker, G.M. (1992) Effects of agricultural practices on field use by invertebrate-feeding birds in winter. *Journal of Applied Ecology* 29, 779–790.
Tzipori, S., Wachsmuth, I.K., Chapman, C., Birner, R., Brittingham, J., Jackson, C. and Hogg, J. (1986) Studies on the pathogenesis of hemorrhagic colitis caused by *Escherichia coli* O157:H7 in gnotobiotic piglets. *Journal of Infectious Diseases* 154, 712–716.
Vernozy-Rozand, C. (1997) A review: detection of *Escherichia coli* O157:H7 and other verocytotoxin producing *Escherichia coli* (VTEC) in food. *Journal of Applied Microbiology* 82, 537–551.
Wallace, J.S. and Jones, K. (1996) The use of selective and differential agars in the isolation of *Escherichia coli O*157 from dairy herds. *Journal of Applied Bacteriology* 81, 663–668.
Wallace, J.S., Stanley, K.N., Currie, J.E., Diggle, P.J. and Jones, K. (1997a) Seasonality of thermophilic *Campylobacter* populations in chickens. *Journal of Applied Microbiology* 82, 219–224.
Wallace, J.S., Cheasty, T. and Jones, K. (1997b) Isolation of verocytotoxin producing *Escherichia coli* O157 from wild birds. *Journal of Applied Microbiology* 82, 399–404.
Walsh, S.M. and Bissonnette, G.K. (1987) Effect of chlorine injury on heat-labile enterotoxin production in enterotoxigenic *E. coli. Canadian Journal of Microbiology* 33, 1091–1096.
Wang, G., Zhao, T. and Doyle, M.P. (1996) Fate of enterohemorragic *Escherichia coli* O157:H7 in bovine feces. *Applied and Environmental Microbiology* 62, 2567–2570.
Whelan, C.D., Monaghan, P., Girdwood, R.W.A. and Fricker, C.R. (1988) The significance of wild birds (*Larus* sp.) in the epidemiology of campylobacter infections in humans. *Epidemiology and Infection* 101, 259–267.
Willis, W.L., Hanner, T.L. and Murray, C. (1991) Evaluation of natural *Campylobacter jejuni* in broiler environments. In: Blankenship, L.C. (ed.) *Colonization Control of Human Bacterial Enteropathogens in Poultry.* Academic Press, New York, pp. 309–314.
Willshaw, G.A., Thirlwell, J., Jones, A.P., Parry, S., Salmon, R.L. and Hickey, M. (1994) Vero cytotoxin-producing *Escherichia coli* O157 in beefburgers linked to an outbreak of diarrhea, hemorrhagic colitis and hemolytic–uremic syndrome in Britain. *Letters in Applied Microbiology* 19, 304–307.
Wilson, J. (1988) *The Birds of Morecambe Bay.* Cicerone Press, Milnthorpe.
Wuethrich, S. (1994) Back on the farm: stopping *E. coli* O157:H7 at its source. *American Society of Microbiology News* 60, 408–410.

Zhao, T., Doyle, M.P. and Besser, R.E. (1993) Fate of enterohemorrhagic *Escherichia coli* O157:H7 in apple cider with and without preservatives. *Applied and Environmental Microbiology* 59, 2526–2530.

Zhao, T., Doyle, M.P., Shere, J. and Garber, L. (1995) Prevalence of *Escherichia coli* O157:H7 in a survey of dairy herds. *Applied and Environmental Microbiology* 61, 1290–1293.

Future Directions, or Where Do We Go from Here?

13

T.H. Pennington

Department of Medical Microbiology, University of Aberdeen, Aberdeen, UK

INTRODUCTION

From time to time, crises occur in a context and with an impact that cause them to have major effects on public policy. The *Escherichia coli* O157 outbreak in central Scotland at the end of 1996 was such an event (Pennington Group, 1997), not only because 21 died and more than 500 fell ill, but because it was yet another dramatic food scare to add to the long list of ones that have dominated the news at regular intervals over the last two decades. It is a widely held view that crises like this one, and others, particularly bovine spongiform encephalopathy (BSE), have not only seriously damaged popular trust in the ability of the present British institutional arrangements to work effectively to protect the public, but have also induced scepticism about the role of 'official' experts and beliefs in 'cover-ups' and the notion that policy-making has been captured by vested interests. These negative perceptions about food policies and their effect on health have caused the UK government to propose a radical reform of the way it approaches food policy and its implementation. It intends to set up a Food Standards Agency, which will operate more openly and at arm's length from government departments (Food Standards Agency, 1998). Its detailed proposals are currently being debated.

OUTBREAKS OF *ESCHERICHIA COLI* O157 IN SCOTLAND

Epidemiologists firmly believe in a hidden hand that causes major food-poisoning outbreaks to start on a Friday afternoon and to develop their full horror over the weekend. The 1996 *E. coli* O157 outbreak in central Scotland was no exception (Ahmed and Donaghy, 1998). The first cases from Wishaw were reported to the Department of Public Health Medicine of Lanarkshire Health Board just after lunchtime on Friday 22 November. By the end of that day, 15 suspect cases had been identified. By the evening, histories had been obtained from nine of the 15 cases. The indications were that eight of these nine had consumed food obtained, either directly or at a church lunch, from a particular butcher's shop – John Barr and Sons – in Wishaw. The possibility of other common exposures could not at this stage be excluded, as a high proportion of the population of Wishaw might patronize this shop in any one week. The number of cases of suspected or confirmed infection continued to increase dramatically (Fig. 13.1). By Sunday 24 November, reports indicated that the distribution of products from Barrs extended into other parts of central Scotland. Cases of infection were subsequently reported in the Forth Valley, Lothian and Greater Glasgow. The distribution chain of meat and meat products was diverse and complex and it took some days for the details on that to be unravelled from a painstaking investigation of the company's records. Some 85 outlets throughout central Scotland were eventually identified as being supplied by the company, making the task of outbreak management and control extremely difficult.

Epidemiological and subsequent microbiological evidence showed that the outbreak comprised several separate but related incidents relating to a lunch (attended by around 100 people) held in Wishaw Parish Church Hall,

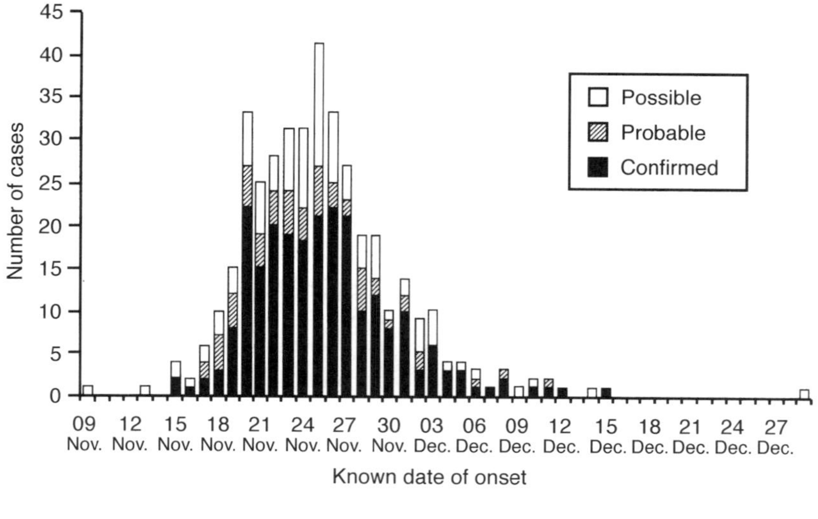

Fig. 13.1. *E. coli* O157 central Scotland outbreak epidemic curve by date of onset of diarrhoea.

a birthday party held in a public house on 23 November 1996 and retail sales in Lanarkshire and the Forth Valley. All isolates of *E. coli* O157 from individuals in the outbreak belonging to phage type 2 had the verocytotoxin gene VT2 and showed indistinguishable profiles by pulsed-field gel electrophoresis.

At the end of the outbreak, 501 cases had been documented (Fig. 13.1); 151 patients had been hospitalized and 21 had died – all aged over 65. These figures make the outbreak one of the world's worst – certainly the worst in mortality, probably the worst in morbidity and in the top three by number of cases.

The Wishaw outbreak is not the only major episode that has been caused by this organism in Scotland. The West Lothian milk outbreak in 1994, with 100 cases (68 confirmed), was also a world record and there have also been infections transmitted by cheese, with a 22-case outbreak in Grampian in the same year. Since 1989, the Scottish Centre for Infection and Environmental Health (SCIEH) has recorded 28 outbreaks – an unenviable record, particularly when account is taken of the fact that most cases of *E. coli* O157 infection are sporadic (73% of the 1744 cases reported to SCIEH between 1990 and 1996). Of even greater concern has been the long-term trend in infection rates. A massive increase has occurred since 1984, when the organism was first seen in Scotland. In that year, only three isolates were made. More than a 100-fold increase has occurred since then and it continues. Annual infection rates for the whole country have risen from 2.24 per 100,000 in 1992 to 9.85 in 1996. That Scotland has a real and particular problem is shown by comparison with data from other countries. Wales probably has the most comprehensive surveillance system anywhere in the world. All acute faecal samples submitted from patients have been screened for *E. coli* O157 since 1990. The average annual rate of laboratory confirmed infections for 1990–1996 was less than 1.5/100,000. In Scotland for the same period, the rate has been greater than 5.

INTERNATIONAL COMPARISONS

Comparison with the rest of the world is not straightforward, for two reasons. First, the surveillance and reporting system in the UK is better developed than just about anywhere else, and comparable data are not often available. Second, the severe illness caused by *E. coli* O157 – with the major complication of the haemolytic uraemic syndrome as a notable feature – is sometimes caused in other countries by different *E. coli* serotypes, such as O111. Routine selective detection methods for these organisms are not yet available. Those comparisons that can be made show, however, that Scotland stands out internationally because of its high incidence of infection (WHO, 1997). Canada, which is the closest rival in incidence rates, approached Scottish levels with 5.3/100,000 in 1991. This fell back to 3.0/100,000 by 1993, but has increased again recently. A recent study there introduced a major caveat to these figures by estimating that, for every symptomatic case reported, between four and nine go unreported. In the USA, more than 100 outbreaks have been reported since 1982. Country-wide laboratory-based surveillance is still being developed there; between 1993 and 1995, the annual average incidence across states was 0.74/100,000, but under-reporting is known to be a significant problem, in part due to inadequate testing. In Japan, the situation is very complex (Izumiya *et al.*, 1997). In 1996, 9451 cases were reported, 1808 patients being hospitalized and 12 died. Many strains of *E. coli* O157 were involved and more than 200 pulsed-field electrophoresis patterns have been identified. What about other smaller countries? Sweden had between zero and three cases per year up till 1995; since then there have been several outbreaks and just over 100 cases in 1995 and in 1996. Denmark has had no outbreaks and an annual incidence of 0.1/100,000 in the years 1989 to 1996. Germany has a problem but is unsure about its scale because of the lack of a nationwide surveillance system. Australia has had two outbreaks, one in 1995 and one in 1996.

These statistics clearly indicate, on the one hand, that *E. coli* O157 and its relatives are causing problems on an increasing scale in many parts of the world and, on the other hand, that a lot more work needs to be done to develop and set up systems to estimate accurately the size of the problem.

This is, of course, not the only unanswered question about the science of *E. coli* O157. Indeed, as more infections are reported, the more uncertainties are uncovered. It is because of this ignorance that no answer can be given to the question, 'Why is *E. coli* O157 such a problem in Scotland?' Although it is known that the organism can live in the intestines of cows and sheep (and a range of other animal species as well, although pigs and chickens do not appear to carry strains pathogenic for humans), it is not clear whether the scale of the human health problem in Scotland relates to higher carriage rates in animals. The role played by other risk factors are equally uncertain. Is the high human incidence due to features of the Scottish diet or cooking practices? *E. coli* O157 is a new organism – it appeared out of the blue in 1982 – and it is almost certain that it is still evolving. It is almost certainly descended from an ordinary *E. coli* that picked up genes for virulence factors from other bacteria (Whittam, 1998). Other serotypes have done this as well – such as *E. coli* O111. Are strains like these, which cause problems in Europe and Australia, going to affect Scotland as well? This is an important question, because these strains are much more difficult to detect in the routine diagnostic laboratory than *E. coli* O157.

A lack of information about the natural history of *E. coli* as a commensal in its natural hosts makes a significant contribution to our difficulties in understanding the biology of *E. coli* O157. This deficit is due to the focusing of research in this topic on aspects that have a direct bearing on the ability of the organism to cause disease in humans and animals, rather than on the biology of carriage itself. Such work that has been done on carriage in healthy hosts raises questions rather than providing answers. Our own work on the *E. coli* flora of a small group of human subjects illustrates this well. We investigated *E. coli* carriage by the members of an Antarctic base. This is a particularly suitable location for long-term studies on the dynamics of carriage and transmission. Its human population is small. Not only do they live in a well-defined environment, but they are isolated from external sources of bacteria for long uninterrupted periods. Sixteen base members were studied for 6 months during the Antarctic winter, when the base was completely isolated from the rest of the world. Sixty *E. coli* electropherotypes (defined by multilocus enzyme electrophoresis) were isolated. Some were isolated repeatedly, often from more than one individual. On the other hand, half were only isolated once. Individuals also varied in their patterns of carriage; some had a simple flora, with only one or two dominant types being repeatedly isolated, whereas others carried, over time, many transient types. Why different *E. coli* types and different individuals behaved in such different ways was not established. Answers to these questions may be relevant to achieving a better understanding of the possible differences in susceptibility of humans and ruminants to infection with *E. coli* O157 and in identifying factors that may be important in the design of control measures – such as the competitive exclusion of *E. coli* O157 by other *E. coli* strains in animal carriers.

In summary, therefore, *E. coli* O157 is a new and evolving pathogen. Consequently, our scientific knowledge about it is imperfect. This deficiency, coupled with ignorance about the natural history of *E. coli* O157 in general, is great enough to significantly impede our ability to predict its behaviour and develop rational, specific, control measures (Advisory Committee on the Microbial Safety of Food, 1995).

These considerations had a major influence on the thinking of the Pennington Group, set up by the Secretary of State for Scotland on 28 November 1996 with a remit 'to examine the circumstances which led to the outbreak in the central belt of Scotland and to advise on the implications for food safety and the general lessons to be learned'. The group was asked to examine the present knowledge of *E. coli*, taking into account scientific research in this area, and the adequacy of present arrangements for, and guidance on, handling food-poisoning outbreaks.

The group concluded (Pennington Group, 1997) that there is no single, simple approach by which the dangers *E. coli* presents can be eradicated. It made recommendations for a range of precautionary, preventive measures and proposals to help in the understanding of the organism and the management and control of outbreaks when they occur, based on the hazard analysis and critical control point (HACCP) system and aimed at minimizing the potential for contamination/cross-contamination with the organism at key stages in the food chain from farm to fork.

A summary of the group's recommendations regarding farms and livestock, slaughterhouses, meat production premises and butchers' shops, controls at the point of consumption, enforcement and surveillance is given in the appendix below.

APPENDIX – SUMMARY OF RECOMMENDATIONS OF THE PENNINGTON GROUP

Farms and livestock

1. There should be an education/awareness programme for farm workers, repeated and updated periodically as appropriate, to ensure they are aware:

(a) of the existence, potential prevalence and nature of *E. coli* 0157;

(b) of the potential for the spread of infection on farms in a number of ways, including notably from faecal material, and of the consequent need for scrupulous personal hygiene;

(c) of the need for care in the use of untreated slurry or manure;

(d) of the absolute requirement for the presentation of animals in an appropriate, clean condition for slaughter.

2. All of this must be backed up by rigorous enforcement by the Meat Hygiene Service at abattoirs.

Slaughterhouses

3. The Meat Hygiene Service should urgently implement its scoring system for clean/dirty animals, should ensure that official veterinary surgeons and the trade are educated and trained in its use and should pursue consistent and rigorous enforcement.

4. The Meat Hygiene Service must take forward urgently, with the help and support of government departments and the industry, the identification and promotion of good practice in slaughterhouses – including specifically in the areas of hide and intestine removal.

5. Abattoir workers should be trained in good hygiene practice during slaughter and the Meat Hygiene Service should concentrate enforcement on slaughter and subsequent handling of carcasses.

6. The HACCP system should be enshrined in the legislation governing slaughterhouses and the transportation of carcasses and meat. Meanwhile, enforcers and the trade should ensure that HACCP principles are observed.

7. The Meat Hygiene Service should be given additional powers to enforce at the abattoir standards for the transportation of meat and carcasses between licensed and non-licensed premises.

8. Further consideration should be given, involving the industry and consumer interests, to the potential use and benefits of end-process treatments, such as steam pasteurization.

9. In line with the approach recommended for more general enforcement, the efforts and resources of the Meat Hygiene Service should be targeted at higher-risk premises – especially those abattoirs with hygiene assessment scores of under 65.

Meat production premises and butchers' shops

10. HACCP (i.e. the approach and all seven principles) should be adopted by all food businesses to ensure food safety. While this is being negotiated into European Union (EU) and domestic legislation, implementation and enforcement of the HACCP principles contained in existing legislation should be accelerated.
11. The government should seek to have HACCP enshrined in the review and consolidation of the vertical EU directives.
12. The government should seek to have all of the HACCP elements negotiated within the horizontal directive.
13. The government should review the application of the Meat Products (Hygiene) Regulations 1994, and the guidance issued subsequently, to clarify the position regarding which premises are intended to be covered by the regulations.
14. Pending HACCP implementation, selective licensing arrangements for premises not covered by the Meat Products (Hygiene) Regulations 1994 should be introduced by new regulations.
15. The licensing arrangements should include appropriate requirements for the documentation of hazard analysis, labelling and record-keeping, to facilitate product recall and temperature control and monitoring. In relation to training, there should be a requirement for all food handlers to have undertaken at least basic food training and for all supervisory staff (and those who run small, one-person operations) to be trained to at least intermediate level. In addition, the licence should cover matters relating to the suitability of premises, equipment and hygiene practices to a level equivalent to that required by the 1994 regulations.
16. In relation to the physical separation requirements of licensing:

(a) There should be separation, in storage, production, sale and display, between raw meat and unwrapped cooked meat/meat products and other ready-to-eat foods. This should include the use of separate refrigerators and production equipment, utensils and, wherever possible, staff;

(b) where the use of separate staff cannot be achieved, alternative standards (such as the completion and implementation by the operator of an HACCP or the provision and use of additional facilities, e.g. for hand-washing in the serving area) might be regarded as sufficient to permit the award of a licence;

(c) where neither (a) nor (b) above can be achieved, the premises concerned should not be permitted to sell both raw and unwrapped cooked meat/cooked meat products (although they may be permitted to sell prewrapped cooked/ready-to-eat meat products prepared elsewhere and brought in for that purpose).

Point of consumption

17. Food-hygiene training should be provided wherever possible within the primary and secondary school curriculum.
18. Guidance and education about food handling and hygiene should be included in all food and catering education and training courses and should be reinforced through periodic advertising and awareness initiatives.
19. Steps should be taken by local authorities to encourage the adoption of HACCP principles in non-registered premises where there is catering for functions for groups of people involving the serving of more than just tea, coffee and confectionery goods.
20. Employers should ensure that food handlers, in particular those working with vulnerable groups and/or in sensitive areas, such as nursing homes and day-care centres, are aware of and implement good hygiene practice. They should be trained in food hygiene, at least to the basic and preferably to the intermediate level.

Enforcement

21. The government should give a clear policy lead on the need for the enforcement of food safety measures and the accelerated implementation of HACCP.
22. The government and local authorities should ensure that there are available suitable and adequate environmental health officer skills and resources to address enforcement and educational awareness issues.
23. The government should consider earmarking local authority funds for these purposes.
24. Local authorities should designate an environmental health officer, with appropriate training, experience and expertise, to head food safety within the authority.

Surveillance

25. The Scottish Office Department of Health should take steps to improve the implementation and monitoring of the recommendations from the Advisory Committee on the Microbiological Safety of Food (ACMSF) and this group on laboratory testing of stool specimens.

26. In discussion with relevant professional groups, a standard case definition and a standard protocol should be agreed for testing and defining clinical cases of infection with *E. coli* O157 and their use promoted in all suspected *E. coli* O157 food-poisoning investigations.
27. On completion of investigations, it should be the responsibility of the Consultant in Public Health Medicine (CPHM) to provide the SCIEH with a minimum data set (in the form of a standard proforma) for all general outbreaks of infectious intestinal disease, including food poisoning.
28. For large (or otherwise significant) outbreaks, a full, written report should be completed and consideration given to its publication. Copies of written reports should go to SCIEH.
29. In particular, there should be written, and published, a full report of the central Scotland outbreak.

REFERENCES

Advisory Committee on the Microbial Safety of Food (1995) *Report on Verocytotoxin-producing* Escherichia coli. HMSO, London.

Ahmed, S. and Donaghy, M. (1998) An outbreak of *Escherichia coli* O157:H7 in Central Scotland. In: Kaper, J.B. and O'Brien, A.D. (eds) Escherichia coli *O157:H7 and Other Shiga Toxin-producing* E. coli *Strains.* ASM Press, Washington, DC, pp. 59–65.

Food Standards Agency (1998) *A Force for Change.* CM 3830, HMSO, London.

Izumiya, H., Terajima, J., Wada, A., Inagaki, Y., Hoh, K.-I., Tamura, K. and Waternabe, H. (1997) Molecular typing of enterohaemorrhagic *Escherichia coli* O157:H7 isolates in Japan by using pulsed-field gel electrophoresis. *Journal of Clinical Microbiology* 35, 1675–1680.

Pennington Group (1997) *Report on the Circumstances Leading to the 1996 Outbreak of Infection with* E. coli *O157 in Central Scotland, with Implications for Food Safety and the Lessons to be Learned.* Stationery Office, Edinburgh.

Whittam, T.S. (1998) Evolution of *Escherichia coli* O157:H7 and other Shiga-toxin producing *E. coli* strains. In: Kaper, J.B. and O'Brien, A.D. (eds) Escherichia coli *O157:H7 and Other Shiga Toxin-producing* E. coli *Strains.* ASM Press, Washington, DC, pp. 195–209.

WHO (1997) *Prevention and Control of Enterohaemorrhagic* Escherichia coli *(EHEC) Infections. Report of a WHO Consultation,* World Health Organization Geneva, *28 April–1 May 1994.*

Index

Note: page numbers in *italics* refer to figures and tables